An Introduction to Glioma

An Introduction to Glioma

Edited by **Matthew Martin**

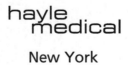

New York

Published by Hayle Medical,
30 West, 37th Street, Suite 612,
New York, NY 10018, USA
www.haylemedical.com

An Introduction to Glioma
Edited by Matthew Martin

International Standard Book Number: 978-1-63241-043-6 (Hardback)

Printed in the United States of America.

Contents

Preface   VII

Part 1   **Introduction**   1

Chapter 1   **Epidemiology of Glioma**   3
Jimmy T. Efird

Chapter 2   **Biological Markers of Recurrence**
and Survival of High-Grade Gliomas:
The Role of Hepatocyte Growth Factor   25
Roberto García-Navarrete, Esperanza García Mendoza,
Alfonso Marhx-Bracho and Julio Sotelo

Chapter 3   **Molecular Etiology of Glioblastomas:**
Implication of Genomic Profiling
From the Cancer Genome Atlas Project   37
Kimberly Ng, Santosh Kesari,
Bob Carter and Clark C. Chen

Chapter 4   **Biomarker Discovery, Validation and Clinical**
Application for Patients Diagnosed with Glioma   49
Kerrie L. McDonald

Part 2   **Gliomagenesis**   77

Chapter 5   **Genomic Abnormalities in Gliomas**   79
Giovanny Pinto, France Yoshioka, Fábio Motta,
Renata Canalle, Rommel Burbano, Juan Rey,
Aline Custódio and Cacilda Casartelli

Chapter 6   **Genetic Diversity of Glioblastoma**
Multiforme: Impact on Future Therapies   103
Franz-Josef Klinz, Sergej Telentschak,
Roland Goldbrunner and Klaus Addicks

Chapter 7   **New Insight on the Role of Transient**
Receptor Potential (TRP) Channels
in Driven Gliomagenesis Pathways   **131**
Giorgio Santoni, Maria Beatrice Morelli,
Consuelo Amantini, Matteo Santoni and Massimo Nabissi

Chapter 8   **Role of the Centrosomal**
MARK4 Protein in Gliomagenesis   **157**
Ivana Magnani, Chiara Novielli and Lidia Larizza

Chapter 9   **The Role of Stem Cells in the Glioma Growth**   **189**
Sergio Garcia, Vinicius Kannen and Luciano Neder

Chapter 10   **Bone Marrow-Derived Cells Support**
Malignant Transformation of Low-Grade Glioma   **201**
Jeffrey P. Greenfield, William S. Cobb,
Caitlin E. Hoffman, Xueying Chen, Prajwal Rajappa,
Chioma Ihunnah, Yujie Huang and David Lyden

Permissions

List of Contributors

Preface

The title of this book is in itself suggestive about the content it covers. It discusses molecular and cell biological aspects of origin and development of glioma, experimental model aspects and systems used for the purpose of diagnosing and treating this anomaly. We hope that this book will provide supportive and relevant information for further understanding the crucial advances in this discipline by experts from various fields associated with glioma.

All of the data presented henceforth, was collaborated in the wake of recent advancements in the field. The aim of this book is to present the diversified developments from across the globe in a comprehensible manner. The opinions expressed in each chapter belong solely to the contributing authors. Their interpretations of the topics are the integral part of this book, which I have carefully compiled for a better understanding of the readers.

At the end, I would like to thank all those who dedicated their time and efforts for the successful completion of this book. I also wish to convey my gratitude towards my friends and family who supported me at every step.

Editor

Part 1

Introduction

Epidemiology of Glioma

Jimmy T. Efird
Center for Health Disparities Research
Department of Public Health
Brody School of Medicine Greenville, North Carolina
USA

1. Introduction

Giomas constitute a broad class of neuroectodermal tumours believed to originate from sustentacular neuroglial cells (Kleihues and Cavenee 2000). Astrocytomas form the largest group of gliomas (>75%) and glioblastoma multiforme (GBM) is the most common type of astrocytoma (CBTRUS 2011). Gliomas that share histologic characteristics with ependymal or oligodendrocyte cells are named ependymomas and oligodendrogliomas, but may not necessarily originate from the aforementioned cell types (Kleihues and Cavenee 2000). Mixed gliomas include those which consist of more than one glia cell type. For example, oligodendroglial glioblastoma multiforme (as defined by some neuropathologists) are GBM tumours with an oligodendroglioma component and generally have a significantly worse clinical outcome than GBM tumours overall (Louis et al 2007). Another mixed glioma is oligoastrocytoma, which contains both oligodendrocyte and astrocyte cells.

The Third Edition of the International Classification of Diseases for oncology (ICD-O-3) is widely used to categorize gliomas by histology (e.g., malignant glioma=9380, ependymoma NOS=9391, astrocytoma=9430, glioblastoma NOS=9440, oligodendroglioma NOS=9450) (Fritz et al 2000). Furthermore, tumours are grouped by site in the ICD-O-3 system using C-codes (e.g., cerebrum=C71.0, frontal lobal=C71.1, temporal lobe=C71.2, parietal lobe=C71.3, occipital lobe=C71.4, ventricle=C71.5, cerebellum=C71.6, spinal cord=C72.0). The World Health Organization (WHO) also has developed a classification index which grades gliomas by disease prognosis (I=best to IV=worst) (Kliehues et al 1993). Recent additions to the "WHO Classification of Tumours" include Grade I - angiocentric gliomas (predominantly occurring in children and young adults in the fronto-parietal cortex, temporal lobe, and hippocampal region), and Grade II – pilomyxoid astrocytoma (typically occurring in infants and children in the hypothalamic/chiasmatic region) (Louis et al 2007). Additionally, WHO has recognized a divergent pattern of gliomas named small cell glioblastoma characterized by EGFR amplification, p16INK4a homozygous deletion, PTEN mutations, and LOH 10q (Louis et al 2007).

2. Incidence and death rates

Gliomas comprise more than 80% of brain tumours (CBTRUS 2011), therefore, descriptive epidemiology about gliomas often is framed in the broader context of brain tumours as a whole.

2.1 Incidence

Overall, brain tumors are relatively rare events. Only 1 in 165 men and women will be diagnosed with cancer of the brain and other nervous system tumours in their lifetime (Altekruse et al 2010). The incidence rate (IR) per 100,000 person-years (100KP-Y) for malignant adult brain tumours ranges from 5.4 (95%CI =4.7-6.1) for the state of Hawaii to 12 (95%CI=12-13) for Wisconsin. IRs by state among children 0-19 years are less variable, ranging from 2 to 4. While geographic differences in IRs might suggest an environmental etiology for brain tumours, ecologic comparisons often do not account for variations in quality of reporting, diagnostic practices, and access/utilization to health care. States falling into the highest quantile for both age-adjusted incidence and death rates (DR) per 100KP-Y include Kentucky (IR=7.9, 95%CI=7.0-8.7; DR=4.9, 95%CI=4.3-5.6), Iowa (IR=7.6, 95%CI=6.7-8.6; DR=5.4, 95%CI=4.6-6.2), and Oregon (IR=7.5, 95%CI=6.7-8.4; DR=5.2, 95%CI=4.5-5.9) (Figures 1 and 2) (NCI State Cancer Profiles 2011). A noticeable cluster of states (depicted in red) with the highest death rates is located along the northern portion of the U.S. from Oregon to Iowa (Figure 2).

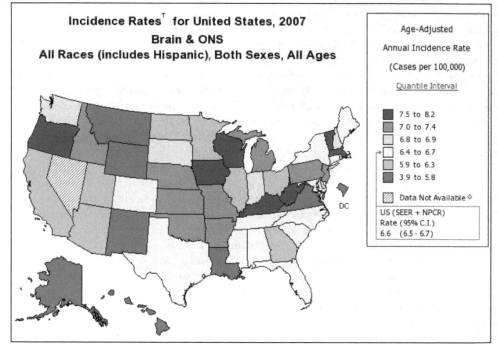

†Age-adjusted (2000 U.S. standard population) cases per 100,000 population per year. ◊Data not available for Nevada.

Fig. 1. Incidence rates (NCI State Cancer Profiles 2011).

Gliomas IRs vary by histology, race, and sex. **Histology**. For example, the age-adjusted rate per 100KP-Y for glioblastoma is 3.19 (95% CI=3.16-3.23) compared with less than 0.2 for anaplastic oligodendroglioma (IR=0.12, 95%CI=0.11-0.13) and protoplasmic/fibrillary astrocytoma (IR=0.11, 95%CI=0.10-0.11) (CBTRUS 2011). **Race**. Whites consistently have higher IR rates than blacks by histologic group (e.g., IR=3.55, 95%CI=3.52-3.59 vs. 1.64, 95%CI=1.57-1.72 for glioblastoma; IR=0.47, 95%CI=0.45-0.48 vs. 0.19, 95%CI=0.17-0.22 for anaplastic astrocytoma; IR=0.29, 95%CI=0.27-0.30 vs. 0.17, 95%CI=0.15-0.19 for ependymoma/anaplastic ependymoma) (CBTRUS 2011). **Sex.** Similarly, men consistently have higher age-adjusted IRs than women by histology (e.g., IR=3.99, 95%CI=3.94-4.04 vs. IR=2.53, 95%CI=2.49-2.57 for glioblastoma; IR=0.48, 95%CI=0.46-0.50 vs. 0.35, 95%CI=0.33-0.36 for anaplastic astrocytoma; and IR=0.27, 95%CI=0.26-0.29 vs. IR=0.25, 95%CI=0.24-0.27 for ependymoma/anaplastic ependymoma), although the latter difference is not statistically significant (CBTRUS 2011). Interestingly, the female prevalence rate (PR) for primary brain tumours per 100KP-Y (PR=264.8) is higher than males (PR=158.7), perhaps attributable to survival bias among women (Porter et al 2010).

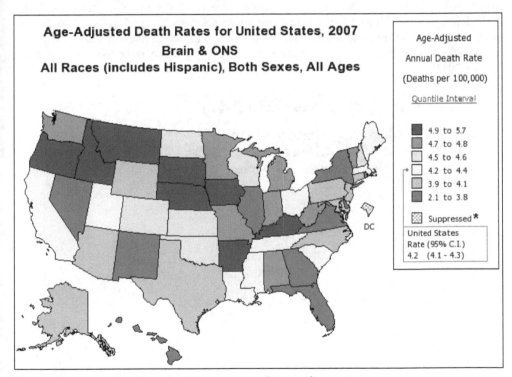

*Counts suppressed since fewer than 16 cases reported in specific area-sex-race category.

Fig. 2. Death rates (NCI State Cancer Profiles 2011).

A higher male (IR=37) to female (IR=2.6) pattern also is observed internationally (Parkin et al 2005), although U.S. rates are higher in both men (IR=7.7, 95%CI=7.5-7.8) and women (IR=5.6., 95%CI=5.5-5.7) compared with international rates (NCI State Cancer Profiles 2011). Less developed countries tend to report lower rates (e.g., Africa, Pacific Islands; IR=3.0 per 100KP-Y for males and 2.1 for females) than more developed countries (e.g., Australia, New Zealand, Europe, North America; IR=5.8 per 100KP-Y for men and 4.1 for females), possibly reflecting less access to modern medical facilities (Parkin et al 2005, CBTRUS 2011). In contrast, the standardized (age, sex, site, year at diagnosis) IR for brain tumours in Japan, a country well known for accessible MR-imaging, is relatively low (2.5 per 100KP-Y person-years) (Matsuda et al 2011). Similarly low rates have been observed in Korea (Lee et al 2010).

2.2 Death rates and survival

The annual number of brain tumour deaths at last count (2007) in the U.S. was n=7,315 for men and 5,919 for women. Age-adjusted rates steadily increased from 1975 to 1991, likely due to advances in neuroimaging, but have decreased linearly thereafter, with recent values on par with 1975 rates (Figure 3) (NCI State Cancer Profiles 2011). Overall DRs are higher among men (DR=5.1, 95%CI=5.0-5.2) than women (DR=3.5, 95%CI=3.4-3.6), however the difference is not statistically significant as was seen for IRs. The lowest DR for men and women combined was observed for the State of Hawaii (DR=2.1, 95%CI=1.4-3.0), which implemented almost complete universal health care coverage in 1994 under the Med-QUEST programme (Hawaii Department of Human Services 2011). However, Hawaii also has the largest non Caucasian population of any state (i.e., 72.8% Asian/Pacific Islander), a factor associated with lower brain tumour incidence and death rates (NCI State Cancer Profiles 2011).

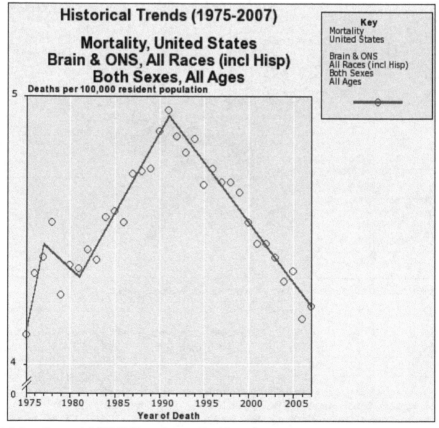

Fig. 3. Mortality trends (NCI State Cancer Profiles 2011).

Survival rates for the majority of malignant gliomas remain disappointingly low, despite decades of advances in surgical, radiation, and chemical therapies, in contrast to improvements in many other cancers. GBMs, for example, typically present as highly aggressive, difficult to treat tumours without clinical, radiologic, or morphologic forewarning of a less virulent precursor tumour (Kanu et al 2009; Ostrom and Barnholtz-Sloan 2011). Secondary GBMs account for only about 10% of all GBMs, based on the presence of IDH1/2 mutations (Ohgaki and Kleihues 2011). The infiltrating nature of these tumours makes treatment difficult. Other obstacles to effective treatment and improved survival include multi-drug resistance, radioresistance, an impermeable blood-brain barrier, a lack of preclinical models, and a rudimentary understanding of neurooncogenetics (Kanu et al 2009).

The relative survival percentages (RSP) for gliomas compared with the general U.S. population vary tremendously by histology and age at diagnosis. For example, the majority of patients diagnosed between age 0-14 years with pilocytic astrocytoma (RSP=97.3%), oligodendroglioma (RSP=95.3), protoplasmic & fibrillary astrocytoma (RSP=84.3%), and mixed glioma (RSP=75.6%) will live beyond 5 years, compared with anaplastic astrocytoma (RSP=32.0%) and glioblastoma (RSP=20.9%) (CBTRUS 2011). In contrast, 5-year relative RSPs are considerably lower across histologic types for those diagnosed between age 45-54 (e.g., RSP=82.4% for pilocytic astrocytoma; RSP=76.8% for oligodendroglioma; RSP=51.1% for mixed glioma; RSP=39.5% for protoplasmic & fibrillary astrocytoma; RSP=28.6% for anaplastic astrocytoma; and RSP=5.6% for glioblastoma). Only 0.8% of patients diagnosed between age 55-64 will be alive after 10 years.

5-Year Relative Survival (whites) by Year of Diagnosis

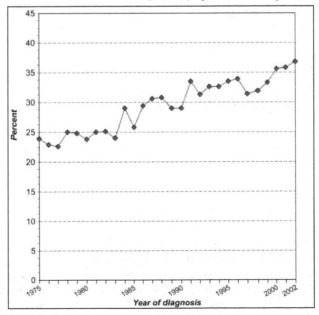

Fig. 4. Survival percent (whites) for cancers of the brain and other nervous system tumours (NCI-SEER 2011).

RSPs also vary by race and sex. Black women (44%) have the highest 5-year RSPs for cancers of the brain and other nervous system tumours, when compared with white women (36.5%), black men (34.8%), and white men (32.6%) (Altekruse et al 2010). When examined by year of diagnosis from 1975 to 2002, whites (Figure 4) consistently have lower 5-year RSPs than blacks independent of sex (Figure 5) (NCI-SEER 2011).

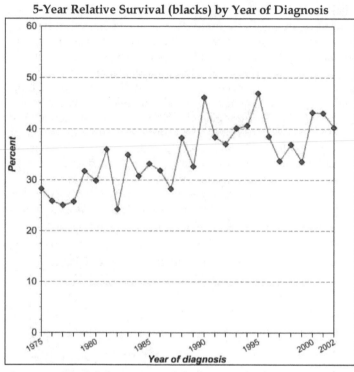

5-Year Relative Survival (blacks) by Year of Diagnosis

Fig. 5. Survival percent (blacks) for cancers of the brain and other nervous system tumours (NCI-SEER 2011).

Among adults, other factors associated with poorer survival include tumour site (frontal, cerebellum, multilobular), and socioeconomic status (less affluent individuals have lower survival rates) (Tseng et al 2006). The latter suggests that socioeconomic inequalities play an important role in glioma outcome, perhaps due to chronic comorbidities, inadequate access and utilization of health care, and longer wait times after surgery for adjuvant therapies (Tseng et al 2006).

While population-based relative survival statistics paint a dismal prognostic picture for certain glioma types, conditional survival rates suggest a more favorable long term outcome for patients who have already survived for a specified amount of time after diagnosis (Table 1) (Porter et al 2011). For Example, a GBM patient has a 70.4% (95%CI=55.6-81.2) relative probability of living 10 years beyond their diagnosis date if they have already survived 5 years. In comparison, the 10-year unconditional probability for GBM is less than 3% (not shown in Table).

Histologic Category	Survival upon 2 years (95%CI)	Survival upon 5 years (95%CI)
Anaplastic astrocytoma	45.4 (38.2-52.3)	73.6 (62.7-81.8)
Anaplastic oligodendroglioma	53.7 (37.8-67.2)	75.6 (51.2-89.0)
Diffuse astrocytoma	53.6 (42.9-63.2)	73.7 (59.6-83.6)
Glioblastoma multiforme	26.2 (20.6-32.1)	70.4 (55.6-81.2)
Hemangioblastoma/hemangioma	93.9 (80.5-98.2)	97.6 (69.3-99.8)
Oligodendroglioma	68.6 (63.1-73.5)	78.5 (72.5-83.3)
Pilocytic astrocytoma	95.9 (92.6-97.8)	99.2 (91.6-99.9)

Table 1. Relative probability of a patient living 10 years beyond their diagnosis date if they have already survived 2 and 5 years.

3. Risk factors

The key epidemiologic determinants of glioma risk include advancing age, male sex, and Caucasian race (Bondy and Wrensch 1996). Few environmental or lifestyle exposures, except for ionising radiation, have been found to be consistently associated with glioma risk. Suspected risk factors include lifestyle behaviors (e.g., smoking, alcohol consumption, coffee drinking), infectious agents (e.g., polyomaviruses, cytomegaloviruses, influenza, varicella zoster, *Toxoplasma gondii*), diet/vitamins (e.g., nitrosamine compounds, vitamin C, vitamin D_3), beauty products (e.g., hair dyes and lighteners, hair waving and straightening chemicals), industrial exposures (e.g., rubber manufacturing, petroleum products), mobile phones, electromagnetic fields, allergies/immunity, agricultural/farm animal exposures, handedness, birth weight/height, and various genetic polymorphisms. While the list is long, methodologic biases are believed to account for the bulk of observed associations. A comprehensive review of factors hypothesized to play a role in the etiology of brain tumors is beyond the intent of the current work and the reader is referred to several recent reviews on the topic (Ostrom and Barnholtz-Sloan 2011; Ohgaki 2009; Fisher et al 2007; Schwartzbaum et al 2006; Ohgaki and Kleihues 2005; Wrensch et al 2002). Rather, the aim of this section is to address the etiology of gliomas in the context of recent publications and current scientific debate on the topic.

3.1 Mobile phones
Mobile (cellular) phones initially appeared on the market in the late 1970's in Japan and soon thereafter were sold in Europe and the U.S. (Bellis 2011). The first commercial wireless call originating in the U.S. occurred on 13 October 1983 (Green 2008).
However, the widespread and frequent use of mobile phones on an affordable scale was not achieved until the earlier 2000's when unlimited usage service contracts became a viable

option to "pay by the minute" billing plans. By the end of 2010 there were approximately 303 million mobile phone subscribers in the U.S., representing 9 times the number in 1995 (CTIA 2011). The World Health Organization estimates 4.6 billion subscribers globally in 2010 (WHO 2011).

The main challenge of epidemiologic studies on mobile phone risk has been the lack of long term, frequent use exposure data (NRPB 2003), especially among users who may be genetically predisposed to brain tumours (Wrensch et al 2009; Shete et al 2009). Population stratification and gene-environment interactions may mask the risk of mobile phone use in insufficiently powered studies. Compounding the situation, the average latency period for many cancers is measured in decades, sometimes as long as 50-60 years, and similarly long intervals may apply to brain tumours (Challis 2007). The flat or declining brain tumour incidence trends observed in the population during the same time period of increasing mobile phone use would seem incongruent if mobile phones are a significant cause of brain tumours (Inskip et al 2010). However, competing risks could explain the effect if brain tumours are caused by more than one factor.

The majority of epidemiologic studies to date generally do not support a causative association between mobile phone use and brain tumours (Ahlbom et al 2009). However, methodologic concerns point to a cumulative underestimation of risk (Kundi 2010). Downward bias may have affected studies that excluded deceased and terminally ill patients, if mobile phone use presumably increases the case fatality rate vis-à-vis enhanced tumor progression. Pre-diagnostic effects of brain tumours may have reduced cell phone use and differentially resulted in lower risk estimates, since referents would not have been affected (NRPB 2003). The use of interviews rather than mailed questionnaire data collection (where it is possible to verify mobile phone use by checking billing records) may have decreased risk estimates due to non-differential exposure misclassification from relying on proxy information. Furthermore, participants tend to underestimate the prevalence of mobile phone use by up to 15% compared with non-participants, leading to a differential reduction in risk estimates for mobile phone use, since participation rates among cases typically are higher than referents by 10-15% (Vrijheid et al 2009; The INTERPHONE Study Group 2010). Risk estimates below unity for brain tumours have been reported in several analyses of mobile phone use (The INTERPHONE Study Group 2010; Inskip et al 2001; Johansen et al 2001; Muscat et al 2000; Hepworth et al 2006). A biologic basis for the results, particularly reports of deceased risk for contralateral use, is ambiguous. In many cases, the inverse associations likely are explained by the aforementioned factors that bias risk estimates in the downward direction. On the other hand, studies in which the participants' status was blinded at interview tended to yield positive risk estimates compared with those who were not blinded (Myung et al 2008).

Two large recent studies have reported increased risks for mobile phone use, especially among heavy users. A multicentric study (13 countries) with 2708 glioma cases and matched referents (age within 5 years, sex, and region of residence within each study centre) observed a 1.40 odds ratio (OR) [95% confidence interval (CI)=1.03-1.89] for glioma among those in the highest mobile phone exposure category (cumulative call time≥1640 hours) compared with the lowest category (never a regular user) (The INTERPHONE Study Group 2010). A subset analysis of the concordance between tumour and preferred side of phone use similarly showed an increased estimated risk among those in the highest decile of cumulative call time (OR=1.55, 95%CI=1.24-1.99). Risk estimates were not reduced for the contralateral side, suggesting against potential reporting bias (Kundi et al 2009). A linear dose response pattern (i.e., consistently increasing risk estimates with dose) is a feature of many but not all known carcinogens and conveys greater weight for a causative association. An upward trend across deciles of cumulative call time was not observed in the above study.

However, in a second recently-conducted study of n=1251 maligant brain tumours (n=1148 gliomas) and n=1267 referents (aged 20-80 years at diagnosis), adjusted estimated risk (age, sex, socioeconomic index, and year of diagnosis) increased with cumulative hours (h) of mobile phone use (none, OR=1.0; 1-100 h, OR=1.2, 95%CI=0.98-1.4; 1001-2000 h, OR=1.5, 95%CI=11.1-2.1; >2000 h, OR=2.5, 95%CI=1.8-3.5) (Hardell et al 2011). Similarly, estimated risk (in the category with >74 hours cumulative use) increased with latency time [years (y) since first use of a cell phone until diagnosis] (none, OR=1.0; >1-5 y, OR=1.0, 95%CI=0.7-1.4; >5-10 y, OR=1.2, 95%CI=0.9-1.6; >10 y, OR=2.7, 95%CI=2.0-3.8), although the linear effect was less pronounce than for cumulative hours of exposure. A key advantage of this study was the use of a mailed questionnaire, which allowed participants to verify responses by checking telephone bills (Kundi 2010). Recall bias could have increased risk estimates in positive studies if more cases than referents believed mobile phone use to be the cause of their brain tumour (Sage and Carpenter 2009; Hepworth et al 2006).

Studies of mobile phone use have been difficult to compare and interpret due to methodologic differences and the paucity of rigorous design. Background levels of electromagnetic radiation (e.g., power lines, fluorescent lights, computer monitors, televisions, and mobile phone base stations) may have confounded studies that did not account for such effects. A recent case-referent study conducted in Japan found a dose-response pattern for increasing exposure to power-frequency magnetic fields (MF) measured in a child's bedroom and brain tumours (<0.1μT, OR=1.0; 0.1 to <0.2 μT, OR=0.74, 95%CI=0.17-3.18; 0.2 to <0.4 μT, OR=1.58, 95%CI=0.25-9.83; ≥0.4 μT, OR=10.9, 95%CI=1.05-113). The OR reported for bedroom MF levels above 0.3 μT, as opposed to above 0.4 μT, was 16 (95%CI=1.85-153). Mobile phones emit both radiofrequency and extremely-low frequency electromagnetic fields (Sage et al 2007). The level of near-field electromagnetic radiation typically emitted on a continuous basis by smart mobile phones ranges from 0.5-0.1 μT (spikes up to 93.5 μT have been recorded during send/receive mode operations), which is above the highest exposure category reported in the Japanese study (Sage et al 2007; Stevenson 2011). Measurements could have been influenced by near-field interference (Silva 2007; Jaffa and Herz 2007), however readings were generally consistent with other independent sources (Sage and Johansson 2007). A large pooled analysis of low-frequency MFs and childhood brain tumors did not observe a dose-response relationship (Kheifets et al 2010). However, inconsistent/imprecise exposure measurements and low participation rates (40%-80%) across studies may have biased results. Furthermore, the actual exposure levels in brain tissue may not necessarily reflect the levels radiated by the mobile phone due to anatomic details and variations in tissue conductivity/permittivity (Kouveliotis et al 2006; Kuster and Balzano 1992).

In March 2010, the Mobile Telecommunications and Health Research Programme (MTHR) initiated funding of a prospective cohort study that will follow approximately 250,000 mobile phone users across 5 European countries for up to 30 years (MTHR 2011; Stewart 2000). While MTHR concludes that short term (less than 10 years) exposure to mobile phone signals does not appear to be associated with an increase in brain and nervous system tumours, they emphasize that there remains "significant uncertainties that can only be resolved by monitoring the health of a large cohort of phone users over a long period of time (MTHR 2011)." Furthermore, the reactions of children to mobile phone emissions may be different and/or stronger than those of adults (as is the case for other environmental exposures such as lead, tobacco smoke, ultraviolet radiation, and ionising radiation) and very little research has been conducted so far to determine whether this is the case (MTHR 2011). No studies on mobile phone use and risk of brain tumours have been planned for the U.S. that are comparable in size and detail to the COSMOS.

The thermal radiation emitted during average mobile phone use is low and generally is not believed to cause direct DNA damage or any other significant deleterious biologic effects on the brain (Wainwright 2000; Johansen et al 2001; Sage and Carpenter 2009; NRPB 2003). However, questions remain regarding the non-thermal effects of non-ionising radiation from mobile phones. Using positron emission tomography (PET), a National Institutes of Health study of 47 participants demonstrated a 7% increase in brain glucose uptake (a measure of metabolic activity) in response to mobile phone signals, supposedly independent of any thermal effects (Volkow et al 2011). The increases in regional glucose metabolism induced by the mobile phone signals were similar in magnitude to those reported after suprathrehold transcranial magnetic stimulation of the sensorimotor cortex. The authors hypothesize that the non-thermal effects on neuronal activity may be mediated by changes in cell membrane permeability, calcium efflux, cell excitability, and/or neurotransmitter release. A significant change in cell proliferation in response to radiofrequency MFs, independent of thermal activity, has been reported in a cell culture experiment involving transformed human epithelial amnion cells (Velizarov et al 1999). Effects demonstrated in other studies include up-regulation of apoptosis genes, induction of reactive oxygen species, changes in protein conformation, the creation of stress proteins, and immune system disturbances (Zhao et al 2007; Sage and Carpenter 2009; NRPB 2003; Valentini et al 2007; Ruediger 2009). Caution is advised when interpreting these effects since numerous contradictory results are present in the literature.

The likelihood that mobile phone use has no impact on the brain is small. Yet, the exact biophysical/biologic mechanism(s), if any, underlying mobile phone effects on neuronal cells, especially in the context of cancer, remains to be confirmed. Additional research is needed to determine if mobile phone use specifically increases brain tumor risk, either independently or in combination with other potential risk factors. Until then, limiting exposure to potentially vulnerable populations (e.g., fetus, children) would seem to be prudent precautionary public health policy, especially given the unknown latency for the development of brain cancer (Kundi et al 2009; Sage and Carpenter 2009). Radiofrequency MF absorption rates are estimated to be two times higher in children than adults, due to the lower thickness of pinna, skin and skull of younger children (Wiart et al 2008). Accordingly, risk may be greater among individuals who use a mobile phone at younger ages, yet few studies have addressed this potential risk group as they age into adulthood. Based on an increased risk for glioma, the WHO/International Agency for Research on Cancer (IARC) has formally classified radiofrequency electromagnetic fields, such as those emitted by wireless communication devices, as "possibly carcinogic to humans (Group 2B) (WHO/IARC 2011)."

3.2 Atopic diseases and farm exposures

Several (Berg-Berkhoff et al 2009; Wigertz et al 2007; Schwartzbaum et al 2003; Hochberg et al 1990; Schlehofer et al 1992; Schlehofer et al 1999; Ryan et al 1992; Brenner et al 2002; Linos et al 2007; Wang and Diepgen 2005; Carrozzi and Viegi 2005) **but not all** (Hagströmer et al

2005; Turner et al 2005; Siegmund et al 2008; Eriksson et al 2005; Cicuttini et al 1997) epidemiologic studies of atopic diseases (e.g., asthma, allergies) have been negatively associated with glioma risk. The protective association has been suggested to reflect increased immune surveillance, although the exact biologic mechanism is unknown (Linos et al 2007; Carrozzi and Viegi 2005). Alterations of the immunological system can enhance the inflammatory response and promote tumor development (Carrozzi and Viegi 2005). The reduced association with allergies also may be due to reverse causality (i.e., immunosuppression induced by the tumor) (Wigertz et al 2007). Glioma patients are known to have an impaired immune system (Dix et al 1999). Interestingly, therapeutic immunity to intracranial tumors has been induced in the laboratory by peripheral immunization with interleukin-4 (IL-4) transduced glioma cells [Okada et al 2001; Benedetti et al 1998].

Farmers have been found to have an increased risk for brain cancer in some studies (Kristensen et al 1996; Reif et al 1989; Wingren et al 1992; Ahlbom et al 1986; Musicco et al 1982; Musicco et al 1988; Brownson et al 1990; Heineman et al 1995), although they generally are healthier than the population-at-large (Kristensen et al 1996; Bråbäck 2002; Population and Public Health Branch (PPHB) 1995; Blair et al 2005; Ronco et al 1992), live longer (Alavanja 1996), and die less frequently from cancer overall (Blair et al 1993). Being raised on a farm (Alfven et al 2006; Ege et al 2007; Riedler et al 2001; Braun-Fahrländer et al 1999; Riedler et al 2000; von Ehrenstein et al 2000; Kilpelainen et al 2000; Klintberg et al 2001; Ernst and Cormier 2000; Remes et al 2003; Leynaert et al 2001; Gassner-Bachmann and Wüthrich 2000; Vercelli 2008) or in a rural area (Godfrey 1975) has been shown to protect against asthma, hay fever, and atopic sensitization. Farm children are exposed to higher concentrations of airborne allergens, but paradoxically become sensitized less frequently and manifest a weaker sensitization response than non-farm controls (Gassner-Bachmann and Wüthrich 2000). The protective effect may be due to a form of "tolerance" that conceivably develops early in life, following repeated exposure to high levels of allergens (e.g., organic dusts, fungi, and endotoxins). Component lipopolysaccharides have been shown to excite Th1 responses and suppress the development of immunoglobulin-E (IgE)-antibodies (Klintberg et al 2001; Bråbäck 2002).

Specific determinants of asthma and atopy in the farm setting remain largely unknown. Any relationship with glioma risk likely is complex and must be interpreted in light of substantial heterogeneity in the protective ability of farming environments and differences in farming practices, especially with respect to microbial exposures (Alfven et al 2006; Ege et al 2007; Vercelli 2008). By self-selection, those who manifest allergies may choose a career path other than farming (i.e., healthy worker effect) (Bråbäck 2002). Farmers represent a diverse group (e.g., dairy, field crop, hog, beef cattle, poultry, fish, marijuana, cotton, and organic), and brain cancer risk, or lack thereof, for farmers could reflect differences in activities and the type, magnitude, and seasonality of exposures. In one report, marijuana smoking was associated with glioma risk, but the study did not specifically examine marijuana farming (Efird et al 2004). Farmers and their families have greater contact with seasonal elements. Season of birth has been associated with adult (Brenner et al 2004; Koch et al 2006; Mainio et al 2006; Efird 2009) and childhood brain tumours (Makino et al 2011; McNally et al 2002; Heuch et al 1998; Yamakawa et al 1979; Hoffman et al 2007; Halperin et al 2004), but the period of greatest risk has varied between studies.

Differences in the definition and the lack of objective measures of atopy should be considered when interpreting the above studies (Wang and Diepgen 2005; Schoemaker et al 2006). Furthermore, there is no definitive trend toward a decreasing risk for glioma with younger ages at onset of the allergic condition, arguing against an immunologic cause for glioma (Schoemaker et al 2006). Paradoxically, increased risk for glioma has been observed in patients with AIDS-related immuno-suppression (Goedert et al 1998; Frisch et al 2001; Grulich et al 1999), but not in those with iatrogenic immuno-suppression (Schiff 2004). Many farm chemicals are classified as probable or likely human carcinogens by the US Environmental Protection Agency (EPA) (e.g., acephate, dichlorvos, dimethoate, lindane, parathion, phosmet, and tetrachlorvinphos) and these agents acting alone or in parallel with decreased atopic sensitization conceivably may increase glioma risk (US Environmental Protection Agency 2003).

3.3 Infectious agents

Polyomaviruses have been detected in the cancerous brain tissue of some patients diagnosed with gliomas (Rollison et al 2003). Polyomaviruses manifest a strong tropism for glial cells in vivo, possibly due to the interaction of glial transcription factors such as Tst-1/Ict6/SCIP with viral promoter sequences (Vasilyera et al 2004). The inoculation of immunologic immature neonate mice with human polyomavirus has been shown to readily cause tumor formation at multiple sites including the brain; older mice do not develop tumors in response to polyoma virus either in the laboratory or by natural infection (Nagashima et al 1984; Zu Rhein and Varakis 1979; London et al 1978; London et al 1983, Sanders 1977; Nagashima et al 1984; Zu Rhein and Varakis, 1979). Similarly, owl and squirrel monkeys injected (intracerebral, subcutaneous, or intravenous) with human JC polyomavirus have developed astrocytomas and glioblastomas (London et al 1978; London et al 1983). Recently, two new members of the *Polyomaviridae family,Karolinska Institutet* Virus (KIPyV) and *Washington Univerisity* virus (WUPyV), have been detected in samples from children with lower respiratory tract disease (Foulongne et al 2008).

Paradoxically, animals are not a permissive host for human JC virus replication, even though integrated JC viral DNA has been identified in the tumors of animals induced with the virus (White et al. 2005; Miller et al, 1984). Though monkeys themselves are not affected, simian virus (SV)-40 (extracted from monkey kidneys) gives cancer to hamsters (Rosenfeld 1962). Human adenovirus type 12 and Rous sarcoma virus are examples of other neuro-oncogenic viruses capable of causing gliomas under laboratory conditions (Zimmerman 1975). Yet, adenovirus in the worst case only causes respiratory disease in humans (Rosenfeld 1962). Some tumor viruses must be injected in animals on the first day of life to be effective, although they may not cause cancer until years later (Bailar and Gurian 1964).

Analogous to human and simian polyomaviruses causing brain tumours in non-permissive rodents, animal polyomaviruses conceivably may cause brain tumours in humans, yet little is understood about the latter topic. Polyomavirus are ubiquous among animals (e.g., cattle, birds, rodents,) (Ashok and Atwood 2006). For example, mouse polyomaviruses (*Mus musculus*) are capable of inducing a wide array of mesenchymal and epithelial cell type cancers in mice (Dawe et al 1987). Exposure to farm animals has been associated in some studies with childhood brain tumours (Efird et al 2003; Bunin et al 1994) but not adult brain tumors (Ménégoz et al 2002).

Epidemiologic evidence in support of a viral/pathogenic etiology for brain tumors remains controversial. In adults, *Toxoplasma gondii* infection has been associated with an increased prevalence of astrocytomas (Schuman et al 1967), while decreased glioma risk has been associated with a history of infections/colds (Schlehofer et al 1999), and chicken pox

(Wrensch et al 2005; Wrensch et al 2001). On the other hand, increased risk for childhood brain tumors has been associated with a history of chicken pox (Bithell et al 1973), influenza (Dickinson et al 2002; Linos et al 1998), measles (Dickinson et al 2002), general viral infections (Fear et al 2001; Linet et al 1996), and neonatal urinary tract infections (Linet et al 1996). A 7.5-fold OR (95% CI=1.3-44.9) for low grade astrocytoma has been observed for neonatal urinary tract infections (Linet et al 1996).

A recent cohort study of 20,132 workers in poultry slaughtering and processing plants, a group with high potential exposures to avian leukosis/sarcoma, reticuloendothesliosis, and Marek's disease viruses, were observed to have a significant excess of brain cancer, compared with the U.S. population (standardized mortality ratio=1.7, 95% CI=1.1-2.4). Although the aforementioned poultry viruses are well established carcinogens in their natural species, it is not known if they cause cancer in humans (Johnson et al 2000).

An infectious etiology for brain tumors is complicated by many factors (Naumova 2006). The same infectious agent may present a different pattern of incidence depending on the host location. A peak evident in the general population may not behave uniformly within certain subpopulations. Temperature, humidity, precipitation, and indoor air quality are among the mitigating factors that may affect the survival and transmissibility of a pathogen. Other factors include poor nutrition, population density, travel, hygiene practices, cultural practices in food consumption/preparation, changes in herd immunity, or evolution of the infectious agent over time. Furthermore, seasonal variation in immune function may increase host susceptibility to infections at certain times of the year (Melnikov et al 1987; Carandente et al 1988).

4. Discussion

The vast majority of glioma cases are idiopathic in origin. Demographic differences in incidence by race, sex, and country suggests that genetics, hormones, and environmental risk factors may play a role in some gliomas. However, study bias (e.g., participation, information, survival), variations in health care access/utilization, residual confounding, and other yet-to-be realized influences may explain the differences in glioma incidence. Complicating matters, the etiology of glioma may be multifactor in nature. That is, several factors operating in unison may cumulatively increase/decrease risk or mask the effect of individual factors when examined in isolation. Additionally, gene-environment and gene-gene interactions may modify underlying risk. Future epidemiologic studies will benefit by improved measures of environmental exposures, more precise statistical methods for detecting interaction effects, and larger multicentre collaborations aimed at better understanding the impact of population stratification.

5. Acknowledgements

Katherine T. Jones (ECU) and Avima Ruder (CDC/NIOSH/DSHEFS) offered valuable comments during the writing of this manuscript. The author also thanks Tamara Sachs for research assistance.

6. References

Ahlbom A, Feychting M, Green A, Kheifets L, Savitz D, Swerdlow A, and ICNIRP (International Commission for Non-Ionizing Radiation Protection) Standing

Committee on Epidemiology. Epidemiology evidence on mobile phones and tumor risk – a review. *Epidemiology* 2009;20:639-652.

Ahlbom A, Navier I, Norell S, Olin R, Spännare R. Nonoccupational risk indicators for astrocytomas in adults. *Am J Epidemiol* 1986;124:334-337.

Alavanja M, Sandler D, McMaster S, Zahm S, McDonnell C, Lynch C, Pennybacker M, Rothman N, Dosemeci M, Bond A, Blair A. The Agricultural Health Study. *Environ Health Perspect* 1996;104:362-369.

Alfven T, Braun-Fahrländer C, Brunekreef B, von Mutius E, Riedler J, Scheynius A, van Hage M, Wickman M, Benz M, Buddle J, Michels K, Schram D, Ublagger E, Waser M, Pershagen G, the PARSIFAL study group. Allergic diseases and atopic sensitization in children related to farming and anthroposophic lifestyle – the PARSIFAL study. *Allergy* 2006;61:414-421.

Altekruse S, Kosary C, Krapcho M, Neyman N, Aminou R, Waldron W, Ruhl J, Howlader N, Tatalovich Z, Cho H, Mariotto A, Eisner M, Lewis D, Cronin K, Chen H, Feuer E, Stinchcomb D, Edwards B (eds). *SEER Cancer Statistics Review, 1975-2007*, National Cancer Institute. Bethesda, MD, http://seer.cancer.gov/csr/1975_2007/, based on November 2009 SEER data submission, posted to the SEER web site, 2010.

Ashok A, Atwood A. Virus receptors and tropism. In: Ahsan N (ed), Polyomaviruses and Human Diseases (Advances in Experimental Medicine and Biology, vol. 577). New York: Springer+Business Media; 2006.

Bailar J, Gurian J. Month of birth and cancer mortality. *J Natl Cancer Inst* 1964;33:237-242.

Berg-Berkhoff G, Schüz J, Blettner M, Münster E, Schlaefer K, Wahrendorf J, Schlehofer B. History of allergic disease and epilepsy and risk of glioma and meningioma (INTERPHONE study group, Germany). *Eur J Epidemiol* 2009;24:433-440.

Bellis M. Selling the cell phone. Part 1: History of cellular phones. http://inventors.about.com/library/weekly/aa070899. Accessed April 2011.

Benedetti S, Di Meco F, Cirenei N, Bruzzone M, Pollo B, Florio N, Caposio L, Colombo M, Cattaneo E, Finocchiaro G. IL-4 gene transfer for the treatment of experimental gliomas. *Adv Exp Med Biol* 1998;451:315-321.

Bithell J, Draper G, Gorbach P. Association between malignant disease in children and maternal virus infections. *Br Med J* 1973;24:706-708.

Blair A, Dosemeci M, Heineman E. Cancer and other causes of death among male and female farmers from twenty-three states. *Am J Ind Med* 1993;23:729-742.

Blair A, Sandler D, Tarone R, Lubin J, Thomas K, Hoppin J, Samanic C, Coble J, Kamel F, Knott C, Dosemeci M, Zahm S, Lynch C, Rothman N, Alavanja M. Mortality among participants in the agricultural health study. *Ann Epidemiol* 2005;15: 279-285.

Bondy M, Wrensch M. Epidemiology of primary malignant brain tumours. *Baillieres Clin Neurol* 1996;5:251-270.

Bråbäck L. Does farming provide protection from asthma and allergies? *Acta Paediatr* 2002;91:1147-1149.

Braun-Fahrländer C, Gassner M, Grize L, Neu U, Sennhauser F, Varonier H, Vuille J, Wäthrich B, and The SCARPOL Team. Prevalence of hay fever and allergic sensitization in farmer's children and their peers living in the same rural community. *Clin Exp Allergy* 1999;29:28-34.

Brenner A, Linet M, Fine H, Shapiro W, Selker R, Black P, Inskip P. History of allergies and autoimmune diseases and risk of brain tumors in adults. *Int J Cancer* 2002;99:252-259.

Brenner A, Linet M, Shapiro W, Selker R, Fine H, Black P, Inskip P. Season of birth and risk of brain tumors in adults. *Neurology* 2004;63:276-281.

Brownson R, Reif J, Chang J, Davis J. An analysis of occupational risks for brain cancer. *Am J Public Health* 1990;80:169-172.

Bunin G, Buckley J, Boesel C, Rorke L, Meadows A. Risk factors for astrocytic glioma and primitive neuroectodermal tumors of the brain in young children: a report from the Children's Cancer Group. *Cancer Epidemiol Biomarkers Prev* 1994;3:197-204.

Carandente F, Angeli A, De Vechi A, Dammacco F, Halberg F. Multifrequency rhythms of immunologic functions. *Chronobiologia* 1988;15:7-23.

Carrozzi L, Viegi G. Allergy and cancer: a biological and epidemiological rebus. *Allergy* 2005;60:1095-1097.

CBTRUS (2011). CBTRUS Statistical Report: Primary Brain and Central Nervous System Tumours Diagnosed in the United States in 2004-2007. Source: Central Brain Tumour Registry of the United States, Hinsdale, IL. website: www.cbtrus.org.

Challis L (Chairperson). Mobile Telecommunications and Health Research Programme Report 2007. MTHR Programme Management Committee. http://www.mthr.org.uk/documents/MTHR_report_2007.pdf. Accessed April 2011.

Cicuttini F, Hurley S, Forbes A, Donnan G, Salzberg M, Giles G, McNeil J. Association of adult glioma with medical conditions, family and reproductive history. *Int J Cancer* 1997;71:203-207.

CTIA (Cellular Telephone Industry Association). Background on CTIA's semi-annual wireless industry survey. http://files.ctia.org/pdf/CTIA_Survey_Year_End_2010_Graphics.pdf . Accessed April 2011.

Dawe C, Freund R, Mandel G, Baller-Hofer K, Talmage D, Benjamin T. Variations in polyoma virus genotype in relation to tumor induction in ,mice-characterization of wild type strains with widely differing profiles. *Am J Pathol* 1987;127:243-261.

Dickinson H, Nyari T, Parker L. Childhood solid tumours in relation to infections in the community in Cumbria during pregnancy and around the time of birth. *Br J Cancer* 2002;87:746-750.

Dix A, Brooks W, Roszman T, Morford L. Immune defects observed in patients with primary malignant brain tumors. *J Neuroimmunol* 1999;100:216-232.

Efird J. Season of birth and risk for adult gliomas (abstract). Brain Tumor Epidemiology Consortium Annual Meeting Abstract Session, The Houstonian Hotel, Houston, Texas, 4-6 April, 2009, Abstract #2.

Efird J, Friedman G, Sidney S, Klatsky A, Habel L. The risk for malignant primary adult-onset glioma ia a large, multiethnic, managed-care cohort: cigarette smoking and other lifestyle behaviors. *J Neuro-Oncol* 2004;68:57-69.

Efird J, Holly E, Preston-Martin S, Mueller B, Lubin F, Filippini G, Peris-Bonet R, McCredie M, Cordier S, Arslan A, Bracci P. Farm-related exposures and childhood brain tumours in seven countries: results from the SEARCH International Brain Tumour Study. *Paediatr Perinat Epidemiol* 2003;17:201-211.

Ege M, Frei R, Bieli C, Schram-Bijkerk D, Waser M, Benz M, Weiss G, Nyberg F, van Hage M, Pershagen G, Brunekreef B, Riedler J, Lauener R, Braun-Fahrländer C, von Mutius E, and the PASIFAL Study team. Not all farming environments protect against the development of asthma and wheeze in children. *J Allergy Clin Immunol* 2007;119: 1140-1147.

Eriksson N, Mikoczy Z, Hagmar L. Cancer incidence in 13811 patients skin tested for allergy. J Investig Allergol Clin Immunol 2005;15:161-166.

Ernst P, Cormier Y. Relative scarcity of asthma and atopy among rural adolescents raised on a farm. Am J Respir Crit Care Med 2000,161,1563-1566.

Fear N, Roman E, Ansell P, Bull D. Malignant neoplasms of the brain during childhood: the role of prenatal and neonatal factors (United Kindom). Cancer Causes Control 2001;12:443-449.

Fisher J, Schwartzbaum J, Wrensch M, Wiemels J. Epidemiology of Brain tumors. Neurol Clin 2007;25:867-890.

Foulongne V, Brieu N, Jeziorski E, Chatain A, Rodière M, Segondy M. KI and WU polyomaviruses in children, France. Emer Infect Dis 2008;14:523-525.

Frisch M, Bigger R, Engels E, Goedert J, for the AIDS-Cancer Match Registry Study Group. Association of cancer with AIDS-related immunosuppression in adults. JAMA 2001;285:1736-1745.

Fritz A, Percy C, Jack A, Shanmugaratnam K, Sobin L, Perkin DM, Whelan S (eds). International Classification of Diseases for Oncology, Third edition. Geneva: World Health Organization; 2000.

Gassner-Bachmann M, Wüthrich B. Farmers' children suffer less from hay fever and asthma. Dtsch Med Wochenschr 2000;125:924-931.

Godfrey R. Asthma and IgE levels in rural and urban communities of The Gambia. Clin Allergy 1975;5:201-207.

Goedert J, Coté T, Virgo P, Scoppa S, Kingma D, Gail M, Jaffe E, Biggar R, for the AIDS-Cancer Match Study Group. Spectrum of AIDS-associated malignant disorders. Lancet 1998;351:1833-1839.

Green E. After just 25 years, cell phones own us. http://www.post-gazette.com/pg/08287/919578-96.stm?cmpid=news.xml. Accessed April 2011.

Grulich A, Wan X, Law M, Coates M, Kaldor J. Risk of cancer in people with AIDS. AIDS 1999;13:839-843.

Hagströmer L, Ye W, Nyrén O, Emtestam L. Incidence of cancer among patients with atopic dermatitis. Arch Dermatol 2005;141:1123-1127.

Halperin E, Miranda M, Watson D, George S, Stanberry M. Medulloblastoma and birth date: evaluation of 3 U.S. datasets. Arch Environ Health 2004;59:26-30.

Hardell L, Carlberg M, Mild K. Pooled analysis of case-control studies on malignant brain tumours and the use of mobile and cordless phones including living and deceased subjects. Int J Oncol 2011;38:1465-1474.

Hardell L, Carlberg M, Mild K. Pooled analysis of two case-control studies on use of cellular and cordless telephones and the risk for malignant brain tumours diagnosed in 1997-2003. Int Arch Occup Environ Health 2006;79:630-639.

Hawaii Department of Human Services. Hawaii Med-QUEST Quality Strategy 2010. http://www.med-quest.us/PDFs/Quality%20Strategy/HI%20MQD%20 Quality%20Strategy%20Approved.pdf. Assessed April 2011.

Heineman E, Gao Y, Dosemeci M, McLaughlin J. Occupational risk factors for brain tumors among women in Shanghai, China. J Occup Environ Med 1995;37:288-293.

Hepworth S, Schoemaker M, Muir K, Swerdlow A, van Tongeren M, McKinney P. BMJ 2006;332:883-887.

Heuch J, Heuch I, Akslen L, Kvåle G. Risk of primary childhood brain tumors related to birth characteristics: a Norwegian prospective study. Int J Cancer 1998;77:498-503.

Hochberg F, Toniolo P, Cole P. Nonoccupational risk indicators of glioblastoma in adults. *J Neurooncol* 1990;8:55-60.

Hoffman S, Schellinger K, Propp J, McCarthy B, Campbell R, Davis F. Seasonal variation in incidence of pediatric medulloblastoma in the United States, 1995-2001. *Neuroepidemiology* 2007;29:89-95.

Inskip P, Hoover R, Devesa S. Brain cancer incidence trends in relation to cellular telephone use in the United States. *Neuro Oncol* 2010;12:1147-1151.

Inskip P, Tarone R, Hatch E, Wilcosky T, Shapiro W, Selker R, Fine H, Black P, Loeffler J, Linet M. Cellular-telephone use and brain tumors. *N Engl J Med* 2001;344:79-86.

Jaffa K, Herz M. Measuring ELF fields produced by mobile phones and personal digital assistants (PDAs). *Bioelectromagnetics* 2007;28:583-584.

Johansson O. Disturbance of the immune system by electromagnetic fields – a potentially underlying cause for cellular damage and tissue repair reduction which could lead to disease and impairment. *Pathophysiology* 2009;16:157-177.

Johansen C, Boice J, McLaughlin, Olsen J. Cellular telephones and cancer – a nationwide cohort study in Denmark. *JNCI* 2001;93:203-207.

Johnson E, Ndetan H, Lo K. Cancer mortality in poultry slaughtering/processing plant workers belonging to a union pension fund. *Environ Res* 2010;110:588-594.

Kanu O, Hughes B, Di C, Lin, Fu J, Bigner D, Yan H, Adamson C. Glioblastoma multiforme oncogenomics and signaling pathways. *Clin Med Oncol* 2009;3:39-52.

Kheifets L, Ahlbom A, Crespi C, Feychting M, Johansen C, Monroe J, Murphy M, Oksuzyan S, Preston-Martin S, Roman E, Saito T, Savitz D, Schüz J, Simpson J, Swanson J, Tynes T, Verkasalo P, Mezei G. A Pooled Analysis Of Extremely Low-Frequency Magnetic Fields And Childhood Brain Tumors. *Am J Epidemiol* 2010;172:752-761.

Kilpelainen M, Terho E, Helenius H, Koskenvuo M. Farm environment in childhood prevents the development of allergies. *Clin Exp Allergy* 2000;30:201-208.

Kliehues P, Burger P, Scheithauer B. The new WHO classification of brain tumours. *Brain Pathol* 1993;3:255-268.

Kleihues P, Cavenee W. *World Health Organization Classification of Tumours. Pathology and genetics of tumours of the nervous system.* IARC: Lyon, 2000.

Klintberg B, Berglung N, Lilga G, Wickman M, van Hage-Hamsten M. Fewer allergic respiratory disorders among farmers' children in a closed birth cohort from Sweden. *Eur Respir J* 2001;17:1151-1157.

Kristensen P, Andersen A, Irgens L, Laake P, Bye A. Incidence and risk factors of cancer among men and women in Norwegian agriculture. *Scand J Work Environ Health* 1996;22:14-26.

Koch H, Klinkhammer-Schalke M, Hofstädter F, Bogdahn U, Hau P. Seasonal patterns of births in patients with glioblastoma. *Chronobiol Int* 2006;23:1047-1052.

Kouveliotis N, Panagiotou S, Varlamos P, Capsalis C. Theoretical approach of the interaction between a human head model and a mobile handset helical antenna using numerical methods. *Progress In Electromagnetics Research, PIER* 2006;65:309-327

Kundi M. Mobile phone use and brain cancer: is the association biased? *Neuroepidemiology* 2010;35:115-116.

Kundi M, Hardell L, Sage C, Sobel E. Electromagnetic fields and the precautionary principle. *Environ Health Perspect* 2009;117:A484-A485.

Kuster N, Balzano Q. Energy absorption mechanisms by biological bodies in the near field of dipole antennas above 300 MHz. *IEEE Trans Vehicle Technol* 1992;41:174-181.

Lee C, Jung K, Yoo H, Park S, Lee S. Epidemiology of primary brain and central nervous system tumours in Korea. *J Korean Neurosurg* 2010;48:145-152.

Leynaert B, Neukirch C, Jarvis D, Chinn S, Burney P, Neukirch F, on behalf of the European Community Respiratory Health Survey. Does living on a farm during childhood protect against asthma, allergic rhinitis, and atopy in adulthood? *Am J Respir Crit Care Med* 2001;164:1829-1834.

Linet M, Gridley G, Cnattingius S, Nicholson H, Martinsson U, Glimelius B, Adami H, Zack M. Maternal and perinatal risk factors for childhood brain tumors (Sweden). *Cancer Causes Control* 1996;7:437-448.

Linos A, Kardara M, Kosmidis H, Katriou D, Hatzis C, Kontzoglou M, Koumandakis E, Tzartzatou-Stathopoulou F. Reported influenza in pregnancy and childhood tumour. *Eur J Epidemiol* 1998;14:471-475.

Linos E, Raine T, Alonso A, Michaud D. Atopy and risk of brain tumors: a meta-analysis. J *Natl Cancer Inst* 2007; 99:1544-1550.

London W, Houff S, Madden D, Fuccillo D, Gravell M, Wallen W, Palmer A, Sever J, Padgett B, Walker D, Zu Rhein G, Ohashi T. Brain tumors in owl monkeys inoculated with a human polyomavirus (JC virus). *Science* 1978;201:1246-1249.

London W, Houff S, McKeever P, Wallen W, Sever J, Padgett B, Walker D. Viral-induced astrocytomas in squirrel monkeys. In: Sever J, Madden (eds), Polyomaviruses and Human Neurological Diseases. New York: Alan R. Liss Inc; 1983.

Louis DN, Ohgaki H, Wiestler O, Cavanee W, Burger P, Jouvet A, Scheithauer B, Kleihues P. The 2007 WHO Classification of Tumours of the Central Nervous System. *Acta Neuro*pathol 2007;114:97-109.

Makino K, Nakamura H, Hide T, Kuratsu J. Risks of primary childhood brain tumors related to season of birth in Kumamoto Prefecture, Japan. *Childs Nerv Syst* 2011;27:75-78.

Mainio A, Hakko H, Koivukangas J, Niemelä A, Räsänen P. Winter birth in association with a risk of brain tumor among a Finnish patient population. *Neuroepidemiology* 2006;27:57-60.

Ménégoz F, Little J, Colonna M, Arslan A, Preston-Martin S, Schlehofer B, Blettner M, Howe G, Ryan P, Giles G, Rodvall Y, Choi W. Contacts with animals and humans as risk factors for adult brain tumours. An international case-control study. *Eur J Cancer* 2002;38:696-704.

National Cancer Institute (NCI). State Cancer Profiles. http://statecancerprofiles.cancer.gov. Accessed April 2011.

Matsuda T, Marugame T, Kamo K, Katanoda K, Ajiki W, Sobue T; The Japan Cancer Surveillance Research Group. Cancer Incidence and Incidence Rates in Japan in 2005: Based on Data from 12 Population-based Cancer Registries in the Monitoring of Cancer Incidence in Japan (MCIJ) Project. *Japan J Clin Oncol* 2011;41:139-47.

McNally R, Cairns D, Eden O, Alexander F, Taylor G, Kelsey G, Birch J. An infectious aetiology for childhood brain tumours? Evidence from space-time clustering and seasonality analyses. *Br J Cancer* 2002;86:1070-1077.

Melnikov O, Nikolsky I, Dugovskaya L, Balitskaya N, Kravchuk G. Seasonal aspects of immunological reactivity of human and animal organism. *J Hyg Epidemiol Microbiol. Immunol.* 1987;31:225-230.

Miller N, McKeever P, London W, Padgett B, Walker D, Wallen W. Brain tumors of owl monkeys inoculated with JC virus contain the JC virus genome. *J Virol* 1984;49:848-856.

Mobile Telecommunications and Health Research (MTHR) Programme. Cohort study of mobile phone use and health (COSMOS). http://www.ukcosmos.org/index.html. Accessed April 2011.

Muscat J, Malkin M, Thompson S, Shore R, Stellman S, McRee D, Neugut A, Wynder E. Handheld cellular telephone use and risk of brain cancer. *JAMA* 2000;284:3001-3007.

Musicco M, Filippini G, Bordo B, Melotto A, Morello G, Berrino F. Gliomas and occupational exposure to carcinogens: case-control study. *Am J Epidemiol* 1982;116: 782-790.

Musicco M, Sant M, Molinari S, Filippini G, Gatta G, Berrino F. A case-control study of brain gliomas and occupational exposure to chemical carcinogens: the risk to farmers. *Am J Epidemiol* 1988;128:778-785.

Myung S, Ju W, McDonnell D, Lee Y, Kazinets G, Cheng C, Moskowitz J. Mobile phone use and risk of tumors: a meta-analysis. *J Clin Oncol* 2009;27:5565-5572.

Nagashima K, Yasui K, Kimura J, Washizu M, Yamaguchi K, Mori W. Induction of brain tumors by a newly isolated JC virus (Tokyo-1 strain). *Am J Pathol* 1984;116:455-463.

National Cancer Institute (NCI) Surveillance Epidemiology and End Results (SEER). Stat Fact Sheets: Brain and Other Nervous System. http://seer.cancer.gov/statfacts/html/brain.html#survival. Accessed April 2011.

National Radiological Protection Board (NRPB). Health effects from radiofrequency electromagnetic fields. Report of an independent advisory group on non-ionising radiation. 2003;14(2):5-177. http://www.hpa.org.uk/web/HPAweb&HPAwebStandard/HPAweb_C/1254510 602951. Accessed April 2011.

Naumova E. Mystery of seasonality: getting the rhythm of nature. *J Public Health Policy* 2006;27:2-12.

Ohgaki H. Epidemiology of brain tumors. In: Verma M, (ed), Methods of Molecular Biology, Cancer Epidemiology, vol. 472. New Jersey: Humana Press; 2009.

Ohgaki H, Kleihues P. Genetic profile of astrocytic and oligodendroglial gliomas. Brain Tumor Pathol [Epub ahead of print] DOI 10.1007.s10014-001-0029-1.

Ohgaki H, Kleihues P. Epidemiology and etiology of gliomas. *Acta Neuropathol* 2005;109:93-108.

Okada H, Villa L, Attanucci J, Erff M, Fellows W, Lotze M, Pollack I, Chambers W. Cytokine gene therapy of gliomas: effective induction of therapeutic immunity to intracranial tumors by peripheral immunization with interleukin-4 transduced glioma cells. *Gene Ther* 2001;8:1157-1166.

Ostrom Q, Barnholtz-Sloan J. Current state of our knowledge on brain tumor epidemiology. *Curr Neurol Neurosci Rep* 2011;11:329-335.

Parkin D, Bray F, Ferlay B, Pisani P. Global cancer statistics, 2002. *CA Cancer J Clin* 2005;55:74-108.

Population and Public Health Branch (PPHB), Health Canada. Farmers at lower risks for many diseases. *Farm Family Health* 1995;3:1-3

Porter K, McCarthy B, Freels S, Kim Y. Prevalence estimates for primary brain tumors in the United States by age, gender, behavior, and histology. *Neuro-Oncology* 2010;12:520-527.

Porter K, McCarthy B, Berbaum M, Davis F. Conditional survival of all primary brain tumor patients by age, behavior, and histology. Neuroepidemiology 2011;36:230-239.

Reif J, Pearce, N, Fraser J. Occupational risks for brain cancer: a New Zealand cancer registry-based study. *J Occup Med* 1989;31:863-867.

Riedler J, Braun-Fahrländer C, Eder W, Schreuer M, Waser M, Maisch S, Carr D, Schierl R, Nowak D, von Mutius E, and the ALEX Study Team. Exposure to farming in early life and development of asthma and allergy: a cross-sectional survey. *Lancet* 2001;358:1129-1133.

Riedler J, Eder W, Oberfeld G, Schreuer M. Austrian children living on a farm have less hay fever, asthma and allergic sensitization. *Clin Exp Allergy* 2000;30:194-200.

Remes S, Iivanainen K, Koskela H, Pekkanen J. Which factors explain the lower prevalence of atopy amongst farmers' children? *Clin Exp Allergy* 2003;33:427-434.

Rollison D, Helzlsouer K, Alberg A, Hoffman S, Hou J, Daniel R, Shah K, Major E. Serum antibodies to JC virus, BK virus, simian 40 virus, and the risk of incident adult astrocytic brain tumors. *Cancer Epidemiol Biomarkers Prev* 2003;12: 460-463.

Ronco G, Costa G, Lynge E. Cancer risk among Danish and Italian farmers. *Br J Ind Med* 1992;49:220-225.

Rosenfeld A. New evidence that cancer maybe infectious. Life Magazine 1962 (June 22);53:2-98.

Ruediger H. Genotoxic effects of radiofrequency electromagnetic fields. *Pathophysiology* 2009;16:89-102.

Ryan P, Lee M, North B, McMichael A. Risk factors for tumors of the brain and meninges: results from the Adelaide Adult Brain Tumor Study. *Int J Cancer* 1992;51:20-27.

Sage C, Carpenter D. Public health implications of wireless technologies. *Pathophysiology* 2009;16:233-246.

Sage C, Johansson O, Sage S. Personel digital assistant (PDA) cell phone units produce elevated extremely-low frequency electromagnetic field emissions. Bioelectromagnetics 2007;28:386-392.

Sage C, Johansson O. Response to comment on "personel digital assistant (PDA) cell phone units produce elevated extremely-low frequency electromagnetic field emissions." *Bioelectromagnetics* 2007;28:581-582.

Sanders F. Experimental carcinogenesis: Induction of multiple tumors by viruses. *Cancer* 1977;40:1841-1844.

Schiff D. Gliomas following organ transplantation: analysis of the contents of a tumor registry. *J Neurosurg* 2004;101:932-934.

Schlehofer B, Blettner M, Preston-Martin S, Niehoff D, Wahrendorf J, Arslan A, Ahlbom A, Choi W, Giles G, Howe G, Little J, Ménégoz F, Ryan P. Role of medical history in brain tumour development. Results from the international adult brain tumour study. *Int J Cancer* 1999;82:155-160.

Schlehofer B, Blettner M, Becker N, Martinsohn C, Wahrendorf J. Medical risk factors and the development of brain tumors. *Cancer* 1992;69:2541-2547.

Schoemaker M, Swerdlow A, Hepworth S, van Tongeren M, Muir K, McKinney P. History of allergies and risk of glioma in adults. *Int J Cancer* 2006;119:2165-2172.

Schuman L, Choi N, Gullen W. Relationship of central nervous system neoplasms to Toxoplasma gondii infection. *Am J Public Health Nations Health* 1967;57:848-856.

Schüz J, Böhler E, Berg G, Schlehofer B, Hettinger I, Schlaefer K, Wahrendorf J, Kunna-Grass K, Blettner M. *Am J Epidemiol* 2006;163:512-520.

Schwartzbaum J, Fisher J, Aldape K, Wrensch M. Epidemiology and molecular pathology of glioma. *Nat Clin Pract Neurol* 2006;2:494-503.

Schwartzbaum J, Jonsson F, Ahlbom A, Preston-Martin S, Lönn S, Söderberg K, Feychting M. Cohort studies of association between self-reported allergic conditions, immune-related diagnoses and glioma and meningioma risk. *Int J Cancer* 2003;106:423-428.

Shete S, Hosking F, Robertson L, Dobbins S, Sanson M, Malmer B, Simon M, Marie Y, Boisselier B, Delattre J, Delattre J, Hoang-Xuan K, El Hallani S, Idbaih A, Zelenika D, Andersson U, Henriksson R, Bergenheim AT, Feychting M, Lönn S, Ahlbom A, Schramm J, Linnebank M, Hemminki K, Kumar R, Hepworth S, Price A, Armstrong G, Liu Y, Gu X, Yu R, Lau C, Schoemaker M, Muir K, Swerdlow A, Lathrop M, Bondy M,Houlston R. Genome-wide association study identifies five susceptibility loci for glioma. *Nat Genet* 2009;41:899–904

Siegmund B, Schlehofer B, Wahrendorf J. Investigation on primary brain tumours and the co-morbidity with diabetes mellitus and atopic diseases in frame of the EPIC study. Brain Tumor Epidemiology Consortium Annual Meeting Abstract Session, German Cancer Research Center, Heidelberg, Germany, 5-7 April 2008, Abstract #5.

Silva M. Measuring ELF fields produced by mobile phones and personal digital assistants (PDAs). *Bioelectromagnetics* 2007;28:580-581.

Stevenson R. Electromagnetic radiation emitted by smart phones. Direct communication 18 April 2011.

Stewart W (Chairperson). Mobile Phones and Health. UK Independent Expert Group on Mobile Phones – 2000. http://www.iegmp.org.uk/report/text.htm. Accessed April 2011.

The INTERPHONE Study Group. Brain tumour risk in relation to mobile telephone use: results of the INTERPHONE international case-control study. *Int J Epidemiol* 2010;39:675-694.

Tseng J, Merchant E, Tseng M. Effects of socioeconomic and geographic variations on survival for adult glioma in England and Wales. *Surg Neurol* 2006;66:258-263.

Turner M, Chen Y, Krewski D, Ghadirian P, Thun M, Calle E. Cancer mortality among US men and women with asthma and hay fever. *Am J Epidemiol* 2005;162:212-221.

US Environmental Protection Agency. April 2003. Chemicals evaluated for carcinogenic potential. Washington, DC, US Environmental Protection Agency, Office of Pesticide Programs, Health Effects Division.

Valentini E, Curcio G, Moroni F, Ferrara M, De Gennaro L, Bertini M. Neurophysiological effects of mobile phone electromagnetic fields on humans: a comprehensive review. *Bioelectromagnetics* 2007;28:415-432.

Vasilyeva I, Shamaev M, Glavatskiy A, Chopick N, Olexenko N, Tsyubko O, Galanta E, Malisheva T. Detection of polyomavirus DNA in human brain tumors. *Exp Oncol* 2004;26:78-80.

Velizarov S, Raskmark P, Kwee S. The effects of radiofrequency fields on cell proliferation are non-thermal. *Bioelectrochem Bioener* 1999;48:177-180.

Vercelli D. Advances in asthma and allergy genetics in 2007. *J Allergy Clin Immunol* 2008;122:267-271.

Volkow N, Tomasi D, Wang G, Vaska P, Fowler J, Telany F, Alexoff D, Logan J, Wong C. Effects of cell phone radiofrequency signal exposure on brain glucose metabolism. *JAMA* 2011;305:808-813.

von Ehrenstein O, von Mutius E, IIIi S, Baumann I, Böhm B, von Kries R. Reduced risk of hay fever and asthma among children of farmers. *Clin Exp Allergy* 2000;30:187-193.

Vrijheid M, Richardson L, Armstrong B, Auvinen A, Berg G, Carroll M, Chetrit A, Deltour I, Feychting M, Giles G, Hours M, Iavarone I, Lagorio S, Lönn S, Mcbride M, Parent M, Sadetzki S, Salminen S, Sanchez M, Schlehofer B, Schüz J, Siemiatycki J, Tynes T,

Woodward A, Yamaguchi N, Cardis E. Quantifying the Impact of Selection Bias Caused by Nonparticipation in a Case–Control Study of Mobile Phone Use. *Ann Epidemiol* 2009;19:33–42.

Wainwright P. Thermal effects of radiation from cellular telephones. *Phys Med Biol* 2000;45:2363-2372.

Wang H, Diepgen T. Is atopy a protective or a risk factor for cancer? A review of epidemiological studies. *Allergy* 2005;60:1098-1111.

White M, Gordon J, Reiss K, Del Valle L, Croul S, Giordano A, Darbinyan A, Khalilu K. Human polyomaviruses and brain tumors. *Brain Res Rev* 2005;50:69-85.

WHO/International Agency for Research on Cancer (IARC). IARC Classifies Radiofrequency Electromagnetic fields as Possible Carcinogenic to Humans. Press Release No. 208, 31 May. IARC: Lyon, France.

Wiart J, Hadjem A, Wong M, Bloch I. Analysis of RF exposure in the head tissues of children and adults. *Phys Med Biol* 2008;53:3681-3695.

Wigertz A, Lönn S, Schwartzbaum J, Hall P, Auvinen A, Christensen H, Johansen C, Klæboe L, Salminen T, Schoemaker M, Swerdlow A, Tynes T, Feychting M. Allergic condition and brain tumor risk. *Am J Epidemiol* 2007;166:941-950.

Wingren G, Axelson O. Cluster of brain cancers spuriously suggesting occupational risk among glassworkers. *Scand J Work Environ Health* 1992;18:85-89.

Wrensch M, Jenkins R, Chang J, Yeh R, Xiao Y, Decker P,Ballman K, Berger M, Buckner J, Chang S, Giannini C, Halder C, Kollmeyer T, Kosel M, LaChance D, McCoy L, O'Neill B, Patoka J, Pico A, Prados M, Quesenberry C, Rice T, Rynearson A, Smirnov I, Tihan T, Wiemels J, Yang P, Wiencke J.Variants in the CDKN2B and RTEL1 regions are associated with high-grade glioma susceptibility. *Nat Genet* 2009;41:905–908

Wrensch M, Minn Y, Chew T, Bondy M, Berger M. Epidemiology of primary brain tumors: current concepts and review of the literature. *Neuro-Oncology* 2002;4:278-299.

Wrensch M, Weinberg A, Wiencke J, Miike R, Barger G, Kelsey K. Prevalence of antibodies to four herpesviruses among adults with glioma and controls. *Am J Epidemiol* 2001;154:161-165.

Wrensch M, Weinberg A, Wiencke J, Miike R, Sison J, Wiemels J, Barger G, DeLorenze G, Aldape K, Kelsey K. History of chickenpox and shingles and prevalence of antibodies to varicella-zoster virus and three other herpesviruses among adults with glioma and controls. *Am J Epidemiol* 2005;161:929-938.

World Health Organization (WHO). Electromagnetic fields and public health: mobile phones. http://www.who.int/mediacentre/factsheets/fs193/en/index.html. Accessed April 2011.

Yamakawa Y, Fukui M, Kinoshita K, Ohgami S, Kitamura K. Seasonal variation in incidence of cerebellar medulloblastoma by month of birth. *Fukuoka Igaku Zasshi* 1979; 70:295-300.

Zhao T, Zou S, Knapp P. Exposure to cell phone radiation up-regulates apoptosis genes in primary cultures of neurons and astrocytes. *Neurosci Lett* 2007;412:34-38.

Zimmerman H. The significance of experimental gliomas for human disease. In: Gliomas Current Concepts in Biology, Diagnosis, and Therapy, Hekmatpanah J (eds). New York: Springer-Verlag; 1975, pp. 6-19.

Zu Rhein G, Varakis J. Perinatal induction of medulloblastomas in Syrian golden hamsters by a human polyoma virus (JC). *Natl Cancer Inst Monogr* 1979;51:205-208,1979.

Biological Markers of Recurrence and Survival of High-Grade Gliomas: The Role of Hepatocyte Growth Factor

Roberto García-Navarrete[1,2,3], Esperanza García Mendoza[1],
Alfonso Marhx-Bracho[2] and Julio Sotelo[1]
[1]*Neuroimmunology Unit, Instituto Nacional de Neurología y Neurocirugía*
[2]*Neurosurgery Department, Instituto Nacional de Pediatría*
[3]*Hospital General Naval de Alta Especialidad, Armada de México*
México

1. Introduction

Malignant gliomas – the most frequent glial tumor of Central Nervous System (CNS) anaplasic astrocytoma and glioblastoma multiforme, are regarded by the World Health Organization as the form of cancer with the worst prognosis in humans. Its biological behavior and severity are associated with increased concentrations of various growth factors, like fibroblastic growth factor (FGF), vascular endothelial growth factor (VEGF), platelet-derived growth factor (PDGF) and hepatocyte growth factor (HGF).

Hepatocyte growth factor (HGF) is a pleomorphic protein with several properties. It was described in 1996 as a protein related to cell proliferation and motility in the rat liver. It has also been associated with morphogenesis of the central nervous system in mammals. HGF has been associated with proliferation of several cell lines, for example carcinoma of colon, stomach, gallbladder, pancreas, and breast. In human gliomas high intratumoral concentrations of HGF and its receptor c-met are associated with poor prognosis; it has also been associated with long-time recurrence of meningioma. In vitro, transfer of the HGF gene increases tumorigenicity, growth, and angiogenesis; interestingly, inhibition of this gene reduces growth rate and malignancy in experimentally induced-glioma in rats.

Human studies have shown that HGF contents in blood (Wen et al. 2011) are closely related with malignancy of glioma; low-grade glioma shows a lower intratumoral concentration of HGF than high-grade glioma.

Recently, we have found HGF directly related in human gliomas to increased angiogenesis, cellular proliferation, resistance to apoptosis induced by gamma radiation, and invasion of healthy tissue along white matter tracts. All of these features are characteristic of malignancy.

In the clinical setting, high HGF levels in cerebrospinal fluid predict mortality and a short disease-free time in patients with malignant glioma, and helps to explain the great variance observed on survival of patients with malignant glioma, suggesting that HGF inhibition strategies could be a useful means of improving survival and disease-free time among glioma patients.

Thus, experimental and clinical findings suggest that HGF is a good target for therapeutic strategies with pharmacogenomic methods and could be useful as a biological marker for monitoring malignant gliomas activity.

2. Malignant glioma

Intracranial neoplasms include a great diversity of tumors with different histopathologic origins, prognoses and treatments: Malignant gliomas such as anaplasic astrocytoma (AA) and glioblastoma multiforme (GM) are the most frequent glial tumors: their incidence is 4/100,000, and they account for 2% of all malignant tumors in adults. Malignant gliomas are associated with poor prognosis; the mean survival time of patients with GM is one year, this gloomy picture has not changed significantly for the last three decades. Similarly, the survival for patients with AA is minor than three years. Therefore, it is of paramount importance to understand the pathophysiology of malignant glial tumors and identify prognostic factors. Both GM and AA have high proliferation and intense vascularity, features closely related with malignant cell growth.

Malignant conditions are related to ability of malignant cells to produce growth factors such as vascular endothelial growth factor (VEGF), platelet derived growth factor (PDGF), and fibroblastic growth factor (FGF) (Arrieta et al., 2002).

Due to their invasive nature, glioblastomas cannot be resected completely by surgery and, despite the progress of neurosurgical techniques and radio/chemotherapy, less than a half of patients survive more than a year, aged subjects have the most significant adverse prognostic factor.

Glioblastoma is the most frequent malignant tumor of the brain, it account for approximately 12–15% of all intracranial neoplasms and 60-75% of astrocytic tumors (Lantos et al., 2002; Lois et al., 2007). In most European and North American countries, the yearly incidence is in the range of 3-4 new cases per 100 000 population (Lois et al., 2007).

2.1 Prognostic factors

Despite progress in surgery, radiotherapy and chemotherapy of brain tumors, the overall survival of patients with glioblastoma remains dismal. Population-based studies from Switzerland and Canada have shown that less than 20% of patients survive more than one year after diagnosis and less than 3% lived longer than 3 years (Lantos et al., 2002; Ohgaki et al., 2007). Clinical trials show a slightly better prognosis, with median survival rates of approximately 12 month; however, they have strong bias toward the recruitment of younger patients and those with higher preoperative Karnofsky performance scores, both are strong predictors of a more favorable clinical outcome.

Virtually all therapy trials have shown that younger glioblastoma patients (<50 years at diagnosis) have a significantly better prognosis (Lois et al., 2007). In a large population-based study, age was the most significant prognostic factor; persisting through all age groups in a linear manner (Ohgaki et al., 2007). Patients with secondary glioblastoma survived significantly longer than those with primary glioblastoma, but this is likely due to their age rather than a reflection of a different biological behavior.

The prognostic value of TP53 mutations in glioblastomas is controversial, it either shows no association or the presence of TP53 mutations was a favorable prognostic factor. In a large population-based study, the presence of TP53 mutations was predictive of longer survival but this was not significant when adjusted for younger age.

There is no consistent correlation of epidermal growth factor receptor (EGFR) amplification with survival largely irrespective of the age at first clinical manifestation. LOH 10 (Lois et al., 2007) is the most frequent genetic alteration in glioblastoma and is associated with reduced survival. The presence of PTEN mutations is not associated with prognosis of glioblastoma patients (Lois et al., 2007).

Since the initial histological description of astrocytic neoplasms, several efforts have been made to identify biomarkers that could predict the biological behavior of the tumor. However, to date only few peptides been identified substances that show a weak association with prognosis.

3. Biological markers of glioblastoma activity

The following paragraphs describe some substances that have been reported as candidates for surveillances of tumor activity by measuring their contents in serum.

A molecular event determining the development of malignancy is the activation of b-catenin, a protein necessary for the alignment and maintenance of epithelial cells by regulating cell growth and cell adhesion. The coexpression of α-catenin reduces the cellular growth and migration induced by EGF on human glioma cells (Ji et al., 2010).

A secreted protein of unknown function, YKL-40 (chitinase-3-like-1), is overexpressed in glioblastoma [4], its presence is associated with LOH 10q (Lois et al., 2007), poorer radiation response, shorter time to tumor progression and reduced overall survival (Ohgaki et al., 2004). It is typically coexpressed with matrix metalloproteinase-9 (MMP-9), and its detection in serum has been used to monitor patients with recurrent tumor growth (Pelloski et al., 2005). One report showed that increased expression of GD3 synthase mRNA, in combination with decreased GalNAcT, correlate with an increased survival of patients with glioblastoma (Hormingo et al. 2006).

3.1 Growth factors

The expression of growth factors and their receptors are associated with glioma malignancy. Thus, their potential therapeutic importance has been demonstrated using specific inhibitors of growth factors in experimental and clinical studies. However, recent results have shown that glioma cells are resistant to this treatment and illustrate the therapeutic difficulties in malignant gliomas.

3.2 Vascular endothelial growth factor

Vascular endothelial growth factor (VEGF) is a signal protein that stimulates vasculogenesis and angiogenesis; VEGF's normal function is to induce growth of vessels during early developmental stages, after injury, at muscle following exercise, and to generate new vessels to bypass blocked arteries. When VEGF is overexpressed, it can contribute to malignant glioma progression. Cancers that express VEGF grow and metastasize, VEGF belongs to platelet-derived growth factor family. They are involved in both, vasculogenesis, the novo, and angiogenesis (Mentlein et al., 2004; Reux et al., 2006).

Within the major growth factors related to angiogenesis, VEGF is one of the most important. In several tumors, VEGF plays a pivotal role for vascularization necessary to supply the malignant tissue with oxygen and nutrients. Human glioma cells are characterized by high production of VEGF, however, functional and autocrine growth stimulatory effects on glioma cells are minor (Reux et al., 2006).

In recurrent GBM trials with temozolomide shown a poor therapeutic response where as VEGF inhibitors as bevacizumab, improve the response rate by 25% to 74%, and the period-free of symptoms increases by 32% to 64%, which is superior to the rate reported for temozolomide alone (Pope et al., 2006; Guiu et al., 2008; Narayana et al., 2009; Nghiemphu et al., 2009; Poulsen et al., 2009; Zuniga et al., 2009). The main effect of VEGF inhibitors is centered on rapid reduction in peritumoral edema, improving corticosteroid use. These studies also indicated that bevacizumab treatment is well tolerated and the risk of intratumoral hemorrhage is low. Toxicity related to bevacizumab therapy in patients with malignant glioma includes hypertension, proteinuria, fatigue, thromboembolic events, and wound-healing delay.

3.2.1 Epidermal growth factor

Epidermal growth factor (EGF), is a prototype member of the EGF-family of peptides which have highly similar structural and functional characteristics. Other peptides include: Transforming Growth Factor-α (TGF-α), amphiregulin, epiregulin, and neuregulin 1-4, all of them related to tyrosine kinase activity which initiates a signal transduction cascade that result in several changes: rise in intracellular calcium contents, increased glycolysis, protein synthesis, DNA synthesis and cell proliferation (Fallon et al., 1984).

EGF is overexpressed in various cancers; malignant glioma, breast, pancreas and liver carcinoma, indicating its main role in malignant cell transformation, tumor occurrence and growth by promoting cell division (Xian et al., 2001). Recent reports show that +61G polymorphism of EGF gene increase the risk for glioma development in European subjects but are a protective factor in Chinese subjects (Tan et al., 2010).

The Epidermal growth factor receptor (EGFR) gene is amplified and overexpressed in approximately 40% of patients with primary GBMs. Increased EGFR signaling drives tumor cell proliferation, invasiveness, motility, angiogenesis, and inhibition of apoptosis. Attempts to identify biomarkers to help predict response to EGFR inhibitors have yielded conflicting results. Currently, there is no convincing evidence of a correlation between EGFR expression in tumoral tissue and prognosis (Van Meir et al., 2010).

3.2.2 Hepatocyte growth factor

Hepatocyte growth factor (HGF), also called scatter factor, is a multifunction protein with strong mitogenic effect on hepatocytes. It was initially isolated as a peptide related to hepatic regeneration. It is considered a reliable indicator of hepatic function alter hepatectomy. This protein is constituted by a heavy chain (60 kD) with four domains and a Light chain (32 kD); it binds through its tirosine-kinase receptor, a product of the proto-oncogene c-Met. Hepatocyte growth factor, secreted by mesenchymal cells, acts as a paracrine effector on different epithelial cells inducing mitogenesis and stimulating cellular motility. It is also a powerful angiogenic factor for endothelial cells in vitro and in vivo. In the liver and kidney, it may have a role as antiapoptotic (Xiao et al., 2001). It is also necessary for embriogenesis as regulator of cell migration and growth. Hepatocyte growth factor is also produced by other cells, such as osteoclasts, participating in the regulation of bone remodeling; its production by monocytes has a role in the regulation of hematopoyesis by stimulation of growth and differentiation of erythroid precursors (Arrieta et al., 2002).

Knockout mice for the HGF gene develop severe abnormalities in the liver, placenta, and nervous system causing fetal death. A direct genetic relation between HGF and cancer has also been recently proposed due to mutations in the catalytic domain of c-Met from patients with renal carcinoma. Overexpression of HGF is present in various cells lines of leukemia and lymphoma and in solid tumors of the breast, prostate, colon, liver, kidney, uterine cervix, endometrium, and bladder (Arrieta et al., 2002). Hepatocyte growth factor also promotes adhesion and migration of cancer cells, due to the high affinity of integrins to their ligands, a phenomenon related to the metastatic tendency of carcinomas (Trussolino et al., 2000; Arrieta et al., 2002).

Normal human astrocytes express HGF and its receptor c-Met (Yamada et al, 1994). Met is a proto-oncogene that when mutated can transform a variety of cell types; the Met receptor is a heterodimer consisting of an extracellular alpha chain and a trans-membrane beta chain, which is a tyrosine kinase, it is widely expressed by epithelial and endothelial cells as well as melanocytes, chondrocytes, skeletal muscle, hematopoietic, lymphoid, and neural cells. The activation of Met by HGF binding is linked to cell growth and survival, including the avoidance of anoikis which is apoptosis induced by insufficient association with cell-matrix, through activation of both the PI3-kinase/PDK/Akt and the Ras/Raf/MEK/ERK pathways and to cell mobility and cytoskeletal organization via activation of the Rho-GTPases, Rho, Rac and CDC (Arrieta et al., 2002).

Activation of Met tyrosine kinase also activates phospholipase C, resulting in the elevation of intracellular calcium and activation of conventional and novel protein kinase C pathways. HGF and Met have been associated with progression, invasiveness and metastasis in a number of neoplasms. Met is expressed in a wide variety of carcinomas, musculoskeletal tumors, soft tissue sarcomas, glioblastoma, astrosarcoma, and several hematopoietic malignancies. HGF Met signaling is a major potential target for the development of cancer therapeutics.

3.2.2.1 Hepatocyte growth factor and malignant gliomas

As HGF, its receptor c-met has been implicated in the genesis, malignant progression, and chemo/radioresistance of multiple human malignancies, including gliomas (Peruzzi et al, 2006; Carapancea et al, 2009; Hadjipanayis et al, 2009a, 2009b). Experimental studies using transient expression of anti-SF/HGF and anti-c-met U1snRNA/ribozymes suppress SF/HGF and c-met expression, c-met receptor activation, tumor cell migration, and anchorage-independent colony formation in vitro. The delivery of U1snRNA/ribozymes to established subcutaneous glioma xenografts via liposome-DNA complexes significantly inhibited tumor growth as well as tumor SF/HGF and c-met expression levels. Histological analysis of tumors treated showed a significant decrease in blood vessel density, increase in activation of the pro-apoptotic enzyme caspase-3, and increase in tumor cell apoptosis. Treatment of animals bearing intracranial glioma xenografts with anti-SF/HGF and anti-c-met U1snRNA/ribozymes substantially inhibited tumor growth and promoted animal survival (Abounander et al, 1999, 2002; Kim et al, 2006).

The use of monoclonal antibodies against the NK23 and NK422 domains of the HGF reduce tumor growth and mitotic rate (Bhargava et al., 1992; Boros et al., 1995; Kimura et al., 1995; Miwa et al., 1997; Neaud et al., 1997; Takeuchi et al 1997; Stella et al., 1999; Grierson et al., 2000; Cao et al, 2001; Brockmann et al, 2003; Burgess et al, 2006); Also, viral transgenes against HGF-RNA reduce invasion of white matter tracts, improving response to radiotherapy (Lal et al, 2005; Chu et al, 2006).

The therapeutic efficacy of SGX523 has recently been proven in human brain tumors. It seems that SGX523 inhibits c-Met, AKT and MAPK phosphorylation, cell proliferation, cell cycle progression, migration and invasion in different human glioblastoma cell lines, glioblastoma primary cells, glioblastoma stem cells and medulloblastoma cell lines. Importantly, oral administration of SGX523 to mice bearing intracranial human glioma xenografts led to inhibition of tumor growth in vivo. This experimental data suggests that c-Met kinase inhibition is a feasible and promising approach for brain tumor therapy (Guessous et al., 2010).

4. HGF and gliomas on clinical setting

Hepatocyte growth factor and its receptor (c-Met) have been detected in normal astrocytes as well as in human gliomas, and other malignant tumors (Koochekpour et al., 1995; Nabeshima et al., 1997; Hirose et al., 1998). In human cultured glioma cells, HGF and c-Met are simultaneously expressed, with an autocrinous effect inducing cell proliferation and migration.

Recent findings suggest that HGF contributes to glioma progression, inducing angiogenesis and expression of additional angiogenic autocrine factors such as VEGF (Laterra et al., 1997; Lamszus et al., 1999; Moriyama et al., 1999; Schmidt et al., 1999). The overexpression of HGF and its receptor c-Met increases cell motility and proliferation of human glioma cells in vitro (Koochekpour et al., 1995).

Intratumoral concentration of HGF in malignant gliomas is greatly increased in comparison with other intracranial tumors and nontumoral brain tissue (Arrieta et al., 2002); it is also related to cell proliferation and peritumoral edema, showing its participation in the pathogenesis of these tumors.

A common cause of failure of treatment of malignant gliomas is resistance to radiotherapy and chemotherapy; the mechanism by which the cell survives to therapeutic attempts involves the production of growth factors that regulate DNA repair and apoptosis. In vitro and in vivo, HGF inhibits drug-induced cytotoxicity and apoptosis in experimental neoplasms treated by radiation, cisplatin, and camptothencin (Bowers et al., 2000); this effect might decrease the therapeutic response of patients with high intratumoral contents of HGF.

There is intense infiltration by microglia in gliomas, which may enhance malignancy by secretion of epidermal growth factor and by inhibition of cytotoxic lymphocytes (Wood et al., 1983); in vitro HGF stimulates the microglial infiltration of gliomas, favoring their growth (Badie et al., 1999).

The direct correlation of cell proliferation with the presence of HGF supports its participation in the promotion of tumoral growth of glioma, as has been shown for other tumors such as breast carcinoma (Lamszus et al., 1997).

The mechanism by which HGF stimulates cell proliferation seems to be related to the tirosine kinase activity of its receptor, which involves Ras and mitosis activation proteins (Arrieta et al., 2002). Such effects can be antagonized by tirosine kinase inhibitors. However, not all HGF effects require phosphorylation of its receptor; for instance, its antiapoptotic effect is independent, suggesting that it could also participate in the genesis of the tumor. The insertion of the HGF gene in human glioma cells increases proliferation of independent colonies in vitro and tumorigenesis in vivo (Laterra et al., 1997).

There are some histological features of malignant glioma associated with prognosis, such as the extent of necrosis or vascular density (Barker et al., 1996). Hepatocyte growth factor is a strong inductor of angiogenesis; its effects are synergistic with other growth factors such as VEGF and bFGF. Intratumoral concentration of HGF shows a direct relation with peritumoral edema, independent of vascular density. Previous studies have shown that HGF increases the permeability of the hematoencephalic barrier, independently of VEGF expression, possibly by the induction of endothelial fenestrations and by the tumoral expression of proteases such as urokinase and extracellular matrix metalloproteinases (Book et al., 1999).

A paracrine loop for HGF effects related with migration of tumor cells along white matter has been described. The increase of HGF in CSF observed may therefore reflect either the transport of HGF from brain parenchyma to the ventricular system or the diffusion of HGF along the subarachnoid space (Garcia-Navarrete et al., 2010).

HGF concentration is closely related with malignancy of glioma; low-grade glioma shows a lower intratumoral concentration of HGF than high-grade glioma. CSF concentrations of HGF greater than 850 pg/ml prior to surgery was predictive of a shorter disease-free time among malignant glioma patients than was observed for patients with a lower concentration (6 ± 0.6 months (95% [CI], 5-7) vs. 9 ± 0.5 months (95% [CI], 8-10), respectively, $p< 0.001$), besides total-gross resection surgery (Garcia-Navarrete et al., 2010). CSF concentration of HGF shows a negative correlation with survival of patients with malignant glioma and explains with high certainty the variance for survival. This suggests that HGF could be a good target candidate for molecular therapy such as RNA interference, by silencing the specific gene for HGF.

Although HGF seems a good target for therapeutic attempts, a phase II study reported the use of a monoclonal antibody against HGF (AMD 102). This study was conducted in patients with histopathologically confirmed diagnosis of GBM, gliosarcoma and history of more than 3 relapses; increases up to 10 times the basal levels of HGF in patients during treatment with AMD did not induce changes in survival time or clinical status as compared with controls (Wen et al., 2011)

5.Conclusions

To date, there is no biological marker that can accurately discern the activity of malignant gliomas. The scientific evidence obtained from experimental studies suggests that Hepatocyte Growth Factor plays a crucial role in the pathophysiology of high-grade gliomas. Findings from clinical studies suggest that HGF may be considered a distinguishing marker of biological activity of malignant gliomas, as it has been consistently demonstrated that the intratumoral, cerebrospinal fluid and serum concentrations are directly associated with prognosis and survival. The results of clinical trials aimed to evaluate the role of inhibitors of HGF or its receptor c-Met have shown disappointing therapeutic results. However, scientific advances in molecular biology could improve the response to treatment with specific inhibitors of HGF metabolism through ingenious genomic manipulations in patients with malignant gliomas.

6. References

Abounader R, Lal B, Luddy C, Koe G, Davidson B, Rosen EM, Laterra J (2002) In vivo targeting of SF/HGF and c-met expression via U1snRNA/ribozymes inhibits glioma growth and angiogenesis and promotes apoptosis. FASEB J. Vol. 16, No. 1, pp. 108-10. PMID - 11729097

Abounader R, Ranganathan S, Lal B, Fielding K, Book A, Dietz H, Burger P, Laterra J (1999). Reversion of human glioblastoma malignancy by U1 small nuclear RNA/ribozyme targeting of scatter factor/hepatocyte growth factor and c-met expression. *J Natl Cancer Inst.* Vol. 91, No. 18, pp. 1548–56. PMID - 10491431

Arrieta O, Garcia E, Guevara P, Garcia-Navarrete R, Ondarza R, Rembao D, Sotelo J. (2002). Hepatocyte growth factor is associated with poor prognosis of malignant gliomas and is a predictor for recurrence of meningioma. *Cancer.* Vol. 15, No. 94, 3210-8. PMID- 12115353

Badie B, Schartner J, Klaver J, Vorphal J. (1999). In vitro modulation of microglia by glioma cells is mediated by hepatocyte growth factor/scatter factor. *Neurosurgery.* Vol. 44, No. 5, pp. 1077–82. PMID - 10232541

Barker FG 2nd, Davis RL, Chang SM, Prados MD. (1996). Necrosis as a prognostic factor in glioblastoma multiforme. *Cancer.* Vol. 77, No. 6, pp. 1161–66. PMID - 8635139

Bhargava M, Joseph A, Knesel J, Halaban R, Li Y, Pang S, Goldberg I, Setter E, Donovan MA, Zarnegar R, Michalopoulos GA, Nakamura T, Faletto D, Rosen EM.. (1992). Scatter factor and hepatocyte growth factor: activities, properties and mechanism. *Cell Growth Differ.* Vol. 3, No. 1, pp.11–20. PMID - 1534687

Boros P, Miller CM. Hepatocyte growth factor: a multifunctional cytokine. *Lancet.* Vol. 345, No. 8945, pp. 293–95. PMID - 7837864

Bowers DC, Fan S, Walter KA, Abounader R, Williams JA, Rosen EM, Laterra J. (2000). Scatter factor/hepatocyte growth factor protects against cytotoxic death in human glioblastoma via phosphatidylinositol 3-kinase- and AKT-dependent pathways. *Cancer Res.* Vol. 60, No. 15, pp. 4277–83. PMID - 10945642

Brockmann MA, Papadimitriou A, Brandt M, Fillbrandt R, Westphal M, Lamszus K (2003) Inhibition of intracerebral glioblastoma growth by local treatment with the scatter factor/hepatocyte growth factor-antagonist NK4. *Clin Cancer Res.* Vol. 9, No.12, pp. 4578–85. PMID - 14555533

Burgess T, Coxon A, Meyer S, Sun J, Rex K, Tsuruda T, Chen Q, Ho SY, Li L, Kaufman S, McDorman K, Cattley RC, Sun J, Elliott G, Zhang K, Feng X, Jia XC, Green L, Radinsky R, Kendall R (2006). Fully human monoclonal antibodies to hepatocyte growth factor with therapeutic potential against hepatocyte growth factor/c-Met-dependent human tumors. *Cancer Res.* Vol. 66, No. 3, pp. 1721–29. PMID - 16452232

Bussolino F, Di Renzo MF, Ziche M, et al. Hepatocyte growth factor is a potent angiogenic factor which stimulated endothelial cell motility and growth. *J Cell Biol.* Vol. 119, No. 2, pp. 629–41. PMID - 1383237

Cao B, Su Y, Oskarsson M, Zhao P, Kort EJ, Fisher RJ, Wang LM, Vande Woude GF (2001). Neutralizing monoclonal antibodies to hepatocyte growth factor/scatter factor (HGF/SF) display antitumor activity in animal models. *Proc Natl Acad Sci USA.* Vol. 98, No. 13, pp. 7443–48. PMID - 11416216

Carapancea M, Alexandru O, Fetea AS, Dragutescu L, Castro J, Georgescu A, Popa-Wagner A, Bäcklund ML, Lewensohn R, Dricu A. (2009). Growth factor receptors signaling in glioblastoma cells: therapeutic implications. *J Neurooncol.* Vol. 92, No. 2, pp. 137-47. PMID - 19043776

Chu SH, Zhu ZA, Yuan XH, Li ZQ, Jiang PC (2006). In vitro and in vivo potentiating the cytotoxic effect of radiation on human U251 gliomas by the c-Met antisense oligodeoxynucleotides. *J Neurooncol.* Vol. 80, No. 2, pp. 143–9. PMID - 16648987

Dreux AC, Lamb DJ, Modjtahedi H, Ferns GA (2006). The epidermal growth factor receptors and their family of ligands: their putative role in atherogenesis. *Atherosclerosis*. Vol. 186, No. 1, pp. 38–53. PMID - 15072443

Fallon JH, Seroogy KB, Loughlin SE, Morrison RS, Bradshaw RA, Knaver DJ, Cunningham DD (1984). Epidermal growth factor immunoreactive material in the central nervous system: location and development. *Science*. Vol. 224, No. 4653, pp. 1107–9. PMID - 6144184

Grierson I, Heathcote L, Hiscott P, Hogg P, Briggs M, Hagan S. (2000). Hepatocyte growth factor/scatter factor in the eye. *Prog Retin Eye Res*. Vol. 19, No. 6, pp. 779–802. PMID - 11029554

Guessous F, Zhang Y, diPierro C, Marcinkiewicz L, Sarkaria J, Schiff D, Buchanan S, Abounader R. (2010). An orally bioavailable c-Met kinase inhibitor potently inhibits brain tumor malignancy and growth. *Anticancer Agents Med Chem*. Vol. 10, No. 1, pp. 28-35. PMID - 20015006

Guiu S, Taillibert S, Chinot O, Taillandier L, Honnorat J, Dietrich PY, Maire JP, Guillamo JS, Guiu B, Catry-Thomas I, Capelle F, Thiebaut A, Cartalat-Carel S, Deville C, Fumoleau P, Desjardins A, Xuan KH, Chauffert B. (2008). Bevacizumab/irinotecan. An active treatment for recurrent high-grade gliomas: preliminary results of an ANOCEF multi-center study. *Rev Neurol (Paris)*. Vol. 164, No. 7, pp. 588–94. PMID - 1856535

Hadjipanayis CG, Van Meir EG. (2009a). Brain cancer propagating cells: biology, genetics and targeted therapies. *Trends Mol Med*. Vol. 14, No. 11, pp. 519-30. PMID - 19889578

Hadjipanayis CG, Van Meir EG. (2009b). Tumor initiating cells in malignant gliomas: biology and implications for therapy. *J Mol Med*. Vol. 87, No. 4, pp. 363-74. PMID - 19189072

Hirose Y, Kojima M, Sagoh M, Murakami H, Yoshida K, Shimazaki K, Kawase T. (1998). Immunohistochemical examination of c-Met protein expression in astrocytic tumors. *Acta Neuropathol (Berl)*. Vol. 95, No. 4, pp. 345–51. PMID - 9560011

Hormigo A, Gu B, Karimi S, Riedel E, Panageas KS, Edgar MA, Tanwar MK, Rao JS, Fleisher M, DeAngelis LM, Holland EC (2006). YKL-40 and matrix metalloproteinase-9 as potential serum biomarkers for patients with high-grade gliomas. *Clin Cancer Res* Vol. 12, No. 19, pp 5698-5704. PMID - 17020973

Ji H, Wang J, Fang B, Fang X, Lu Z. (2010). a-Catenin inhibits glioma cell migration, invasion, and proliferation by suppression of b-catenin transactivation. *J Neurooncol*. (Epub ahead of print). PMID - 20872274

Kim KJ, Wang L, Su YC, Gillespie GY, Salhotra A, Lal B, Laterra J (2006). Systemic anti-hepatocyte growth factor monoclonal antibody therapy induces the regression of intracraneal glioma xenografts. *Clin Cancer Res*. Vol. 12, No. 4, pp. 1292–98. PMID - 16489086

Kimura F, Miyazaki M, Suwa T, Kakizaki S, Itoh H, Kaiho T, Ambiru S, Shimizu H, Togawa A. (1996). Increased levels of human hepatocyte growth factor in serum and peritoneal fluid after partial hepatectomy. *Am J Gastroenterol*. Vol. 91, No. 1, pp. 116–21. PMID - 8561110

Koochekpour S, Jeffers M, Rulong S, Taylor G, Klineberg E, Hudson EA, Resau JH, Vande Woude GF. (1997). Met and hepatocyte growth factor/scatter factor expression in human gliomas. *Cancer Res.* Vol. 57, No. 23, pp. 5391–98. PMID - 9393765

Lal B, Xia S, Abounader R, Laterra J (2005). Targeting the c-Met pathway potentiates glioblastoma responses to gamma-radiation. *Clin Cancer Res.* Vol. 11, No. 12, pp. 4479–86. PMID - 15958633

Lamszus K, Jin L, Fuchs A, Shi E, Chowdhury S, Yao Y, Polverini PJ, Laterra J, Goldberg ID, Rosen EM. (1997). Scatter factor stimulates tumor growth and tumor angiogenesis in human breast cancers in the mammary fat pads of nude mice. *Lab Invest.* Vol. 76, No. 3, pp. 339–53. PMID - 9121117

Lamszus K, Laterra J, Westphal M, Rosen E. (1999). Scatter factor/ hepatocyte growth factor (SF/HGF) content and function in human gliomas. *Int J Dev Neurosci.* Vol. 17, No. 5-6, pp. 517–30. PMID - 10571413

Lantos PL, Louis DN, Rosenblum MK, Kleihues P (2002). Tumours of the Nervous System. *Oxford University Press*: London.

Laterra J, Rosen E, Nam M, Ranganathan S, Fielding K, Johnston P. (1997). Scatter factor/hepatocyte growth factor expression enhances human glioma tumorigenicity and growth. *Biochem Biophys Res Commun.* Vol. 235, No. 3, pp. 743–7. PMID - 9207232

Louis D.N., Ohgaki H., Wiestler O.D., Cavenee W.K. (2007) WHO Classification of Tumours of the Central Nervous System. *IARC*: Lyon 2007.

Mentlein R, Forstreuter F, Mehdorn HM, Held-Feindt J. (2004). Functional significance of vascular endothelial growth factor receptor expression on human glioma cells. *J Neurooncol.* Vol. 67, No. 1-2, pp. 9-18. PMID - 15072443

Miwa Y, Harrison PM, Farzaneh F, Langley PG, Williams R, Hudges RD. Plasma levels and hepatic mRNA expression of transforming factor-beta 1 in patients with hepatic fulminant failure. *J Hepatol.* Vol. 27, No. 5, pp. 780–88. PMID - 9382963

Moriyama T, Kataoka H, Koono M, Wakaisaka S. (1999). Expression of hepatocyte growth factor/scatter factor and its receptor c-Met in brain tumors: evidence for a role in progression of astrocytic tumors. *Int J Mol Med.* Vol. 3, No. 5, pp. 531–36. PMID - 10202187

Nabeshima K, Shimao Y, Sato S, Kataoka H, Moriyama T, Kawano H, Wakisaka S, Koono M. (1997). Expression of c-Met correlates with grade of malignancy in human astrocytic tumours: an immunohistochemical study. *Histopathology.* Vol. 31, No. 5, pp. 436–43. PMID - 9416484

Narayana A, Kelly P, Golfinos J, Parker E, Johnson G, Knopp E, Zagzag D, Fischer I, Raza S, Medabalmi P, Eagan P, Gruber ML. (2009). Antiangiogenic therapy using bevacizumab in recurrent high-grade glioma: impact on local control and patient survival. *J Neurosurg.* Vol. 110, No. 1, pp. 173–180. PMID - 18834263

Neaud V, Faouzi S, Guirouilh J, Le Bail B, Balabaud C, Bioulac-Sage P, Rosenbaum J. (1997). Human hepatic myofibroblast increase invasiveness of hepatocellular carcinoma cells: evidence for a role of hepatocyte growth factor. *Hepatology.* Vol. 26, No. 6, pp. 1458–66. PMID - 9397985

Nghiemphu PL, Liu W, Lee Y, Than T, Graham C, Lai A, Green RM, Pope WB, Liau LM, Mischel PS, Nelson SF, Elashoff R, Cloughesy TF. (2009). Bevacizumab and chemotherapy for recurrent glioblastoma: a single-institution experience. *Neurology*. Vol. 72, No. 14, pp. 1217–22. PMID - 19349600

Oblinger JL, Pearl DK, Boardman CL, Saqr H, Prior TW, Scheithauer BW, Jenkins RB, Burger PC, Yates AJ (2006). Diagnostic and prognostic value of glycosyltransferase mRNA in glioblastoma multiforme patients. *Neuropathol Appl Neurobiol*. Vol. 32, No. 4, pp. 410-18. PMID - 16866986

Ohgaki H, Dessen P, Jourde B, Horstmann S, Nishikawa T, Di Patre PL, Burkhard C, Schuler D, Probst-Hensch NM, Maiorka PC, Baeza N, Pisani P, Yonekawa Y, Yasargil MG, Lutolf UM, Kleihues P (2004). Genetic pathways to glioblastoma: a population-based study. *Cancer Res*, Vol. 64, No. 19, pp. 6892-99. PMID - 15466178

Ohgaki H, Kleihues P (2007). Genetic pathways to primary and secondary glioblastoma. *Am J Pathol*, Vol. 170, No. 5, pp 1445-53. PMID - 17456751

Pelloski CE, Mahajan A, Maor M, Chang EL, Woo S, Gilbert M, Colman h, Yang H, Ledoux A, Blair H, Passe S, Jenkins RB, Aldape KD (2005). YKL-40 expression is associated with poorer response to radiation and shorter overall survival in glioblastoma. *Clin Cancer Res*. Vol. 11, No. 9, pp. 3326-34. PMID - 15867231

Peruzzi, B. and Bottaro, D.P. (2006). Targeting the c-Met signaling pathway in cancer. *Clin. Cancer Res*. Vol. 12, No. 12, pp. 3657-60. PMID - 16778093

Pope WB, Lai A, Nghiemphu P, Mischel P, Cloughesy TF. (2006). MRI in patients with high-grade gliomas treated with bevacizumab and chemotherapy. *Neurology*. Vol. 66, No. 8, pp. 1258–60. PMID - 16636248

Poulsen HS, Grunnet K, Sorensen M, Olsen P, Hasselbalch B, Nelausen K, Kosteljanetz M, Lassen U. (2009). Bevacizumab plus irinotecan in the treatment patients with progressive recurrent malignant brain tumours. *Acta Oncol*. Vol. 48, No. 1, pp. 52–58. PMID - 19031176

Schmidt NO, Westphal M, Hagel C, Ergün S, Stavrou D, Rosen EM, Lamszus K. (1999). Levels of vascular endothelial growth factor, hepatocyte growth factor/scatter factor and basic fibroblast growth factor in human gliomas and their relation to angiogenesis. *Int J Cancer*. Vol. 84, No. 1, pp. 10-18. PMID - 9988225

Stella MC, Comoglio PM. (1999). HGF: a multifunctional growth factor controlling cell scattering. *Int J Biochem Cell Biol*. Vol. 31, No. 12, pp. 1357–62. PMID - 10641789

Takeuchi E, Nimura Y, Nagino M, Kurumiya Y, Maeda A, Kamiya J, Kondo S, Kanai M, Miyachi M, Uesaka K, Yoshida S. (1997). Human hepatocyte growth factor in bile: an indicator of posthepatectomy liver function in patients with biliary tract carcinoma. *Hepatology*. Vol. 26, No. 5, pp. 1092–99. PMID - 9362347

Tan D, Xu J, Li Y, Lai R. (2010). Association between +61G polymorphism of the EGF gene and glioma risk in different ethnicities: a meta-analysis. *Tohoku J Exp Med*. Vol. 222, No. 4, pp. 229-35. PMID – 21123997

Trusolino L, Cavassa S, Angelini P, Andó M, Bertotti A, Comoglio PM, Boccaccio C. (2000). HGF/scatter factor selectively promotes cell invasion by increasing integrin avidity. *FASEB J*. Vol. 14, No. 11, pp. 1629–40. PMID - 10928998

Van Meir EG, Hadjipanayis CG, Norden AD, Shu HK, Wen PY, Olson JJ.. (2010). Exciting New Advances in Neuro-Oncology: The Avenue to a Cure for Malignant Glioma. *CA Cancer J Clin*. Vol. 60, No. 3, pp 166–193. PMID - 20445000

Wen PY, Schiff D, Cloughesy TF, Raizer JJ, Laterra J, Smitt M, Wolf M, Oliner KS, Anderson A, Zhu M, Loh E, Reardon DA. (2011). A phase II study evaluating the efficacy and safety of AMG 102 (rilotumumab) in patients with recurrent glioblastoma. *Neuro Oncol.* Vol. 13, No. 4, pp. 437-46. PMID - 21297127

Wood GW, Morantz RA. (1983). Depressed T lymphocyte function in brain tumor patients: monocytes as suppressor cells. *J Neurooncol.* Vol. 1, No. 2, pp. 87–94. PMID - 6236289

Xian CJ, Li L, Deng YS, Zhao SP, Zhou XF. (2001). Lack of effects of transforming growth factor-alpha gene knockout on peripheral nerve regeneration may result from compensatory mechanisms. *Exp Neurol.* Vol. 172, No. 1, pp. 182-8. PMID - 11681850

Xiao G, Jeffers M, Bellacosa A, Mitsuuchi Y, Vande Woude G, Testa J. (2001). Anti-apoptotic signaling by hepatocyte growth factor/Met via the phosphatidylinositol 3-kinase/Akt and mitogen activated protein kinase pathways. Proc Natl Acad Sci. Vol.98, No. 1, pp. 247–52. PMID - 11134526

Yamada T, Tsubouchi H, Daikuhara Y, Prat M, Comoglio PM, McGeer PL, McGeer (1994). Immunohistochemistry with antibodies to hepatocyte growth factor and its receptor protein (c-Met) in human brain tissues. *Brain Res.* Vol. 637, No. 1-2, pp. 308–12. PMID - 8180811

Zuniga RM, Torcuator R, Jain R, Anderson J, Doyle T, Ellika S, Schultz L, Mikkelsen T.. (2009). Efficacy, safety and patterns of response and recurrence in patients with recurrent high-grade gliomas treated with bevacizumab plus irinotecan.*J Neurooncol.* Vol. 91, No. 3, pp. 329–36. PMID - 18953493

Molecular Etiology of Glioblastomas: Implication of Genomic Profiling From the Cancer Genome Atlas Project

Kimberly Ng.[1], Santosh Kesari[2], Bob Carter[3,4] and Clark C. Chen[1,5]

[1]*Department of Radiation Oncology, Dana-Farber Cancer Institute, Boston, MA*
[2]*Department of Neurology, Moores UCSD Cancer Center, UCSD,*
[3]*Center for Theoretic and Applied Neuro-Oncology,*
University of California San Diego, San Diego, CA
[4]*Department of Surgery, Division of Neurosurgery,*
University of California San Dieog, San Diego, CA
[5]*Division of Neurosurgery, Beth Israel Deaconess Medical Center, Boston, MA*
USA

1. Introduction

In the landmark review by Hanahan and Weinberg[1], the authors distilled the essence of cancer into six distinct phenotypes, including evasion of apoptosis, self-sufficiency in growth signals, insensitivity to anti-growth signals, tissue invasion and metastasis, limitless replicative potentials, and sustained angiogenesis. The widely accepted paradigm suggests that cancer arises as a result of mutations or epigenetic events, which alter function of genes critical for attaining these phenotypes. These gene functions are intimately linked to the regulation of developmental processes[2], their aberrant function in tumor inevitably lead to cell states that resemble stages during normal development. These cell states can be captured using genomic technologies to define distinct molecular subtypes. With the advent of The Genome Cancer Atlas project for glioblastoma[3,4], we now have a glimpse of the genetic events underlying glioblastoma pathogenesis as well as distinct molecular subtypes. In this review, the genomic profiles of glioblastoma will be reviewed in the context of the properties described by Hanahan and Weinberg. Molecular subtypes of glioblastoma will be discussed in the context of developmental biology and the cell of origin.

2. Glioblastoma

Glioblastoma is the most common form of primary brain tumor, with dismal prognosis. The incidence of this tumor is fairly low, with 2-3 cases per 100,000 people in Europe and North America. Despite its rarity, overall mortality related to glioblastoma is comparable to the more prevalent tumors[5]. This is, in large part, due to the near uniform fatality of the afflicted patients. Indeed, glioblastoma is one of the most aggressive of the malignant tumors. Without treatment, the median survival is approximately 3 months[6]. The current standard of treatment involves maximal surgical resection followed by concurrent radiation therapy and chemotherapy with the DNA alkylating agent, temozolomide[7]. With this regimen, the median survival is approximately 14 months. For nearly all affected, the treatments available remain palliative.

Studies carried out over the past three decades suggest that glioblastomas, like other cancers, arise secondary to the accumulation of genetic alterations. These alterations can take the form of epigenetic modifications, point mutations, translocations, amplifications, or deletions, and modify gene function in ways that deregulate cellular signaling pathways leading to the cancer phenotype[1]. The exact number and nature of genetic alterations and deregulated signaling pathways required for tumorogenesis remains an issue of debate[8], although it is now clear that CNS carcinogenesis requires multiple disruptions to the normal cellular circuitry[3, 4].

3. The Cancer Genome Atlas (TCGA) project

The Cancer Genome Atlas (TCGA) is a comprehensive and coordinated effort to catalogue the genetic and epigenetic changes in the cancer genome, with goals of identifying those responsible for carcinogenesis. The project constitutes a joint effort of the National Human Genome Research Institute (NHGRI), National Cancer Institute (NCI), and the U.S. Department of Health and Human Services, and collects tumor specimen from major cancer centers spanning across the continental U.S. The project aims to provide the genomic profile of 500 specimens of various cancer types using state-of-the-art platforms for sequencing, microRNA, mRNA, single-nucleotide polymorphisms, and methylation profiling.

TCGA started as a pilot project in 2006 with focus on glioblastoma as the first cancer type for study. With the success of the pilot project, TCGA plans to expand its efforts to aggressively pursue 20 or more additional cancers. This article will review the major insights derived from the TCGA in the context of the cancer phenotypes proposed by Hanahan and Weinberg[1].

4. The cancer phenotype

The aggregate of cancer research investigation spanning the past three decades suggest that cancer is a genetic disease characterized by mutations or epigenetic events that abrogate or compromise regulatory circuitry governing cell proliferation and homeostasis[8]. In the landmark review by Hanahan and Weinberg[1], the authors distilled the essence of these regulatory circuits into six distinct phenotypes, including evading apoptosis, self-sufficiency in growth signals, insensitivity to anti-growth signals, tissue invasion and metastasis, limitless replicative potentials, and sustained angiogenesis. The following section will review the TCGA findings pertinent to these phenotypes.

4.1 Self-sufficiency in growth signals – The Receptor Tyrosine Kinase (RTK)/Phospholnosital 3 Kinase (PI3K) signaling cascade

Active cellular proliferation in normal cells requires signals from its environment. These signals typically involve the binding of a transmembrane receptor to growth factors, extracellular matrix components, or cell surface components. This mitogenic signaling process is under stringent regulation in normal cells. Typically, multiple ligand-receptor interactions in a permissive cellular state are required before cellular proliferation can take place. This regulation minimizes the probability of dysregulated, autonomous cell growth[1,9]. The importance of growth factors in biology was recognized by a Nobel Prize in Physiology or Medicine to Stanley Cohen and Rita Levi-Montalcini in 1986. Subsequent identification that many oncogenes participate in cellular signaling related to growth factor function was also awarded a Nobel Prize in Physiology or Medicine (to Michael Bishop and Harold Varmus in 1989).

To abridge this stringent growth regulation, tumors often mutate the transmembrane receptors or their downstream effectors in ways that constitutively activate the pathway. The pathway most commonly mutated to achieve this end in glioblastoma involves the RTK-PI3K pathway[9,10]. RTKs are cell surface receptors that are normally activated only in response to growth factor binding[9]. Results from the TCGA revealed that nearly all glioblastomas harbor activating mutations or amplifications in genes required for this signaling cascade[3,4,11,12]. Epidermal Growth Factor Receptor (EGFR) and Platelet Derived Growth Factor Receptor (PDGFR) are two prototypical members of RTK[3, 4, 12].

For EGFR and PDGFR, binding of the growth factor to the ligand leads to homo- or hetero-dimerization of the receptor. This dimerization facilitates autophosphorylation of the cytoplasmic domains of the dimerized receptor at select tyrosine residues[9]. The phosphorylated tyrosine residue, in turn, recruits and binds to other signaling proteins to the cell membrane. In some cases, the phospho-tyrosine bound proteins serve as a platform for the recruitment of other effector proteins. In other cases, the bound protein undergoes a conformational change upon binding to the RTK and becomes activated in the process[9].

One of the critical cellular kinases that become activated upon binding to RTK is PI3K[13]. PI3Ks catalyze the phosphorylation of a critical component of the cell surface, phosphatidylinositol-4,5-isphosphate (PI(4,5)P2). This phosphorylation generates phosphatidylinositol-1,4,5-isphosphate (PI(1,4,5)P3), which in turn serves as a docking site for pro-proliferative down-stream effector proteins[10]. Thus, RTK activation transforms the cell membrane into a catalytic surface populated with a high density of pro-mitotic signaling molecules, ultimately leading to cell proliferation.

Expectedly, gene functions that inhibit the generation of this pro-proliferative "catalytic surface" function as tumor suppressors. For instance, the hydrolysis of (PI(1,4,5)P3) into (PI(4,5)P2) is catalyzed by a phosphatase termed Phosphatase and Tensin Homology (PTEN). PTEN inactivating mutations have been identified in up to 50% of tumor specimens[14]. Similarly, one of the effector proteins recruited to a phosphorylated RTK is Ras. Ras encodes a monomeric G-protein that cycles between an active form bound to GTP and an inactive form that binds to GDP[15]. It functions as a critical component of the pro-proliferative "catalytic surface". Through a series of protein-protein interactions, RTK activation catalyzes the exchange of GDP for GTP in Ras, initiating signals required for cellular proliferation. The protein encoded by neurofibromatosis 1 (NF1) functions to catalyze the exchange of GTP for GDP in Ras, consequently preventing cell proliferation. In this context, it is not surprising that NF1 patients are predisposed to gliomagenesis[16]. The TCGA results showed that approximately 20% of glioblastomas harbor loss of function mutations in NF1[3,4]. TCGA additionally revealed gain of function mutations in K-ras have also been identified in glioblastoma specimens[3].

4.2 Insensitivity to anti-growth signals – The RB axis

In addition to receiving pro-growth signals from their environment, cells also receive multiple anti-proliferative signals to prevent cell growth. These anti-growth signals, like their pro-mitotic counterparts, are sensed by the binding of transmembrane receptors to soluble factors, extracellular matrix components, or cell surface components.

Most of these anti-proliferative signals operate at the G1 phase of the cell cycle to trigger either 1) entry into a transient quiescent (G0) state or 2) entry into a post-mitotic, differentiated state. The importance of cell cycle regulation in biology was recognized by a Nobel Prize in Physiology or Medicine to Leland Hartwell, Tim Hunt, and Sir Paul Nurse in 2001.

At the molecular level, nearly all of these signals converge at the retinoblastoma protein (RB) [1]. In quiescent cells, the RB protein is hyper-phosphorylated. This form of RB binds and sequesters the E2F family of transcription factors[17]. The genes transcribed by these transcription factors are essential for the G1-S transition of the cell cycle[18]. Phosphorylation of RB releases the sequestered E2F transcription factors and allows for cell growth. During normal cell cycle progression, induction of cyclin D1 and its associated cyclin-dependent kinases, CDK4 and CDK6, at the G1-S transition is responsible for the phosphorylation of RB. The kinase activity of the CDK4/6-cyclin D complex is under complex regulation, including the critical negative regulators CDKN2A (p16[Ink4a]), CDKN2B, and CDKN2C. TCGA results showed that mutations and gene amplifications disrupting RB function are found in approximately 80% of glioblastomas, suggesting the critical importance of escaping anti-growth signals[3,4]. Additionally, single nucleotide polymorphisms in the *CDKN2A* and *CDKN2B* have been identified as risk factors for glioma development[19,20].

4.3 Evading apoptosis – The p53 axis

Apoptotic programs are inherent in all normal cells. These programs are activated by a number of physiologic signals during development and/or in response to cellular stress. Since the tumor state is associated with cellular stress capable of activating apoptosis (e.g. increased oxidative stress, increased DNA damage accumulation), inactivation of these programs constitute a critical step during carcinogenesis. The importance of apoptosis as a fundamental biologic process was recognized by a Nobel Prize in Physiology or Medicine awarded to Sydney Brenner, Robert Horvitz, and John Sulston in 2002.

The regulation of apoptotic pathways is highly complex[21]. Broadly speaking, there are two pathways of apoptosis that converge on the activation of effector proteases (termed caspases), which ultimately trigger the pathognomonic DNA fragmentation, cell shrinkage, and membrane blebbing. The intrinsic cell death pathway (often termed the mitochondrial apoptotic pathway) involves the release of cytochrome c from the mitochondrial membrane space[22]. Binding of cytochrome c to a protein termed apoptosis protease-activating factor 1 (APAF-1), in turn, initiates the caspase cascade. In contrast, the extrinsic apoptotic pathway operates independently of mitochondria and is activated by direct signaling from cell surface receptors to the effector caspase[23].

Both intrinsic and extrinsic apoptotic programs are profoundly influenced by the p53 tumor suppressor protein[24]. *TP53* encodes a transcription factor that regulates gene sets critical for cell cycle progression and apoptosis. Under normal conditions, p53 is a short-lived protein[25]. In response to cellular stress (for instance, DNA damage or oncogene expression), p53 undergoes post-translational modifications and protein-protein interactions that enhance its stability and transcriptional activity[25]. Key among the transcripts regulated by p53 are pro-apoptotic genes (including BAX and Puma) that facilitate both the intrinsic and extrinsic pathway[24]. Additionally, p53 interact with a number of anti-apoptotic proteins to inhibit their function[24].

There are several lines of evidence that point to the importance of the p53 axis in glioblastoma pathogenesis. In the TCGA database, mutations that inactivate this axis are found in greater than 70% of glioblastoma specimens[3,4]. Patients harboring germ-line mutations in *TP53* are afflicted with cancer predisposition including increased risk for glioblastoma[26]. Finally, inactivation of p53 is required for glioma formation in genetically defined murine models[27].

4.4 Replicative potential

The definition of cancer as a continuous growing entity implies that normal cells exhibit a limited capacity for proliferation. Indeed, estimates based on tissue culture work suggest that most normal cells have the capacity for 50 doublings [28]. Studies over the past three decades suggest that the main reason for this limited life span involve progressive shortening of chromosomes due to loss of telomeres. Telomeres consist of thousands of six base pair sequence element of repeats that are located at the ends of every chromosome. Because of the inability of DNA polymerases to replicate the 3' ends of chromosomal DNA, approximately 60 base pairs of the telomeric sequence is lost with each replicative cycle[29]. With progressive erosion of the telomeric sequence, the unprotected chromosomal ends participate in aberrant fusion events that inevitably result in cell death[30].

To overcome this inherent limitation, most cancer cells activate an enzyme called telomerase. Telomerase is a reverse transcriptase capable of elongating telomeres[31]. Various mechanisms are employed by tumors to activate telomerase in order to sustain continued cell growth. Elizabeth Balckburn, Carol Greider, and Jack Szostak were awarded the Nobel Prize in Physiology or Medicine in 2009 for their discovery of telomerase.

With regards to glioblastomas, single nucleotide polymorphisms in two genes encoding components of the telomerase (*RTEL1* and *TERT*) have been identified as risk factors for glioma development[19, 20]. Additionally, elevated expression level of *TERT* in glioblastoma is associated with decreased patient survival [32]. These studies suggest a critical importance of telomeric biology in glioblastoma growth and survival.

Angiogenesis. The intense proliferation of cancer cells require continued supply of oxygen and nutrients. Due to inherent limitations on the distance that oxygen and macromolecules can travel, virtually all cells in a tissue reside with 100 um of a capillary. In xenograft model systems, solid tumors can only proliferate up to a size of 1-2 mm without development of new blood supply[33]. Thus, angiogenesis necessarily constitutes a pre-requisite during solid tumor progression.

One way by which cancer cells signal angiogenesis is by secretion of soluble factors that bind to receptors present on the surface endothelial cells. A key soluble factor that functions in such capacity is the Vascular Endothelial Growth Factor (VEGF). VEGF binds to RTKs on the surface of endothelial cells to facilitate their proliferation – leading to angiogenesis[34]. In normal cells, transcription of VEGF and other pro-angiogenic signaling factors are under strict regulation. The induction of Hypoxia Inducible Factor I (HIF1) is a pivotal element in this regulatory network[35]. HIF1 encodes a dimeric transcription factor consisting of two subunits: HIF1α and HIF1β. HIF1β is constitutively expressed irrespective of oxygen concentration, whereas HIF1α levels increase dramatically in response to hypoxia. The underlying mechanism for this regulation is that HIF1α is hydroxylated by HIF Prolyl-4-Hydroxylase (HPH) in the presence of di-oxygen (O_2), iron, and α-ketoglutarate. The hydroxylated HIF1α is targeted for proteasome degradation. Without molecular oxygen,

HIF1α is not hydroxylated and is free to dimerize with HIF1β to activate the transcription of downstream pro-angiogenetic factors.

Integrated analysis of genomic data in glioblastoma revealed recurrent mutations in the R132 residue of isocitrate dehydrogenase 1 (IDH1)[4], a gene largely responsible for the production of α-ketoglutarate. The TCGA data revealed that the IDH1 mutation is predominantly found in one particular molecular subtype of glioblastoma[12, 36] (see following section on **molecular subtypes**). The wildtype IDH1 normally functions as a homodimer that converts isocitrate to α-ketoglutarate[37]. Biochemical characterization of the R132 mutated IDH1 revealed that it functions in a dominantly negative fashion to inhibit the process. Expectedly, glioblastoma harboring the R132 IDH1 mutation harbor decreased levels of α-ketoglutarate. Given the importance of α-ketoglutarate in HIF1α degradation, one would anticipate increased HIF1α accumulation and increased VEGF secretion in glioblastoma harboring the IDH1 mutation. These observations were confirmed in a panel of primary glioblastoma specimens[38]. Thus, the IDH1 mutation constitutes an example of how glioblastoma subverts the endogenous molecular circuit to facilitate angiogenesis. It should be noted that the effect of the IDH1 mutation appears pleiotropic. Another study revealed that the R132 mutant IDH1 proteins exhibits a gain-of-function phenotype by generating R(-)-2-hydroxyglutarate, a carcinogenic metabolite[39].

In glioblastomas without IDH1 mutation, alternate mechanisms are utilized to facilitate angiogenesis. It is somewhat intuitive that during normal development, periods of cellular proliferation must be coordinated with angiogenesis. Indeed, a large body of work suggests that gene functions that facilitate cell-autonomous growth or insensitivity to growth inhibition and apoptosis also tend to facilitate angiogenesis[40, 41]. It is likely that most glioblastoma cells attain angiogenesis by aberrant activation of such coordinated developmental programs. For instance, EGFR activation has been shown to up-regulate VEGF in both HIF dependent and independent manner[42]. Inactivation of Rb increases VEGF expression and angiogenesis in vivo[40]. Similarly, p53 normally up-regulates thrombospondin 1, an inhibitor of angiogenesis[43]; inactivation of p53 can facilitate angiogenesis by ablation of this up-regulation.

4.5 Invasion and metastasis

The ability to invade and metastasize constitutes the fundamental distinction between benign and malignant tumors. It is important to note that invasion refers not just to distortion of normal tissue secondary to tumor growth. Instead, it refers to a coordinated set of cellular activities to destroy and migrate into the surrounding normal tissue. Metastasis refers to the capacity to travel via circulation to a distant tissue site[33]. Glioblastoma is unique in that while it is one of the most invasive of cancers, it rarely metastasizes outside of the central nervous system.

It is a truism that cancer cells generally retain some general properties of the cell of origin. Since glioblastoma originates from astrocytes, which normally possess significant migratory capacity, the invasive nature of glioblastoma would be anticipated. During normal development, astrocytes migrate in a centripetal manner to establish a scaffold for neuroblasts[44]. Additionally, in response to injury, astrocytes migrate to the affected region to form a gliotic scar[45]. This migratory capacity is the phenotypic expression of carefully orchestrated interactions between cellular cytoskeletal proteins, cell adhesion molecules, and extracellular matrix[33].

To date, the TCGA has not uncovered gain of function mutations in these proteins. However, enhanced invasive properties have been associated with mutations establishing autonomous growth or suppressing apoptosis. For instance, aberrant EGFR activation results in increased expression and phosphorylation of cell adhesion molecules that ultimately lead to increased invasiveness[46]. Similarly, the p53 mutation drives cancer invasiveness by facilitating the recycling of integrin, a class of cell surface receptor that interacts with extracellular matrix during cell migration[47].

The aggregate of the data suggest that both angiogenesis and cell migratory properties are intimately integrated into a master circuitry controlled by critical proteins that dictate cellular response to growth or apoptotic signals. In this context, mutations facilitating self-autonomous growth or suppression of apoptosis also contribute to angiogenesis and cell invasion.

4.6 Cross-talk between canonical pathways
The conceptualization of distinct pathways contributing to the various critical phenotypes constitutes a simplification aimed to consolidate distinct biological concepts. The reality is that pathways mediating the cancer phenotype exhibit high degrees of cross-talk and functional redundancy. For instance, EGFR hyperactivation is associated with increased tumor growth (replicative potential), angiogenesis, and increased tumor motility [48]. Similarly, many genes mediating cell motility, telomere function, and angiogenesis are under transcriptional regulation by p53 and RB associated E2Fs[49].

5. Pathway of glioblastoma progression

It was previously thought that glioblastoma arises from the acquisition of a defined set of mutations that occur in a particular temporal order. This model is largely grounded on the framework established in colon cancer, where a series of genetic alterations characterizes different phases of neoplastic progression[50]. The framework is supported by the observation that Grade II astrocytomas typically harbor mutations in p53; Grade III astrocytomas harbor activating mutations/amplifications of CDKN2A (p16[Ink4a]); and Grade IV astrocytomas harbor mutations in PTEN and EGFR[51]. This data was interpreted to mean that glioblastoma results from sequential inactivation of the p53, RB, and RTK/PI3K axes.

While such a paradigm may hold true for a subset of the secondary glioblastomas, the picture emerging from the genomic characterization of primary glioblastomas reveals a much more dynamic process[3,4]. The profile of somatic mutations in different glioblastomas is highly variable. These results suggest that most glioblastomas evolve along a multitude of pathways in response to differing selective pressures to achieve the phenotypes described by Hanahan and Weinberg[52]. This somewhat stochastic model of cancer progression further implies that mutations critical at one juncture in the neoplastic process may lose relevance as additional mutations are acquired. Thus, while a mutational profile constitutes an archeological profile of the history of the neoplasm, extrapolating therapeutic targets from such a profile may be challenging.

6. Molecular subtypes

Genome-scale gene expression profiling using microarray technology have revealed distinct molecular subtypes within tumors previously classified as glioblastomas [12, 53-55]. The number of subtypes varies depending on the study, however, three subtypes consistently appear across independent studies and reflect distinct biologic and clinical behaviors [12, 55, 56]. Importantly, the transcript signature parallels those obtained during distinct stages in neural development, suggesting the tumor may have arisen from different stages of neurogenesis[55].

The first subtype is termed pro-neural. The transcript signature resembles those of neuro-blasts and oligodendrocytes derived from fetal and adult brain[55]. This subtype harbors molecular and clinical features that closely mirror those previously classified as secondary glioblastomas. Molecularly, pro-neural glioblastomas harbor mutations classically associated with the secondary subtype, including p53 and PDGFR[12]. Accordingly, grade II and III gliomas harbor molecular signatures most reminiscent of the pro-neural subtype[55]. Clinically, this subtype typically affects younger patients, is associated with improved overall survival[55], and responds poorly to concurrent radiation/temozolomide treatment upon disease progression[12]. Interestingly, mutations in the isocitrate dehydrogenase 1 gene (*IDH1*), a metabolic protein required for conversion of isocitrate to a-ketoglutamate during the citric acid cycle, is frequently observed in pro-neural glioblastomas (see section on glioblastoma predisposition syndromes). The molecular basis of how this mutation contributes to the cancer phenotype remains an active area of investigation.

Classical (also termed proliferative by some authors) constitutes the second molecular subtype. Transcript signature in the classical subtype resembles those observed in transit amplifying neural progenitor cells[55] and murine astrocytes[12]. This subtype is exclusively found in WHO grade IV tumors and constitutes a form of primary glioblastoma[57]. Molecularly, this subtype is characterized by amplification of (or activating mutations in) EGFR and CDKN2A (p16[Ink4a]). Genes involved in pathways highly active in neural stem and progenitor cells (including the Notch and Sonic hedgehog pathway) are highly expressed in the classical subtype).[58] The patients afflicted are typically older than those with the pro-neural subtype. Relative to the other subtype, patients afflicted with the classical subtype exhibit the worst prognosis, but the best therapeutic response to concurrent radiation/temozolomide treatment.

The mesenchymal subtype makes up the final category. The transcript signature in the mesenchymal subtype mirrors those observed in the neural stem cells of the forebrain[55] and cultured astroglial cells[59]. Most cultured glioblastoma cell lines exhibit transcript signatures that fall into this subtype. Molecularly, the subtype is characterized by inactivating NF1 and PTEN mutations[12]. This subgroup also has the highest expression of angiogenesis markers including VEGF (Vascular Epithelial Growth Factor) transcripts and highest density of microvascular proliferation[12]. The patients afflicted are typically older than those with the pro-neural subtype. Relative to the other subtypes, mesenchymal glioblastomas exhibit clinical response similar to the classical subtype, and a trend toward slightly improved prognosis and response to radiation/temozolomide therapy[12].

There is significant debate with regards to the origin of the distinct molecular subtypes. On one extreme is the thought that the subtypes originate from the same cell type with differences driven by distinct signaling pathways. The other extreme suggests that subtypes are determined by the same signaling pathways activated in a different cell of origin. The observation that the same canonical pathways are altered irrespective of subtype would tend to support the latter hypothesis. However, it is conceivable that different genes thought to participate in the same canonical pathway may modulate processes distinct of that pathway. Such functions may contribute to the distinct molecular subtypes. Still, it is conceivable that differences in signaling and cell of origin both contribute to subtype formation. This critical debate awaits experimental resolution.

7. Summary

The past three decades of work in cancer research has generated a sophisticated conceptual framework for the process of neoplastic transformation. The framework suggests that genetic and epigenetic events inactivating critical pathways that regulate several key aspects of cellular function are an etiology. These cellular functions can be categorized as self-sufficiency in growth signaling, evasion of apoptosis, insensitivity to anti-growth signals, tissue invasion, and limitless replicative potential and angiogenesis. This framework has largely been validated by a large scale, high-throughput characterization of the genomic and epigenomic landscape in glioblastomas. The picture emerging from these analyses suggests that most glioblastomas evolve along a multitude of pathways in response to differing selective pressures to achieve the cancer phenotypes. Transcript based analysis revealed distinct subtypes with potential implications with regards to the cell of origin. The dynamic interplay of growth dysregulation and the cell of origin during the neoplastic transformation process harbors vital implications with regards to therapeutic development.

8. References

[1] Hanahan D, Weinberg RA. The hallmarks of cancer. *Cell.* Jan 7 2000;100(1):57-70.

[2] Zelenka PS. Proto-oncogenes in cell differentiation. *Bioessays.* Jan 1990;12(1):22-26.

[3] TCGA. Comprehensive genomic characterization defines human glioblastoma genes and core pathways. *Nature.* Oct 23 2008;455(7216):1061-1068.

[4] Parsons DW, Jones S, Zhang X, et al. An integrated genomic analysis of human glioblastoma multiforme. *Science.* Sep 26 2008;321(5897):1807-1812.

[5] Wen PY, Kesari S. Malignant gliomas in adults. *N Engl J Med.* Jul 31 2008;359(5):492-507.

[6] Walker MD, Alexander E, Jr., Hunt WE, et al. Evaluation of BCNU and/or radiotherapy in the treatment of anaplastic gliomas. A cooperative clinical trial. *J Neurosurg.* Sep 1978;49(3):333-343.

[7] Stupp R, Mason WP, van den Bent MJ, et al. Radiotherapy plus concomitant and adjuvant temozolomide for glioblastoma. *N Engl J Med.* Mar 10 2005;352(10):987-996.

[8] Stratton MR, Campbell PJ, Futreal PA. The cancer genome. *Nature.* Apr 9 2009;458(7239):719-724.

[9] Schlessinger J. Cell signaling by receptor tyrosine kinases. *Cell.* Oct 13 2000;103(2):211-225.

[10] Hennessy BT, Smith DL, Ram PT, Lu Y, Mills GB. Exploiting the PI3K/AKT pathway for cancer drug discovery. *Nat Rev Drug Discov.* Dec 2005;4(12):988-1004.

[11] Stommel JM, Kimmelman AC, Ying H, et al. Coactivation of receptor tyrosine kinases affects the response of tumor cells to targeted therapies. *Science.* Oct 12 2007;318(5848):287-290.

[12] Verhaak RGW, Hoadley KA, Purdom E, et al. Integrated genomic analysis identifies clinically relevant subtypes of glioblastoma characterized by abnormalities in PDGFRA, IDH1, EGFR, and NF1. *Cancer Cell.* Jan 19 2010;17(1):98-110.

[13] Cantley LC. The phosphoinositide 3-kinase pathway. *Science.* May 31 2002;296(5573):1655-1657.

[14] Li J, Yen C, Liaw D, et al. PTEN, a putative protein tyrosine phosphatase gene mutated in human brain, breast, and prostate cancer. *Science.* Mar 28 1997;275(5308):1943-1947.

[15] Downward J. Targeting RAS signalling pathways in cancer therapy. *Nat Rev Cancer.* Jan 2003;3(1):11-22.

[16] Walker L, Thompson D, Easton D, et al. A prospective study of neurofibromatosis type 1 cancer incidence in the UK. *Br J Cancer.* Jul 17 2006;95(2):233-238.

[17] Knudsen ES, Wang JY. Targeting the RB-pathway in cancer therapy. *Clin Cancer Res.* Feb 15 2010;16(4):1094-1099.

[18] Buchkovich K, Duffy LA, Harlow E. The retinoblastoma protein is phosphorylated during specific phases of the cell cycle. *Cell.* Sep 22 1989;58(6):1097-1105.

[19] Shete S, Hosking FJ, Robertson LB, et al. Genome-wide association study identifies five susceptibility loci for glioma. *Nat Genet.* Aug 2009;41(8):899-904.

[20] Wrensch M, Jenkins RB, Chang JS, et al. Variants in the CDKN2B and RTEL1 regions are associated with high-grade glioma susceptibility. *Nat Genet.* Aug 2009;41(8):905-908.

[21] Fan TJ, Han LH, Cong RS, Liang J. Caspase family proteases and apoptosis. *Acta Biochim Biophys Sin (Shanghai).* Nov 2005;37(11):719-727.

[22] Lowe SW, Cepero E, Evan G. Intrinsic tumour suppression. *Nature.* Nov 18 2004;432(7015):307-315.

[23] Ashkenazi A, Dixit VM. Apoptosis control by death and decoy receptors. *Curr Opin Cell Biol.* Apr 1999;11(2):255-260.

[24] Haupt S, Berger M, Goldberg Z, Haupt Y. Apoptosis - the p53 network. *J Cell Sci.* Oct 15 2003;116(Pt 20):4077-4085.

[25] Harris CC. p53 tumor suppressor gene: from the basic research laboratory to the clinic--an abridged historical perspective. *Carcinogenesis.* Jun 1996;17(6):1187-1198.

[26] Li FP, Fraumeni JF, Jr. Soft-tissue sarcomas, breast cancer, and other neoplasms. A familial syndrome? *Ann Intern Med.* Oct 1969;71(4):747-752.

[27] Holland EC. Gliomagenesis: genetic alterations and mouse models. *Nat Rev Genet.* Feb 2001;2(2):120-129.

[28] Hayflick L. The Limited in Vitro Lifetime of Human Diploid Cell Strains. *Exp Cell Res.* Mar 1965;37:614-636.

[29] Zhang X, Mar V, Zhou W, Harrington L, Robinson MO. Telomere shortening and apoptosis in telomerase-inhibited human tumor cells. *Genes Dev.* Sep 15 1999;13(18):2388-2399.

[30] Artandi SE, Chang S, Lee SL, et al. Telomere dysfunction promotes non-reciprocal translocations and epithelial cancers in mice. *Nature.* Aug 10 2000;406(6796):641-645.

[31] Cohen SB, Graham ME, Lovrecz GO, Bache N, Robinson PJ, Reddel RR. Protein composition of catalytically active human telomerase from immortal cells. *Science.* Mar 30 2007;315(5820):1850-1853.

[32] Alonso MM, Fueyo J, Shay JW, et al. Expression of transcription factor E2F1 and telomerase in glioblastomas: mechanistic linkage and prognostic significance. *J Natl Cancer Inst.* Nov 2 2005;97(21):1589-1600.

[33] Leber MF, Efferth T. Molecular principles of cancer invasion and metastasis (review). *Int J Oncol.* Apr 2009;34(4):881-895.

[34] Veikkola T, Alitalo K. VEGFs, receptors and angiogenesis. *Semin Cancer Biol.* Jun 1999;9(3):211-220.

[35] Sharp FR, Bernaudin M. HIF1 and oxygen sensing in the brain. *Nat Rev Neurosci.* Jun 2004;5(6):437-448.

[36] Yan H, Parsons DW, Jin G, et al. IDH1 and IDH2 mutations in gliomas. *N Engl J Med.* Feb 19 2009;360(8):765-773.

[37] Yan H, Bigner DD, Velculescu V, Parsons DW. Mutant metabolic enzymes are at the origin of gliomas. *Cancer Res.* Dec 15 2009;69(24):9157-9159.

[38] Zhao S, Lin Y, Xu W, et al. Glioma-derived mutations in IDH1 dominantly inhibit IDH1 catalytic activity and induce HIF-1alpha. *Science.* Apr 10 2009;324(5924):261-265.

[39] Dang L, White DW, Gross S, et al. Cancer-associated IDH1 mutations produce 2-hydroxyglutarate. *Nature.* Dec 10 2009;462(7274):739-744.

[40] Gabellini C, Del Bufalo D, Zupi G. Involvement of RB gene family in tumor angiogenesis. *Oncogene.* Aug 28 2006;25(38):5326-5332.

[41] Hoeben A, Landuyt B, Highley MS, Wildiers H, Van Oosterom AT, De Bruijn EA. Vascular endothelial growth factor and angiogenesis. *Pharmacol Rev.* Dec 2004;56(4):549-580.

[42] Haley JD, Gullick WJ, eds. *EGFR Signaling Networks in Cancer Therapy.* New York: Humana Press; 2008.

[43] Rak J, Mitsuhashi Y, Sheehan C, et al. Oncogenes and tumor angiogenesis: differential modes of vascular endothelial growth factor up-regulation in ras-transformed epithelial cells and fibroblasts. *Cancer Res.* Jan 15 2000;60(2):490-498.

[44] Jacobsen CT, Miller RH. Control of astrocyte migration in the developing cerebral cortex. *Dev Neurosci.* Mar-Aug 2003;25(2-4):207-216.

[45] Ridet JL, Malhotra SK, Privat A, Gage FH. Reactive astrocytes: cellular and molecular cues to biological function. *Trends Neurosci.* Dec 1997;20(12):570-577.

[46] Micallef J, Taccone M, Mukherjee J, et al. Epidermal growth factor receptor variant III-induced glioma invasion is mediated through myristoylated alanine-rich protein kinase C substrate overexpression. *Cancer Res.* Oct 1 2009;69(19):7548-7556.

[47] Muller PA, Caswell PT, Doyle B, et al. Mutant p53 drives invasion by promoting integrin recycling. *Cell.* Dec 24 2009;139(7):1327-1341.

[48] Nakamura JL. The epidermal growth factor receptor in malignant gliomas: pathogenesis and therapeutic implications. *Expert Opin Ther Targets.* Apr 2007;11(4):463-472.

[49] Sherr CJ, McCormick F. The RB and p53 pathways in cancer. *Cancer Cell.* Aug 2002;2(2):103-112.

[50] Vogelstein B, Fearon ER, Hamilton SR, et al. Genetic alterations during colorectal-tumor development. *N Engl J Med.* Sep 1 1988;319(9):525-532.

[51] Gladson CL, Prayson RA, Liu WM. The pathobiology of glioma tumors. *Annu Rev Pathol.* 2010;5:33-50.

[52] Salk JJ, Fox EJ, Loeb LA. Mutational heterogeneity in human cancers: origin and consequences. *Annu Rev Pathol.* 2010;5:51-75.

[53] Nutt CL, Mani DR, Betensky RA, et al. Gene expression-based classification of malignant gliomas correlates better with survival than histological classification. *Cancer Res.* Apr 1 2003;63(7):1602-1607.

[54] Liang Y, Diehn M, Watson N, et al. Gene expression profiling reveals molecularly and clinically distinct subtypes of glioblastoma multiforme. *Proc Natl Acad Sci U S A.* Apr 19 2005;102(16):5814-5819.

[55] Phillips HS, Kharbanda S, Chen R, et al. Molecular subclasses of high-grade glioma predict prognosis, delineate a pattern of disease progression, and resemble stages in neurogenesis. *Cancer Cell.* Mar 2006;9(3):157-173.

[56] Brennan C, Momota H, Hambardzumyan D, et al. Glioblastoma subclasses can be defined by activity among signal transduction pathways and associated genomic alterations. *PLoS One.* 2009;4(11):e7752.

[57] Mischel PS, Shai R, Shi T, et al. Identification of molecular subtypes of glioblastoma by gene expression profiling. *Oncogene.* Apr 17 2003;22(15):2361-2373.

[58] Bar EE, Chaudhry A, Lin A, et al. Cyclopamine-mediated hedgehog pathway inhibition depletes stem-like cancer cells in glioblastoma. *Stem Cells.* Oct 2007;25(10):2524-2533.

[59] Gunther HS, Schmidt NO, Phillips HS, et al. Glioblastoma-derived stem cell-enriched cultures form distinct subgroups according to molecular and phenotypic criteria. *Oncogene.* May 1 2008;27(20):2897-2909.

Biomarker Discovery, Validation and Clinical Application for Patients Diagnosed with Glioma

Kerrie L. McDonald

Cure For Life Neuro-oncology Group, University of NSW
Australia

1. Introduction

Combined radiotherapy and chemotherapy with the alkylating agent, temozolomide plus an additional six cycles of temozolomide has been the mainstay of treatment for patients diagnosed with glioblastoma for the past 6 years. Clinically, high variability in the response to this treatment is typically observed, with some patients enjoying progression free survival for longer than others. However, tumour relapse is inevitable in the majority of patients. Local tumour recurrence, occurring within 2-3cm of the original resection cavity (the area exposed to radiation treatment) is most frequently observed. *Relapsed glioblastomas are typically unmanageable with median survival after recurrence of only a few months (Brandes et al. 2001).* Numerous chemotherapeutic agents have been trialled in patients with recurrent glioblastomas and include enzastaurin (Wick et al. 2010), immunotherapeutic targeting of EGFRvIII (Sampson et al. 2011), cilengitide (trial ongoing) (Reardon et al. 2011), NovoTTF-100A (trial ongoing), gefitinib (Uhm et al. 2010), imatinib (Dresemann et al. 2010), bevacizumab plus irinotecan (Vredenburgh et al. 2007). Only bevacizumab has shown promise for the treatment of recurrent glioblastoma, although the benefits of such a drug are still debatable. The Food and Drug Administration (FDA) in the USA approved bevacizumab for GBM under its accelerated approval process. However in Europe, the Committee for Medicinal Products for Human Use (CHMP) adopted a negative opinion.

As new therapeutic regimes are developed, it is paramount that we develop a strategy for identifying the patients that will show a positive response to treatment. The recognition and validation of biomarkers of clinical response is important for several reasons: to avoid unnecessary toxicity in patients that fail to respond to the particular treatment; to reduce the colossal cost to healthcare which is typically associated with targeted therapy and most importantly, to better understand drug resistance. This improved knowledge could lead to new strategies to overcome the initial resistance and identify synergistic drug combinations.

1.1 Prognostic and predictive biomarkers

Hopes for progressing curative treatment programs for cancer patients centre on the development and successful implementation of personalised medicine. Personalised medicine hinges on biomarkers which are highly sensitive and highly specific in revealling information that is relevant for diagnosis, prognosis and therapy. The most sought after biomarkers are the ones that can identify which patients are at high risk of tumour relapse and developing cytotoxicity to specific chemotherapeutic agents. The use of biomarkers to identify patients who don't respond to treatment early could confer enormous benefits for patients diagnosed with glioblastoma, especially considering the short survival time. Many biomarkers have shown excellent utility in survival prognostication but not necessarily at the level of influencing an oncologist's decision to administer a specific drug or alter the treatment schedule (Figure 1). In addition, another challenge in oncology is the translation of prospective biomarkers from the lab into validated diagnostic tests.

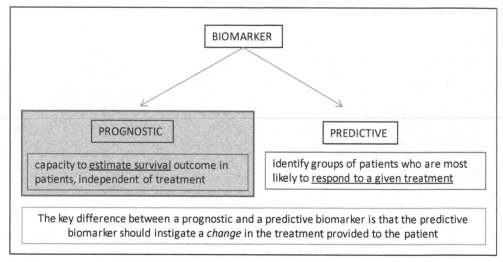

Fig. 1. Schematic overview of the key difference between biomarkers with prognostic and predictive qualities. Prognostic markers are more common in glioblastoma.

Most biomarkers often have both prognostic and predictive value. There is no strict rule when it comes to what constitutes a biomarker. A marker can consist of genomic and proteomic patterns, single genes or proteins, chromosomal abnormalities, epigenetic signatures, aberrant microRNA as well as imaging changes observed on a MRI or PET scan. A **prognostic marker** has the capacity to **estimate survival** outcome in patients, independent of treatment. The genetic profiling of large tumour cohorts with comprehensive clinical and survival data have promoted the discovery of novel molecular biomarkers associated with survival, in addition to traditional clinical and morphological features. Examples of biomarkers with prognostic significance include amplification of Epithelial Growth Factor Receptor (EGFR) (Shinojima et al. 2003; Layfield et al. 2006; Kaloshi et al. 2007; Gan et al. 2009; Inda et al. 2010), over-expression of chitinase-3-like-1 (CH3L1 or YKL-40) (Hormigo et al. 2006; Pelloski et al. 2007), osteopontin (Sreekanthreddy et al. 2010), loss of phosphatase and tensin homolog (PTEN) (Hill et al. 2003; Parsa et al. 2007) and mutations in the tumour suppressor protein, p53 (Shiraishi et al. 2002; Ruano et al. 2009). Prognostic biomarkers have great utility in the clinic. Not only do these markers present as potential therapeutic targets but they can be used to pool groups of glioma with similar genetic profile. This enrichment of the test population leads to increased homogeneity and a much more uniform response to treatment (Figure 2).

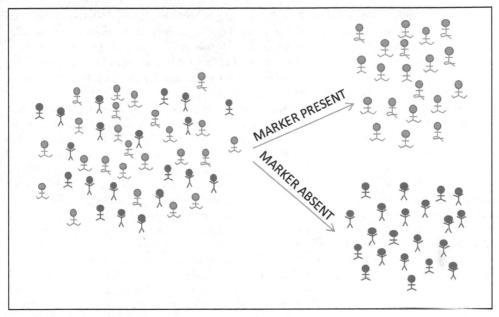

Fig. 2. Molecular diagnostics allows for the identification of GBM subgroups with similar genetic profile. This enrichment allows for a more uniform tumour response.

Much more difficult to identify are biomarkers with **predictive power** in the context of a specific therapy. Predictive biomarkers are markers which can be used to identify groups of patients who are most likely to respond to a given treatment. The key difference between a prognostic and a predictive biomarker is that the predictive biomarker should instigate a *change* in the treatment provided to the patient (Figure 1). Estrogen Receptor (ER) status in patients with breast cancer strongly predicts treatment response to tamoxifen (Kurokawa et al. 2000; Hu&Mokbel 2001). Additionally, patients with variant forms of the gene CYP2D6 (also called simply 2D6) may not receive full benefit from tamoxifen because of the slow metabolism of the tamoxifen prodrug into its active metabolite 4-hydroxytamoxifen (Goetz 2010; Stingl et al. 2010; de Souza&Olopade 2011). Approximately 60% of malignant melanomas harbour the BRAF mutation. Although patients with the damaged BRAF are non-responsive to the KRAS/BRAF inhibitor, sorafenib, response to the second-generation drug called PLX4720 is favourable (Whittaker et al. 2010). Improved outcomes have also been reported in patients with non-small cell lung cancer (NSCLC) harbouring EGFR mutations treated with the tyrosine kinase inhibitors (TKI) erlotinib and gefitinib (Kim et al. 2008; Paz-Ares et al. 2010).

In a highly heterogeneous tumour such as glioblastoma, the search for predictive markers to treatment for use in clinical trials and in every day clinic has been disappointing.

1.2 Molecular subtypes of glioblastoma

Most centres around the world use the World Health Organisation (WHO) grading of tumours of the central nervous system (Fuller&Scheithauer 2007). Glioma grade is defined by the presence or absence of histopathological features, namely: nuclear pleomorphism, mitoses, proliferative index and necrosis and/or microvascular proliferation. A significant limitation to this histopathology-based analysis is its inability to detect functional differences occurring on the subcellular level. This is evidenced by the high variability observed in the clinical outcomes in patients with the same diagnosis and differences in response to therapy. To advance survival times and clinical treatment of these patients with an, on average, dismal prognosis molecular markers with capacity to take into consideration the high molecular heterogeneity are needed in the clinic.

The wide spectrum of molecular difference in glioblastoma is evident from global expression studies, in particular, the molecular cataloguing project: The Cancer Genome Atlas (TCGA) (2008). Surveying the mutational environment of glioblastoma revealed that aberrations occur most commonly in genes whose protein products regulate the core cell growth signalling pathways that are already known to be important such as EGFR, PTEN, p53 and CDKN2A. What this survey did reveal was the extent of genomic complexity. Each tumour harbours different mutations. In addition, we are beginning to appreciate that the core pathways of cancer are not linear, rather complex and interacting. Given this complexity, it is very unlikely that a single genetic change will predict treatment response.

Gene expression profiling has provided an opportunity to further define prognostic and predictive factors (Settle&Sulman 2011). Gene signatures have successfully categorised glioblastomas that histologically appear indistinguishable, into molecular subgroups which often have very different clinical outcomes (Colman et al. 2010; Verhaak et al. 2010). Based on survival associated genes, 76 high grade gliomas were classified into the broad genotology groups; proneural, mesenchymal and proliferative (Phillips et al. 2006). The use of larger and multiple datasets have refined these subtypes into two broad groups, proneural and mesenchymal angiogenic (Colman et al. 2010). Overexpression of a mesenchymal gene expression signature and loss of a proneural signature are associated with a poor prognosis group. By subtyping glioblastoma into mesenchymal and proneural subtypes, the sameness of patient populations is improved. In addition, the genes belonging to each group provides biologists hints for therapeutic targeting. For example, the mesenchymal subtype of glioblastoma is over-represented by genes involved in angiogenesis and invasion (Colman et al. 2010). This subgroup of patients is more responsive to bevacizumab. Mutation in the isocitrate dehydrogenase 1 (IDH1) gene is strongly associated with the proneural subtype of glioblastoma and a much better prognosis (Noushmehr et al. 2010). Increasing evidence suggests that proneural glioblastomas have a different histogenic origin which is further supported by the recent discovery of a glioma-CpG island methylator phenotype (G-CIMP) (Noushmehr et al. 2010). Both IDH1mt and the G-CIMP have a higher incidence in secondary GBMs which arise from a prior, lower grade lesion. MGMT promoter methylation, G-CIMP and mutations in IDH1 are all prognostic. Although a correlation between proneural GBM subtypes and specific treatment has not been determined, it has been suggested by a few studies that chemotherapy agents such as temozolomide and others targeted at cell growth may not be as effective for this group as previously thought (Verhaak&Valk 2010).

2. Prognostic biomarkers in glioma

Molecular markers identified to hold prognostic significance in glioma include loss of heterozygosity of the chromosomal arms 1p and 19q (LOH 1p/19q), methylguanine methyltransferase (MGMT) promoter methylation, mutations in the isocitrate dehydrogenase 1 (IDH1) gene, mutations in TP53, loss of PTEN activity, amplification of

EGFR, presence of the EGFR delta variant (EGFRvIII) and overexpression of chitinase 3-like 1 (YKL40). Gene profiling and cross validation in multiple independent datasets has resulted in the separation of glioblastoma into two major subgroupings: proneural and mesenchymal. The proneural tumours have a much better survival outlook and can be further characterised by the presence of a glioma CpG island methylation phenotype (gCIMP).

Extensive reviews of EGFR, PTEN and TP53 are covered elsewhere. This discussion will focus on LOH 1p/19q, MGMT promoter methylation and mutations in IDH.

2.1. Loss of heterozygosity 1p and 19q

A hallmark of oligodendroglial tumours is the co-deletion of the chromosomal arms 1p and 19q corresponding to an unbalanced translocation t(1;19) (q10;p10). This can be readily detected using Fluorescence In situ hybridisation (FISH) (Figure 3). LOH at 1p19q is observed in up to 69% of grade II and grade III (anaplastic) oligodendrogliomas and is far more common in 'pure' oligodendroglioma than astrocytoma and mixed oligoastrocytoma (Barbashina et al. 2005). LOH of 1p19q confers a clear survival advantage in anaplastic oligodendroglioma and mixed oligoastrocytoma however the survival advantage conferred for grade II lesions is less clear (Laigle-Donadey et al. 2005; Jenkins et al. 2006; Walker et al. 2006) . Whether the co-deletion mediates a prognostic advantage or results in a heightened sensitivity to radiation and chemotherapy is unknown. In general, oligodendrogliomas with LOH at 1p19q represent a group of highly chemosensitive gliomas, especially to the combination of procarbazine, lomustine (CCNU), and vincristine (PCV).

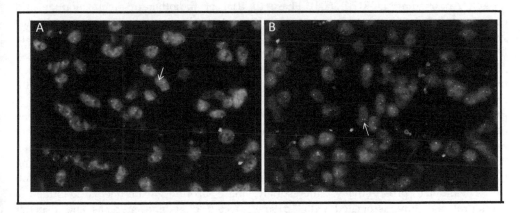

Fig. 3. Representative photomicrographs of loss of 1p (A) and loss of 19q (B) chromosomal arms detected using FISH. Arrow indicates only one chromosome copy instead of the expected two. Photomicrographs were kindly donated by Dr Michael Buckland, Department of Neuropathology, University of Sydney.

The standard treatment for anaplastic oligodendrogliomas consists of complete surgical removal where possible followed by radiation therapy and chemotherapy, typically with temozolomide because it is well tolerated. It is generally accepted that chemotherapy is of value in the treatment of patients with anaplastic oligodendrogliomas (Mokhtari et al. 2011).

Because of the potential toxicity to the CNS, many clinicians have suggested that radiotherapy treatment may be better reserved for progressive disease. Treatment with temozolomide is now favoured over PVC treatment because of its low toxicity. Studies treating anaplastic oligodendroglioma patients with temozolomide have also found that the presence of LOH at 1p/19q is a favourable predictive marker (Brandes et al. 2006; Mikkelsen et al. 2009; Ramirez et al. 2010). This could also be because the majority of oligodendrogliomas harbouring LOH at 1p/19q also show methylation in the promoter region of MGMT. Clinical studies have been designed to establish whether combining or adding chemotherapy to radiotherapy is of benefit to oligodendroglioma patients or whether these patients could benefit from upfront chemotherapy (without radiotherapy).

Two large prospective trials have shown little benefit for adding adjuvant PVC before radiotherapy (Cairncross et al. 2006) or after radiotherapy (van den Bent et al. 2006). To address whether treatment of oligodendrogliomas with chemotherapy alone is feasible and safe, the NOA-04 Phase III trial compared radiotherapy versus chemotherapy with either PCV or temozolomide as initial therapy in 318 patients with anaplastic gliomas (WHO grade 3) (randomly assigned 2:1:1 to receive radiotherapy (arm A) or chemotherapy with either PCV (arm B1) or temozolomide (arm B2)) (Wick et al. 2009). The clinical relevance of 1p/19q codeletion, O^6-methylguanine DNA-methyltransferase (MGMT) promoter methylation, and IDH1 mutations in codon 132 in these tumours were also measured and analysed. This important trial confirmed that there was no survival difference in administering initial radiotherapy or initial chemotherapy (Wick et al. 2009). One very important finding to emerge from the study was the presence of mutations in IDH1 provided the best prognostic model. An ongoing EORCT 26081 Phase III trial of radiotherapy, temozolomide and concomitant and adjuvant temozolomide in patients with anaplastic oligodendrogliomas with 1p/19q codeletions will further confirm what the optimal treatment for these tumours is (more information below).

The gene products that are affected as a result of LOH remain under investigation and may include mediators of cytotoxic resistance or may represent an early oncogenic lesion still retaining sensitivity to genotoxic agents or insults. Microarray technology has been used to profile gene expression in oligodendrogliomas to look for putative tumour suppressor gene candidates and genes which could mediate the observed chemosensitivity using a variety of microarray platforms (Mukasa et al. 2002; Nutt et al. 2003; Mukasa et al. 2004; Tews et al. 2006; Tews et al. 2007; Ducray et al. 2008). These studies have identified some interesting gene candidates located on the 1p and 19q chromosomal arms however none have gone on to be validated prospectively. Interestingly, these profiling experiments identified a proneural signature associated with 1p19q codeleted oligodendrogliomas and a better survival outcome (Phillips et al. 2006). In contrast, the mesenchymal signature is more commonly associated with glioblastoma (discussed in more detail below). Noteworthy is the absence of EGFR amplifications in the proneural group. Ducray and colleagues compared 1p19q codeleted gliomas to EGFR-amplified gliomas and found that the proneural gene internexin (INA) which encodes neurofilament-interacting protein was significantly differentially expressed (Ducray et al. 2009). The prognostic significance of INA was further assessed and confirmed in the prospective, randomized EORTC 26951 trial of adjuvant PVC (Mokhtari et al. 2011). INA strongly correlated with 1p19q codeletion, mutated IDH1 and MGMT promoter methylation.

2.2 MGMT

The O^6-methylguanine-DNA methyltransferase gene, *MGMT*, located on chromosome 10q26.1 encodes a DNA repair protein that restores mutagenic O^6-alkylguanine to normal guanine within genomic DNA. O^6-alkylguanines can pair erroneously with thymine during DNA replication, resulting in G:C>A:T transitions, as well as causing cross-links between adjacent strands of DNA, both of which can lead to neoplastic transformation (Gerson 2004). MGMT thus protects cells from the toxic and carcinogenic effects of alkylating agents and is absent in many types of human malignancy. Loss of MGMT protein expression is frequently associated with transcriptional silencing of the MGMT gene by methylation of its CpG island promoter in various neoplasia, (Esteller et al. 1999) as exemplified by 35-55% of gliomas (Silber et al. 1998; Esteller et al. 2000; Nakamura et al. 2001; Kamiryo et al. 2004; Paz et al. 2004; Brell et al. 2005; Hegi et al. 2005). However, several large studies of glioma have shown the correlation between immunohistochemical loss of MGMT and promoter methylation is not always correlative (Preusser et al. 2008; Cao et al. 2009; Hawkins et al. 2009; Mellai et al. 2009).

Alkylating drugs such as temozolomide are used in chemotherapy for the targeted cell death of rapidly-replicating neoplastic cells and MGMT expression is a key factor in conferring resistance to these agents. In 2005, a new treatment regime was developed and tested in a randomised, phase III clinical trial whereby the alkylating agent, temozolomide was combined with radiotherapy (RT) in concurrent treatment followed by an additional 6 cycles of Temozolomide for newly diagnosed glioblastoma (Stupp et al. 2005). This was the first trial to achieve a clinically meaningful and statistically significant overall median survival benefit of 2.5 months when compared to radiotherapy alone. More compelling were the two-year survival rates with 26% of patients treated with concurrent treatment still alive after two years compared with just 10.4% for patients treated with radiotherapy alone. These survival benefits were still apparent after 5 years of follow-up (Stupp et al. 2009).

The molecular basis for the differential response of glioblastoma patients to temozolomide has been recognized. Temozolomide is an oral alkylating chemotherapy which is spontaneously converted into its active metabolite and readily crosses the blood-brain barrier. The primary mode of action of temozolomide is to damage the DNA by introducing alkyl adducts. These cause genetic mutations as well as cross-links between DNA strands that inhibit DNA replication and thereby trigger cell death. Thus alkylating agents target rapidly replicating neoplastic cells. However, while temozolomide introduces alkyl adducts into DNA, MGMT reverses them. Thus tumour cells expressing MGMT are chemoresistant to this class of drugs (Pegg 1990). In a companion laboratory study to the phase III trial combining radiotherapy with temozolomide, Hegi et al. demonstrated a pronounced positive survival response in patients whose tumours had lost MGMT by promoter methylation. Strikingly, patients whose tumours were MGMT-methylated demonstrated extended overall and progression-free survival compared to those whose tumours were unmethylated, and therefore MGMT methylation was postulated to be a positive predictor of patient response to alkylating agents (Esteller et al. 2000; Hegi et al. 2005). Since these seminal reports in 2005, the standard of care for patients diagnosed with glioblastoma has comprised surgery with maximal feasible resection and radiotherapy with concurrent and adjuvant temozolomide. Yet widespread adoption of MGMT methylation as a marker of response to temozolomide in clinical practice has not transpired.

2.2.1 Routine testing for MGMT methylation

While MGMT methylation could be routinely used as a prognostic/predictive marker in glioblastoma, there is so far no consensus on the method to be applied. Assessment of MGMT promoter methylation is difficult due to the complex nature of the techniques involved. To detect methylation, bisulfite treatment of the DNA is required, a process that may result in degradation of DNA and subsequent low success rates in PCR. This is further compounded by the fact that the most commonly available tissue for assessment is formalin fixed paraffin embedded (FFPE), and the DNA subsequently extracted from this tissue is usually fragmented, again making PCR more difficult.

Promoter methylation analysis by qualitative methyl-specific polymerase chain reaction (MSP) or semi-quantitative methyl-specific polymerase chain reaction (SQ-MSP), especially from FPPE tissue is technically demanding. MSP is the more limited because the methylation status of only a few CpG sites (i.e., those interfering with the PCR primer binding) can be interrogated at once. The technique also has the drawback of providing only a qualitative indication of the methylation status of the sites. Karayan-Tapon (Karayan-Tapon et al. 2010) evaluated MGMT promoter methylation using MSP, SQ-MSP and pyrosequencing. The best predictive value for overall survival was obtained by *pyrosequencing*. Pyrosequencing technology is a technique that generates a quantitative measure of methylation and automatically calculates and reports percent methylation for each CpG site in the studied sequence, thus allowing detection of partially methylated CpG sites.

There are other methodologies for assessing the promoter methylation of MGMT. The testing needs to be resolved for MGMT to be used routinely in the clinic and perhaps a surrogate marker of MGMT such as another protein product readily visualised by immunohistochemistry or a polymorphism detected in blood may be the way forward.

2.2.2 Strategies to overcome MGMT activity

With the recognition that an unmethylated MGMT promoter is associated with a poorer response to temozolomide, strategies have evolved to circumvent the resistance that MGMT confers. Combination therapy with multiple chemotherapeutic drugs known to deplete MGMT (specifically procarbazine and temozolomide) has been successfully assessed in a Phase I trial (Newlands et al. 2003) but as yet has not been shown to confer a benefit in survival. O^6 benzylguanine (O^6BG), a substrate for MGMT, has also been used to decrease MGMT levels. However, systemic administration of O^6BG has been associated with significant toxicity, thereby necessitating a reduction in chemotherapy dose (Quinn et al. 2002; Quinn et al. 2005). A recent case report of local administration of O^6BG, allowing the systemic effects to be avoided, shows some promise (Koch et al. 2007).

Alteration of temozolomide dosing regimens from the usual method of 5 days of treatment every 28 days to more frequent, lower-dose treatment has been evaluated. Protracted temozolomide exposure may reduce MGMT activity. Brock and colleagues demonstrated safety of a low dose of temozolomide for up to 49 consecutive days, however the efficacy of this lower dose is unclear (Brock et al. 1998). Depletion of peripheral mononuclear MGMT has been demonstrated with more prolonged dosing regimens and unfortunately this has been associated with profound lymphocytopaenia and opportunistic infections (Tolcher et al. 2003; Wick et al. 2004; Wick&Weller 2005). More recent evidence suggest that daily dosing may be associated with improved outcome (Buttolo et al. 2006). Additionally, a dosing regimen of 14 days of treatment out of every 28 days has not only been shown to lead to a progression free survival benefit, outcome with this treatment regimen was not significantly associated with MGMT promoter methylation (Wick et al. 2007).

Treating patients with continuous 50mg/m² at relapse after a standard temozolomide schedule of 150-200mg/m² resulted in a PFS6 of 47-57% (Perry et al. 2008). The efficacy and safety of this continuous dose-intense temozolomide schedule for recurrent GBM was tested in a multicenter, phase II study, RESCUE. Overall, PFS6 in 116 patients with recurrent GBM was 24% (Perry et al. 2010). Not surprisingly, the best responding patients were those who were treated with conventional chemoradiotherapy. However, what was interesting was the similar benefit to treatment recorded in the patients who experienced early progression on standard therapy (Perry et al. 2010).

2.3 IDH mutations

The Cancer Genome Atlas (TCGA) efforts made the initial breakthrough discovery that 11% of glioblastomas harbour point mutations in cytoplasmic and mitochondrial NADP+-dependent isocitrate dehydrogenases 1 and 2 (IDH1 and IDH2) (Balss et al. 2008; Parsons et al. 2008; Dang et al. 2009). The normal function of the IDH enzymes is to convert isocitrate into α-ketoglutarate. Mutations, specifically at the arginine 132 (R132) codon, are more frequently observed in low grade and anaplastic gliomas and secondary glioblastomas (50-93%) than mutations found in IDH2 [arginine 172 (R172) codon] (3-5%). No gliomas have been found to have point mutations in both IDH1 and IDH2 (Yan et al. 2009).

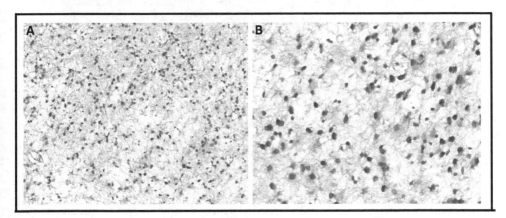

Fig. 4. Representative photomicrographs of IDH1 mutations detected with the Anti-Human IDH1 R132H Mouse Monoclonal Antibody (DIA-H09M) at x20 magnification (A) and x40 (B) Photomicrographs were kindly donated by Dr Michael Buckland, Department of Neuropathology, University of Sydney.

Hartmann and colleagues used an antibody which specifically detected the R132 mutation in IDH1 allowing assessment with simple immunohistochemistry (Hartmann et al. 2010). (Figure 4). The mutation was detected in 72% low grade astrocytomas (AII; n=227); 64% anaplastic astrocytomas (AA; n=228); 82% low grade oligodendroglioma (OII; n=128); 70% anaplastic oligodendroglioma (AO; n=174); 82% low grade oligoastrocytomas (OAII; n=76); 66% anaplastic oligoastrocytoma (AOA; n=177) and 9% glioblastoma (GBM; n=521). What was most significant about this study was the progression free and overall survival curves.

In order of most favourable to poor survival: (1) AA with IDH1 mutation, (2) GBM with IDH1 mutation, (3) AA with IDH1 wild type and (4) GBM with IDH1 wild type. Routine testing for IDH1 mutations will have clinical ramifications regarding histological diagnosis and treatment schemes. The IDH1 mutation is of greater prognostic relevance than histopathological diagnosis according to the World Health Organisation (WHO) classification system (Hartmann et al. 2010). Subsidised treatment schemes approved for glioblastoma such as concomitant radiotherapy and temozolomide and bevacizumab (USA only) may need to be revised to allow anaplastic gliomas with IDH1 wild type status to be treated.

Mutations of the codons in IDH1 and 2 lead to a loss in the production of α-ketoglutarate and a gain of the catalytic activity to produce 2-hydroxyglutarate (2-HG) (Xu et al. 2011). 2-HG levels are highly elevated in IDH-mutated cancers and lead to genome wide histone and DNA methylation alterations (Xu et al., 2011; Dang et al., 2009). Hypermethylation at a large number of loci have been associated with IDH-mutated glioma suggesting that IDH mutation is associated with a distinct DNA methylation phenotype (Noushmehr et al. 2010; Christensen et al. 2011). GoldenGate array methylation data was obtained from 131 glioma patients (all types and histological grades) to interrogate methylation patterns associated with IDH mutation and survival. IDH1 mutations were present in 60% of tumours. Distinct differences between the numbers of significantly differentially hypermethylated loci were noted in IDH mutant tumours compared to IDH wild type tumours. Specific to IDH mutant tumours, cellular signalling pathways were hypermethylated whilst metabolism and biosynthesis pathways were hypermethylated (Christensen et al. 2011). This might be compensatory for the metabolic stress related to the mutation.

In a series of elegant *in vitro*-based experiments, Yan's group transformed human oligodendroglial (HOG) cells with IDH1-R132 or treated cells with 2-HG (Yan et al. 2009). They noted changes in gene expression common to both IDH1-R132 cells and 2-HG-treated cells when compared to IDH1-wildtype and untreated cells, implying that these changes were the result of increased 2HG (Reitman et al. 2010; Reitman&Yan 2010). However, reductions in glutamate and several glutamate-related metabolites were observed exclusively in the IDH1-R132 cells. Particular attention was paid to reduced levels of a common dipeptide in the brain, N-acetyl-aspartyl-glutamate (NAAG), however its contribution to pathogenesis remains unclear (Reitman et al. 2011).

Recently, IDH mutations have been shown to be tightly associated with the presence of a glioma CpG island methylator phenotype (gCIMP) (Noushmehr et al. 2010). CIMPs are characterised by highly concordant DNA methylation of a subset of loci. Improved survival was observed in gliomas with IDH1 mutation and positive for gCIMP suggesting that there are molecular features within gCIMP gliomas that encourage a less aggressive phenotype. CIMP positive colon cancers also have a better prognosis. It is not known whether glioma cells acquire the mutation in IDH1 which then leads to genome histone and DNA methylation patterns, reflected by the presence of a gCIMP or that transcriptional silencing of gCIMP targets may provide the optimal environment for gliomas to acquire the mutation (genomic instability) (Noushmehr et al. 2010).

Gliomas with IDH1 mutations as well as the presence of gCIMP displayed significantly better overall survival (median survival: 2.9 years) compared to all other patients (median survival: 1.04 years). The favourable survival observed in IDH1 mutation-gCIMP positive gliomas may be because these tumours are highly represented in the proneural subset of gliomas. Clinically, the prognostic utility of IDH1 mutations emerged in the NOA-04 trial.

IDH1 mutations conferred a significantly longer time to treatment failure (TTF) which was independent of histology, treatment, codeletion of 1p and 19q and MGMT promoter methylation status (Wick et al. 2009). IDH1 mutations as well as the gCIMP represent a significant breakthrough in how we diagnose patients. Testing for IDH1 mutations has quickly translated into routine diagnostic use. No doubt, IDH1 mutations and perhaps the gCIMP will be used to stratify patients for future clinical trials. Attention has shifted to examining therapeutic targets for IDH1 as well as the possibility of inducing mutations in IDH1 in GBMs that don't possess the mutation.

3. Use as predictive biomarkers

Biomarkers which can foretell whether patients are resistant to a certain treatment and predict drug sensitivity are urgently needed. The success rate of matching biomarkers with treatments has been less than satisfactory. Fewer than 100 biomarkers have been validated for routine clinical practice, despite the publication of more than 150,000 claimed biomarkers. Impeding the successful translation of biomarkers into the clinical setting is non-standardised biological specimen and clinical data collection, particularly clinical information pertaining to drug sensitivity and progression free survival. In addition, far greater numbers of tumour specimens from patients treated uniformly may be needed to be analysed than what we previously assumed.

The only biomarker with reported predictive value is MGMT promoter methylation. As discussed earlier in the MGMT section, the role of MGMT is to protect cells from alkylating damage specifically by removing the alkyl adducts from the O^6 position of guanine and the O^4 position of thymine and effectively restoring the DNA bases and prevent TMZ-induced cell death. However, the present NOA-04 trial does not support the suggestion that *MGMT* promoter methylation is simply predictive for response to alkylating chemotherapy (Wick et al. 2009). NOA-04 showed a striking difference in PFS between patients with versus without *MGMT* promoter methylation who were treated with radiotherapy alone. Thus *MGMT* promoter hypermethylation in anaplastic gliomas may be regarded as (1) a prognostic marker for good outcome in patients treated with radiotherapy or (2) predictive for response to radiotherapy itself.

The most significant issue with implementing MGMT promoter methylation as a predictive test for TMZ therapy is that there is currently no alternative treatment strategy available for those patients with unmethylated MGMT tumours. Until alternative treatments are available and the MGMT test is more reliable and robust, will clinicians consider MGMT promoter methylation as a predictive test.

4. Use of biomarkers in clinical trials

Co-deletion of the chromosomal arms 1p and 19q is a requirement for entry of anaplastic gliomas into the CODEL study which is assessing the role of concomitant and adjuvant temozolomide added to standard radiotherapy and has temozolomide monotherapy in an observation arm. A phase III randomized sister study to CODEL, CATNON, examines radiotherapy with or without concurrent and/or adjuvant temozolomide in patients with non-1p/19q deleted anaplastic gliomas (Figure 5). This type of dual study design allows for the patient populations to be enriched in a specific marker, yet it doesn't exclude either tumour types (codeleted and nondeleted 1p/19q). All specimens will also be tested for MGMT promoter methylation.

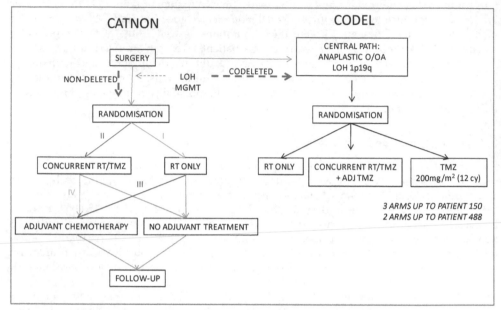

Fig. 5. Overview of the CATNON and CODEL trials

A phase I/IIa trial examined the effectiveness of adding cilengitide to concurrent chemoradiotherapy (Stupp et al. 2010). This study demonstrated the effectiveness of cilengitide but also showed that there was a clear survival benefit in the patients with MGMT promoter methylation (Stupp et al. 2010). The phase III CENTRIC trial (recruitment closed in Feb, 2011) restricted recruitment to newly diagnosed GBM patients with confirmed MGMT methylation. An additional two phase II trials sponsored by the pharmaceutical company, EMD Serono, are designed to treat patients with unmethylated MGMT: CORE (Cilengitide, Temozolomide, and Radiation Therapy in Treating Patients with Newly Diagnosed Glioblastoma and Unmethylated Gene Promoter Status) and ExCentric. CORE (trial still open; May 2011) examines the efficacy of increasing the dose schedule of cilengitide (2000mg twice weekly and 2000mg five times per week) versus standard concurrent chemoradiotherapy (without cilengitide). The ExCentric trial (recruitment open, May 2011) has taken a much different approach. In this trial, procarbazine is added to the concurrent schedule of radiotherapy, TMZ, cilengitide and patients will be treated adjuvantly for an additional 6 cycles with the triple cocktail of cilengitide, TMZ and procarbazine. The patients have so far shown excellent toleration of this combination.

The RTOG-0825 examines the effect of bevacizumab administered with radiotherapy compared to conventional concurrent chemoradiotherapy (TMZ) in primary GBM. All patients enrolled in this study will be tested for MGMT promoter methylation. Unique to this study, however, all samples will be prospectively tested with the nine-gene profile which separates the proneural GBM from the mesenchymal-angiogenic GBM (Colman et al. 2010). It is becoming mandatory for future trial design to incorporate molecular inclusion criteria to identify the poorly responding patients from the patients who benefit.

5. Targeted therapies for glioblastoma

Molecular targeted therapies specifically inhibit amplified or aberrant proteins that drive tumour cell growth. The key to targeted therapy is identifying a target whose *inhibition will stop the growth of the tumour cell*. Whilst this field has rapidly developed, our understanding at the molecular level of the precise role that potential targets have in tumorigenesis and the survival dependence that tumours have on these components has not progressed at the same rate. Unlike melanoma, lung and breast cancer, glioblastoma lacks significant driver mutations which are present in ample abundance and in all tumours. The TCGA analysis revealed a wide spectrum of molecular variation in glioblastoma. TCGA used global gene expression analysis to show aberrations occurred more commonly in genes whose protein products regulated the core cell growth signalling pathways that were already known to be important such as EGFR, PTEN, p53 and CDKN2A. One pathway which is frequently dysregulated is the receptor tyrosine kinase (RTK)/phosphatidylinositol 3-kinase (PI3K)/Akt/mammalian target of rapamycin (mTOR) cascade. Approximately 86% of clinical samples analysed by the TCGA with both copy number and sequencing data had a genetic alteration in the RTK/PI3K pathway (Parsons et al. 2008). In addition, genetic alterations in two other core pathways; RB (87%) and TP53 (78%) were documented. At the time (3 years ago now) it was reasonable to suggest that all tumours be sequenced and the genetic aberrations be documented before selecting the targeted therapy. For example, for tumours with alterations in CDKN2A or CDKN2C or amplifications in CDK4 or CDK6, a CDK inhibitor should be recommended. Unfortunately, we underestimated the extent of genomic complexity and it is very doubtful that therapies targeted to a single genetic change will ever be effective. A range of molecular targeted drugs applied in combination or in addition to each other is needed (Jansen et al. 2010). In clinical practice, the multi-drug approach is currently limited by intellectual property. Most likely the efficacy of two drugs may require two competing pharmaceutical companies to work together.

To understand why our current single targeted therapies are ineffective, it is useful to examine the earlier clinical studies with EGFR- and VEGF-targeted drugs. We can also glean value from trials using targeted therapy in other cancers. Even when the target of interest is much more prominent such as KRAS or BRAF, valuable lessons can still be learnt.

5.1 Targeting the RTK/PI3K pathway

In a study of 49 patients with recurrent glioblastoma, tumour shrinkage was evident in 9 patients (25%) (Mellinghoff et al. 2005). Logically, it was of great interest to better understand the underlying molecular biology of these 9 responders. Pre-treatment tissue was only available for 7 of the responding patients and 19 patients who did not respond. The authors found coexpression of EGFRvIII and PTEN sensitised glioblastoma to erlotinib and correctly validated this finding in tissue samples from different institutions undergoing similar treatment (n=33) (Mellinghoff et al. 2005). Unfortunately, the relationship between EGFRvIII and intact PTEN co-expression did not translate to the subsequent prospective phase I/II trials (Brown et al. 2008; van den Bent et al. 2009). No relationship between aberrations in the RTK core and the EGFR inhibitor, lapatinib (Thiessen et al. 2010) or addition of erlotinib with the mTOR inhibitor, sirolimus (Reardon et al. 2010) were linked with response.

5.2 Targeting angiogenesis

The development of anti-angiogenic agents for glioblastoma have been promising and include bevacizumab (Vascular endothelial growth factor [VEGF] antibody), cediranib (VEGF receptor antagonist), cilengitide (mentioned previously; integrin antagonist) and Enzastaurin (Protein Kinase-C-β-antagonist).

The preclinical and clinical data for cediranib treatment in glioblastoma looked very promising (Dietrich et al. 2009; Gerstner et al. 2011). Unfortunately, the International Multicentre Phase III trial, REGAL was negative. The REGAL study compared the use of cediranib alone, cediranib in combination with lomustine and lomustine plus placebo. In the 325 patients with recurrent GBM studied, only 16% treated with cediranib monotherapy were alive and progression free at 6 months (APF6) compared to 34.5% in the combination group and 24.5% in the lomustine plus placebo group (results reported by T. Batchelor at the Society of Neuro-oncology Annual Meeting, 2010; (Ahluwalia 2011)). Akin to cediranib, preclinical and studies of enzastaurin showed good anti-glioma activity but failed to show any significant benefits when trialled in a phase III study comparing enzastaurin to lomustine. Although less toxicity was observed with enzastaurin, no significant differences in median progression free survival and overall survival were observed (Wick et al. 2011). The humanized antibody, Bevacizumab (Avastin), has received the most attention, with Food and Drug Administration (FDA) approval for use in recurrent GBM in the USA. No such approvals have been obtained in Europe and Australia. This is predominantly because there is only a modest overall survival benefit of 7.8-9.2 months suggesting a further improvement of efficacy is needed. Numerous phase II studies have shown modest survival benefits with bevacizumab either as a monotherapy or in combination with irinotecan (Chinot et al. 2011; Jakobsen et al. 2011; Lai et al. 2011; Prados et al. 2011; Reardon et al. 2011). Consistent to all trials examining bevacizumab efficacy is the reduction of steroids for patients and valuable palliation with preservation of key performance status (KPS), supporting a role for bevacizumab as a therapy in late stage disease (Hofer et al. 2011). Whether bevacizumab results in true glioma cell destruction or is it merely its ability to control the perivascular leak, resulting in better symptom control (associated with improvement of gadolinium MRI) needs to be elucidated.

An issue consistent with all trials of cediranib, enzastaurin and bevacizumab is their testing on recurrent glioblastoma as opposed to primary glioblastoma. Recurrent glioblastoma are already highly refractory to treatment and the potential benefits of these drugs may be missed. New studies are investigating bevacizumab up front with standard radiation therapy and temozolomide. This has shown to be well tolerated (Vredenburgh et al. 2011) and it is a strategy that the RTOG-0825 trial has incorporated (discussed previously).

With all of these targeted therapies, it would seem obvious that the more target present, the more efficacious the drug. Unfortunately, this has not been the case. For example, why patients with high expression of VEGF have not shown strong response to bevacizumab? These issues pertaining to biomarkers in targeted therapy trials will be discussed in turn below:

5.3 Many retrospective analyses of single arm investigations are performed in small and often heterogeneous cohorts of patients

The co-expression of EGFRvIII and PTEN was first discovered in an initial test set consisting of 49 recurrent GBM treated with either gefitinib (n=37) or erlotinib (n=12). 26 patients with clear-cut evidence of a response or tumour progression had sufficient tissue for molecular analysis. Hence, just over half of the originally small cohort was analysed for molecular biomarkers. The validation study used a different tissue type entirely as only paraffin-embedded slides were available. Again, this material was untreated tumour tissue, not the recurrent lesion. The validation set was extremely underpowered (n=33) with only 8 responders identified in this dataset. It is imperative that collaborations between different institutes and countries work together to increase the power of these biomarker studies.

5.3.1 A lack of standardisation in the methods used for marker measurement

Assays for biomarkers need to be reliable. The assay needs to give identical results if repeated in the same or in another laboratory. The result needs to be the same, even when different methodologies are used. And finally, we need to ask whether the test provides added value to clinical practice. This has often been a strong criticism of studies incorporating MGMT promoter methylation (as discussed previously) and unfortunately the same issues surround biomarkers for targeted therapies. The original study by Mellinghoff and colleagues used immunohistochemistry (IHC) to assess PTEN expression (Mellinghoff et al. 2005). The problem with this approach is the antibody used does not detect the full length PTEN protein. Should mutations arise in the C-terminal end of the protein, these would go undiscovered using IHC assay. IHC for EGFR is also contentious. EGFR overexpression in GBM is generally driven by EGFR amplification. The scoring of EGFR IHC can be variable and different antibodies have different specificities to the EGFR protein. Amplification of EGFR or more specifically gain of copy number is most commonly detected by fluorescence in situ hybridization (FISH) and can be routinely performed in most histopathological laboratories. What is puzzling is the lack of sequencing of both EGFR and PTEN genes in the subsequent phase I/II clinical trials assessing TKIs. The most frequent mutant form of EGFR is EGFR Variant III (EGFRvIII or EGFR delta) which is missing the ligand –binding domain resulting in the constitutive activation of the EGFR-phosphoinositide 3-kinase pathway. IHC specific to the EGFRvIII mutant form is highly specific as too is the commonly used RT-PCR method. However, there are additional missense mutations encoding extracellular EGFR that have been shown to drive oncogenesis in vitro and can be inhibited by small-molecular tyrosine kinase inhibitors.

The original pre-clinical/clinical study sequenced all exons and flanking intronic sequences for EGFR (kinase domain), the HER2/neu (kinase domain) and all exons of PTEN. FISH was also performed to detect EGFR amplification and RT-PCR was used to amplify EGFR (1044-bp product) and EGFRvIII (243-bp product). In addition, EGFR and PTEN were examined with IHC (Mellinghoff et al. 2005). 26 of the 49 patients underwent sequencing, which included 6 patients who showed a response to erlotinib. No mutations were found. Van den Bent and colleagues assessed the benefits of erlotinib compared to temozolomide or cumustine in recurrent GBM in a randomized phase II study (van den Bent et al. 2009). Obtaining full data for all patients in this study was problematic. From 100 patients, PTEN expression could be determined in 82 patient cases and pAKT in 64 patients. Like the Mellinghoff study, no mutations in EGFR were detected, however only exons 19 to 21 were assessed. Although an association between EGFRvIII and EGFR amplification with poor overall survival was shown, no correlation between response and the co-expression of PTEN and EGFR was measured (van den Bent et al. 2009). In fact, no significant activity of erlotinib was observed. In another study of 65 patients, erlotinib efficacy was assessed in combination with temozolomide (Prados et al. 2009). Again no association with EGFRvIII and PTEN and response was measured, however in this study, MGMT promoter methylation was associated with better response. EGFR was measured with FISH and IHC, PTEN and EGFRvIII were analysed by IHC. No mutational analysis of EGFR was undertaken. Reardon and colleagues assessed the combination of erlotinib with a mTOR inhibitor, sirolimus in recurrent GBM (Reardon et al. 2010). Again, EGFR, EGFRvIII, PTEN, PI3K and pS6 were assessed by IHC and no association for these markers with clinical response was found. Mutational analysis was not conducted. Moreover, the general methodologies did not differ in the studies addressing erlotinib and response and the Phase II studies could not validate the findings of Mellinghoff et al.

Elegant biomarker studies have been associated with the anti-angiogenic drugs. Attention has focused predominantly on secreted factors and imaging modalities. Interleukin 6 (IL-6) is over-expressed in the majority of gliomas and functions as an immune regulator and an autocrine growth factor (Saidi et al. 2009). High starting levels of IL-6 may influence the efficacy of bevacizumab as it provides redundancy for the VEGF/VEGFR pathway and promotes an immune response that stimulates angiogenesis by non-VEGF mechanisms. Sorenson et al. reported the combination of MRI imaging (measured changes in vascular permeability/flow [K^{trans}] and changes in microvessel volume) and circulating collagen IV levels in plasma to be predictive of outcome in glioblastoma patients treated with cediranib (Sorensen et al. 2009). The level of circulating endothelial progenitor cells (cEPCs) and viable circulating endothelial cells (cECs) has also been shown to correlate with response (Sorensen et al. 2009). The ability to identify changes in a tumour's perfusion offers the potential to predict growth or regression. Dynamic susceptibility-weighted contrast-enhanced (DSC) MR imaging can be used to measure relative cerebral blood volume (rCBV) as a surrogate marker of perfusion. A pilot study of 16 patients with recurrent glioblastoma and treatment with bevacizumab found that MR perfusion imaging showed a significantly improved correlation with time to progression (Sawlani et al. 2011). Studies from Tsien (Tsien et al. 2011) and Server (Server et al. 2011)- both show positive results for this scan in patients with PsPD. Only changes in the hypoxia inducing factor (HIF) 2 alpha [$HIF2\alpha$] have been shown to be promising surrogates of response to anti-angiogenic therapies (Mao et al. 2011).

5.3.2 Methodologies chosen in the study may not represent a comprehensive analysis of multiple components of a specific pathway

None of the studies examining erlotinib have comprehensively analysed the downstream components involved in EGFR signalling. Additional testing of PI3K and PS6 were added in some studies. It is very common for glioblastomas to have dysregulated signalling cascades downstream of EGFR, particular the negative feedback loops. Several growth factor pathways are also triggered. It's not economically feasible in most instances to assess all aspects of the RTK/PI3K/AKT/mTOR signalling cascade. However, a new system of testing drugs and identifying which subtypes of glioblastoma are susceptible to the drug could be to use human glioblastoma xenograft panels serially passaged in nude mice. This model allows tumour burden to be monitored non-invasively and rapid assessment of biological pathways (Prasad et al. 2011).

Feedback mechanisms also pose an issue with targeted therapies blocking angiogenesis. Tumours frequently recur after treatment with cediranib and bevacizumab and are refractory to further treatments. There have been different theories postulated as to why this "rebound" effect occurs. Tumours may switch to VEGF-independent angiogenic pathways or vessel co-option. A commonly held theory is that recurrent glioblastomas switch their growth pattern after anti-VEGF treatment (di Tomaso et al. 2011). The tumour cells are exposed to an increased hypoxic environment leading to increased migration, invasion, heightened glycolysis and increased PI3K pathway activation. Combining bevacizumab with anti-glycolytic agents or PI3K inhibitors might be more effective. Tumour-initiating CD133+ve cells are radio-resistant and can self renew to reform tumours, suggesting that these cells are responsible for tumour relapse (Liu et al. 2009). More significantly, exposure to bevacizumab inhibited the maturation of tumour endothelial progenitors into the endothelium but not the differentiation of CD133+ cells into progenitor cells (Wang et al. 2011). This fundamental study showed that there is a dynamic balance between the CD133+ cell population and tumour cells and we need to target the endothelial transition as well as VEGF.

5.3.3 Not all mutations within a given gene are screened

In simplistic terms, the plethora of TKIs are designed to be effective on patients harbouring EGFR mutations. However, in the majority of studies exploring gefitinib and erlotinib, the EGFR gene is not fully sequenced to identify variants and mutations. TCGA analyses have identified a high diversity of genes mutated within glioblastoma. As prices drop with Next Generation sequencing, capabilities to better define precise genetic aberrations associated with response to a specific treatment will improve. Copy number aberrations (amplifications and deletions) and structural aberrations (intra-chromosomal rearrangements- inversions, inverted/tandem duplications) are not detected using traditional Sanger sequencing in the lab. Our ability to assess these aberrations must improve at the rate that new targeted therapies are flooding the market. BRAF is a commonly deleted gene in approximately 8% of solid tumours, however over 30 different mutations in the BRAF gene have been implicated in cancer (Dienstmann&Tabernero 2011; Puzanov et al. 2011).

5.3.4 A pathway-centric approach is needed

As eluded to in our discussion of multiple pathways and feedback loops in any given target, we need to develop ways to target multiple points of a pathway akin to attacking the Achilles heel of the tumour. Recent data suggest that miRNA expression is tightly coordinated, and that each miRNA may target numerous messages. Thus, a specific miRNA has the potential to regulate several members of an entire signalling pathway. miRNAs negatively regulate their targets by one of two mechanisms: either by near perfect binding to the mRNA target and induction of miRNA-associated, multiprotein RNA-induced-silencing complex (miRISC), which results in accelerated mRNA decay (Yekta 2004; Wu 2006) or by less perfect binding to the target mRNA 3′-UTR and inhibition of translation through a RISC complex similar to, or identical with, the complex recruited in RNA interference (RNAi) (Humphreys et al. 2005; Pillai et al. 2005; Esquela-Kerscher&Slack 2006).

miR-7 directly regulates the expression of EGFR in glioblastoma and has also been shown to directly attenuate the activation of AKT and ERK1/2 (extracellular signal-regulated kinase) indicating its ability to co-ordinately regulate EGFR signalling (Webster et al. 2009). We also showed that miR-124a attenuated glioblastoma migration and invasion at multiple points of the pathway (Fowler et al. 2011). New technologies are currently being developed to facilitate the use of miRNAs as a realistic therapeutic option. Until then, combination treatments and developing inhibitors which can affect a multiplicity of targets are critical.

5.3.5 Differing response criterion

The inability to accurately define endpoints from clinical trials makes the evaluation of new therapies subjective and significantly delays treatment development. At present overall survival (OS) and 6 month progression free survival (PFS6) are two defined end points accepted in most clinical trials testing for new GBM therapies. PFS6 relies on a combination of gadolinium enhanced MRI imaging and potentially subjective clinical evaluation. Seizures, depression and steroid induced myopathy can all influence clinical signs and symptoms. Since 1990, the MacDonald criterion has been used as an objective radiologic assessment of response in GBM. This two dimensional measurement has been mainstay for evaluating tumour response and is based upon measurements of the enhancing tumour area (the product of the maximal cross-sectional enhancing diameters) (Macdonald et al. 1990). With the advance of treatments administered to patients with GBM, the MacDonald Criteria has a number of important limitations. The MacDonald criteria does not discriminate measurable disease from non-measureable disease, cannot identify non-tumour related increases in enhancement and provides no use for the evaluation of anti-angiogenic drugs. Bevacizumab can cause accelerated regression of VEGF driven angiogenesis and rapid resolution of gadolinium MRI changes in responding patients. There is concern however as to whether anti-VEGF therapy results in true glioma cell destruction or their ability to control the perivascular leak, resulting in better symptom control (associated with improvement of gadolinium MRI).

An international working group was formed to review and improve the response assessment criteria for high grade gliomas, coined Response Assessment in Neuro-Oncology (RANO) (Wen et al. 2010). The guidelines have devised a better standardisation of how clinicians measure response, which will ultimately result in a more uniform assessment of disease status across different centres. Unfortunately, the new RANO guidelines do not address the persistent problem of the irregularity of gliomas and the difficulty of measuring tumours treated with anti-angiogenic drugs, suggesting that volumetric measurements that count all enhancing and non-enhancing voxels may prove more accurate in the future.The RANO working party acknowledges that an important area of future research is the need to *develop advanced novel MRI techniques.*

5.3.6 Inadequate tissue

Biobanks or biorepositories play a critical role in the evolution of biomarkers, targets and targeted therapies. Five years ago, the NCI announced their plans to enlist dozens of bio-repositories in the USA to provide large tumour numbers and use high-throughput DNA sequencing and computational biology to produce with new methods of detecting and treating cancers. Unfortunately sub-standard tissue and data collection provided a significant road block to the Cancer Genome Atlas effort. Biorepositories remain underfunded and unappreciated. Despite billions of dollars poured into cancer research, innovation in the field of biobanking is sadly lacking. Standard operating procedures (SOPs) are not consistent between sites, and sometimes differ within single institutes. Methodologies for preserving tissue vary and times between tumour removal and time of processing fluctuate. Significant genetic changes can occur between the time of tissue removal from the body and time of processing. The collection of tissue has to be taken seriously and investments need to be urgently made to promote basic, translational and clinical research as well as social gain in terms of improved cancer care and economic development.

Collection and storage of frozen tissue is critical for biomarker development. Many of our current biomarker assays are performed on Formalin Fixed Paraffin Embedded (FFPE) tissue. This type of tissue, whilst preserving morphology for diagnosis, induces problems for downstream molecular applications. High quality RNA is difficult to obtain from FFPE tissue and PCR amplification from FFPE DNA is limited to products of less than 200 base pairs. It is also difficult to control the processes leading up to tissue fixation. In a first class Neuro-oncology centre in Australia, FFPE blocks were being sent to Central Headquarters for MGMT methylation detection. Unfortunately, a sizeable batch of tissues were non-determinative (could not be amplified). Tissue from surgeries performed on a Friday were fixed in formalin, however the laboratory was unattended over the weekend, resulting in the tissue submerged in formalin for up to 72 hours (routinely, formalin should be removed after 24 hours).

Another issue that we are not taking into careful consideration are the molecular changes acquired in the tumour *after* treatment. Many biomarker studies are performed on tumour obtained at initial surgery event. This tissue has not been exposed to treatment. However, the majority of novel treatments are tested at the time of recurrence. Changes in chromosome aberrations and mismatch repair proteins have been detected in paired tumour specimens (primary and relapsed). Careful consideration of the tissue and its relevance to the clinical circumstance of the patient is required.

6. Future directions for biomarker development

To advance personalised medicine, a co-operative effort between cancer researchers and clinicians is urgently needed. There is very little collaboration between scientists working on targeted therapies such as the TKIs and anti-angiogenics...what worked, what didn't? Specific consideration needs to be paid to increasing sample sizes, sequencing entire genes, implementing robust methodologies and taking a holistic approach to understanding pathways. Cancer is multifaceted and we urgently need to unravel these complexities. Two prospective biomarker trials have been encouraging: the I-SPY 2 (investigation of serial studies to predict your therapeutic response with imaging and molecular analysis 2) for women with locally advanced breast cancer (Barker et al. 2009) and BATTLE (Biomarker Integrated Approaches of Targeted Therapy for Lung Cancer Elimination) for pre-treated patients with non-small cell lung cancer (NSLC) (Kim 2011). Both trials employ an adaptive phase II/III clinical trial design. The I-SPY 2 is performed as a neo-adjuvant trial. A core biopsy is provided and tested for Estrogen Receptor (ER), Progesterone Receptor (PR), Human Epidermal Growth Factor Receptor 2 (HER2) and MammaPrint status (a gene signature known to be predictive of outcome). Based upon the marker outcomes, the patients will be stratified into two arms of a standard neoadjuvant regime: paclitaxel (plus trastuzumab [Herceptin] for HER2+ patients followed by doxorubicin (Adriamycin) and cyclophosphamide (Cytoxan). Five new drugs will be trialled in the other arms (each being added to the standard therapy). Patients are currently being recruited. The BATTLE trial takes on a very similar adaptive design but differs in its examination of samples from post-treated NSLC. Key drugs and associated biomarkers (Erlotinib/EGFR; Vandetanib/VEGFR; Erlotinib + bexarotene/ Retinoid + EGFR and Sorafenib/ KRAS/BRAF) were tested both as an equal randomisation design and an adaptive randomisation design. This trial confirmed that tumours harbouring mutations in KRAS/BRAF showed a disease control of 79% when treated with sorafenib but only 14% of the patients responded to erlotinib. Conversely, sorafenib, although active against wild type or mutated KRAS, had worse disease control in patients with EGFR mutations. A limitation in applying these adaptive trial designs to glioblastoma will be adequate numbers. Additionally, the BATTLE trial identified that grouping mutations together were less predictive than individual markers. This may also impact on a highly heterogenous cancer such as glioblastoma. Nevertheless, these trials show that, with a highly integrated team of multidisciplinary investigators, better overall survival in glioblastoma is achievable.

7. Acknowledgements

I would like to acknowledge the support and financial assistance from the Cure For Life Foundation and the Cancer Institute NSW.

8. References

(2008). Comprehensive genomic characterization defines human glioblastoma genes and core pathways. *Nature*, Vol. 455, No. 7216, (Oct 23) pp. 1061-1068.

Ahluwalia, M. S. (2011). 2010 Society for Neuro-Oncology Annual Meeting: a report of selected studies. *Expert Rev Anticancer Ther*, Vol. 11, No. 2, (Feb) pp. 161-163.

Balss, J., et al. (2008). Analysis of the IDH1 codon 132 mutation in brain tumors. *Acta Neuropathol*, Vol. 116, No. 6, (Dec) pp. 597-602.

Barbashina, V., et al. (2005). Allelic losses at 1p36 and 19q13 in gliomas: correlation with histologic classification, definition of a 150-kb minimal deleted region on 1p36, and evaluation of CAMTA1 as a candidate tumor suppressor gene. *Clin Cancer Res*, Vol. 11, No. 3, (Feb 1) pp. 1119-1128.

Barker, A. D., et al. (2009). I-SPY 2: an adaptive breast cancer trial design in the setting of neoadjuvant chemotherapy. *Clin Pharmacol Ther*, Vol. 86, No. 1, (Jul) pp. 97-100.

Brandes, A. A., et al. (2001). Changing boundaries in the treatment of malignant gliomas. *Expert Rev Anticancer Ther*, Vol. 1, No. 3, (Oct) pp. 357-370.

Brandes, A. A., et al. (2006). Temozolomide 3 weeks on and 1 week off as first-line therapy for recurrent glioblastoma: phase II study from gruppo italiano cooperativo di neuro-oncologia (GICNO). *Br J Cancer*, Vol. 95, No. 9, (Nov 6) pp. 1155-1160.

Brell, M., et al. (2005). Prognostic significance of O6-methylguanine-DNA methyltransferase determined by promoter hypermethylation and immunohistochemical expression in anaplastic gliomas. *Clin Cancer Res*, Vol. 11, No. 14, (Jul 15) pp. 5167-5174.

Brock, C. S., et al. (1998). Phase I trial of temozolomide using an extended continuous oral schedule. *Cancer Research*, Vol. 58, No. 19, (Oct 1) pp. 4363-4367.

Brown, P. D., et al. (2008). Phase I/II trial of erlotinib and temozolomide with radiation therapy in the treatment of newly diagnosed glioblastoma multiforme: North Central Cancer Treatment Group Study N0177. *J Clin Oncol*, Vol. 26, No. 34, (Dec 1) pp. 5603-5609.

Buttolo, L., et al. (2006). Alternative schedules of adjuvant temozolomide in glioblastoma multiforme: A 6-year experience. *Journal Of Clinical Oncology*, Vol. 24, No. 18, (Jun 20) pp. 60S-60S.

Cairncross, G., et al. (2006). Phase III trial of chemotherapy plus radiotherapy compared with radiotherapy alone for pure and mixed anaplastic oligodendroglioma:

Intergroup Radiation Therapy Oncology Group Trial 9402. *J Clin Oncol*, Vol. 24, No. 18, (Jun 20) pp. 2707-2714.

Calin, G. A., et al. (2002). Frequent deletions and down-regulation of micro- RNA genes miR15 and miR16 at 13q14 in chronic lymphocytic leukemia. *Proc Natl Acad Sci U S A*, Vol. 99, No. 24, (Nov 26) pp. 15524-15529.

Cao, V. T., et al. (2009). The correlation and prognostic significance of MGMT promoter methylation and MGMT protein in glioblastomas. *Neurosurgery*, Vol. 65, No. 5, (Nov) pp. 866-875; discussion 875.

Chinot, O. L., et al. (2011). AVAglio: Phase 3 trial of bevacizumab plus temozolomide and radiotherapy in newly diagnosed glioblastoma multiforme. *Adv Ther*, Vol. 28, No. 4, (Apr) pp. 334-340.

Christensen, B. C., et al. (2011). DNA methylation, isocitrate dehydrogenase mutation, and survival in glioma. *J Natl Cancer Inst*, Vol. 103, No. 2, (Jan 19) pp. 143-153.

Colman, H., et al. (2010). A multigene predictor of outcome in glioblastoma. *Neuro Oncol*, Vol. 12, No. 1, (Jan) pp. 49-57.

Conti, A., et al. (2009). miR-21 and 221 upregulation and miR-181b downregulation in human grade II-IV astrocytic tumors. *J Neurooncol*, Vol. 93, No. 3, (Jul) pp. 325-332.

Dang, L., et al. (2009). Cancer-associated IDH1 mutations produce 2-hydroxyglutarate. *Nature*, Vol. 462, No. 7274, (Dec 10) pp. 739-744.

de Souza, J. A. and O. I. Olopade (2011). CYP2D6 genotyping and tamoxifen: an unfinished story in the quest for personalized medicine. *Semin Oncol*, Vol. 38, No. 2, (Apr) pp. 263-273.

di Tomaso, E., et al. (2011). Glioblastoma recurrence after cediranib therapy in patients: lack of "rebound" revascularization as mode of escape. *Cancer Res*, Vol. 71, No. 1, (Jan 1) pp. 19-28.

Dienstmann, R. and J. Tabernero (2011). BRAF as a Target for Cancer Therapy. *Anticancer Agents Med Chem*, Vol. 11, No. 3, (Mar 1) pp. 285-295.

Dietrich, J., et al. (2009). Cediranib: profile of a novel anti-angiogenic agent in patients with glioblastoma. *Expert Opin Investig Drugs*, Vol. 18, No. 10, (Oct) pp. 1549-1557.

Dresemann, G., et al. (2010). Imatinib in combination with hydroxyurea versus hydroxyurea alone as oral therapy in patients with progressive pretreated glioblastoma resistant to standard dose temozolomide. *J Neurooncol*, Vol. 96, No. 3, (Feb) pp. 393-402.

Ducray, F., et al. (2009). alpha-Internexin expression identifies 1p19q codeleted gliomas. *Neurology*, Vol. 72, No. 2, (Jan 13) pp. 156-161.

Ducray, F., et al. (2008). Anaplastic oligodendrogliomas with 1p19q codeletion have a proneural gene expression profile. *Mol Cancer*, Vol. 7, No., pp. 41.

Esquela-Kerscher, A. and F. J. Slack (2006). Oncomirs - microRNAs with a role in cancer. *Nat Rev Cancer*, Vol. 6, No. 4, (Apr) pp. 259-269.

Esteller, M., et al. (2000). Inactivation of the DNA-repair gene MGMT and the clinical response of gliomas to alkylating agents. *N Engl J Med*, Vol. 343, No. 19, (Nov 9) pp. 1350-1354.

Esteller, M., et al. (1999). Inactivation of the DNA repair gene O6-methylguanine-DNA methyltransferase by promoter hypermethylation is a common event in primary human neoplasia. *Cancer Res*, Vol. 59, No. 4, (Feb 15) pp. 793-797.

Fowler, A., et al. (2011). miR-124a is frequently down-regulated in glioblastoma and is involved in migration and invasion. *Eur J Cancer*, Vol. 47, No. 6, (Apr) pp. 953-963.

Fuller, G. N. and B. W. Scheithauer (2007). The 2007 Revised World Health Organization (WHO) Classification of Tumours of the Central Nervous System: newly codified entities. *Brain Pathol*, Vol. 17, No. 3, (Jul) pp. 304-307.

Gan, H. K., et al. (2009). The EGFRvIII variant in glioblastoma multiforme. *J Clin Neurosci*, Vol. 16, No. 6, (Jun) pp. 748-754.

Gerson, S. L. (2004). MGMT: its role in cancer aetiology and cancer therapeutics. *Nat Rev Cancer*, Vol. 4, No. 4, (Apr) pp. 296-307.

Gerstner, E. R., et al. (2011). Infiltrative patterns of glioblastoma spread detected via diffusion MRI after treatment with cediranib. *Neuro Oncol*, Vol. 12, No. 5, (May) pp. 466-472.

Goetz, M. P. (2010). Update on CYP2D6 and its impact on tamoxifen therapy. *Clin Adv Hematol Oncol*, Vol. 8, No. 8, (Aug) pp. 536-538.

Hartmann, C., et al. (2010). Patients with IDH1 wild type anaplastic astrocytomas exhibit worse prognosis than IDH1-mutated glioblastomas, and IDH1 mutation status accounts for the unfavorable prognostic effect of higher age: implications for classification of gliomas. *Acta Neuropathol*, Vol. 120, No. 6, (Dec) pp. 707-718.

Hawkins, N. J., et al. (2009). MGMT methylation is associated primarily with the germline C>T SNP (rs16906252) in colorectal cancer and normal colonic mucosa. *Mod Pathol*, Vol. 22, No. 12, (Dec) pp. 1588-1599.

Hegi, M. E., et al. (2005). MGMT gene silencing and benefit from temozolomide in glioblastoma. *N Engl J Med*, Vol. 352, No. 10, (Mar 10) pp. 997-1003.

Hill, C., et al. (2003). Genetic markers in glioblastoma: prognostic significance and future therapeutic implications. *Adv Anat Pathol*, Vol. 10, No. 4, (Jul) pp. 212-217.

Hofer, S., et al. (2011). Clinical outcome with bevacizumab in patients with recurrent high-grade glioma treated outside clinical trials. *Acta Oncol*, Vol. 50, No. 5, (Jun) pp. 630-635.

Hormigo, A., et al. (2006). YKL-40 and matrix metalloproteinase-9 as potential serum biomarkers for patients with high-grade gliomas. *Clin Cancer Res*, Vol. 12, No. 19, (Oct 1) pp. 5698-5704.

Hu, J. C. and K. Mokbel (2001). Does c-erbB2/HER2 overexpression predict adjuvant tamoxifen failure in patients with early breast cancer? *Eur J Surg Oncol*, Vol. 27, No. 4, (Jun) pp. 335-337.

Humphreys, D. T., et al. (2005). MicroRNAs control translation initiation by inhibiting eukaryotic initiation factor 4E/cap and poly(A) tail function. *Proc Natl Acad Sci U S A*, Vol. 102, No. 47, (Nov 22) pp. 16961-16966.

Inda, M. M., et al. (2010). Tumor heterogeneity is an active process maintained by a mutant EGFR-induced cytokine circuit in glioblastoma. *Genes Dev*, Vol. 24, No. 16, (Aug 15) pp. 1731-1745.

Jakobsen, J. N., et al. (2011). Irinotecan and bevacizumab in recurrent glioblastoma multiforme. *Expert Opin Pharmacother*, Vol. 12, No. 5, (Apr) pp. 825-833.

Jansen, M., et al. (2010). Molecular pathology in adult gliomas: diagnostic, prognostic, and predictive markers. *Lancet Neurol*, Vol. 9, No. 7, (Jul) pp. 717-726.

Jenkins, R. B., et al. (2006). A t(1;19)(q10;p10) mediates the combined deletions of 1p and 19q and predicts a better prognosis of patients with oligodendroglioma. *Cancer Res*, Vol. 66, No. 20, (Oct 15) pp. 9852-9861.

Ji, J., et al. (2009). MicroRNA expression, survival, and response to interferon in liver cancer. *N Engl J Med*, Vol. 361, No. 15, (Oct 8) pp. 1437-1447.

Kaloshi, G., et al. (2007). FABP7 expression in glioblastomas: relation to prognosis, invasion and EGFR status. *J Neurooncol*, Vol. 84, No. 3, (Sep) pp. 245-248.

Kamiryo, T., et al. (2004). Correlation between promoter hypermethylation of the O6-methylguanine-deoxyribonucleic acid methyltransferase gene and prognosis in patients with high-grade astrocytic tumors treated with surgery, radiotherapy, and 1-(4-amino-2-methyl-5-pyrimidinyl)methyl-3-(2-chloroethyl)-3-nitrosourea-b ased chemotherapy. *Neurosurgery*, Vol. 54, No. 2, (Feb) pp. 349-357; discussion 357.

Karayan-Tapon, L., et al. (2010). Prognostic value of O6-methylguanine-DNA methyltransferase status in glioblastoma patients, assessed by five different methods. *Journal of neuro-oncology*, Vol. 97, No. 3, pp. 311-322.

Kefas, B., et al. (2009). The neuronal microRNA miR-326 acts in a feedback loop with notch and has therapeutic potential against brain tumors. *J Neurosci*, Vol. 29, No. 48, (Dec 2) pp. 15161-15168.

Kim, E., Herbst RS, Wistuba II, Lee IJ, Blumenschein GR, Tsao A, Stewart DJ, Hicks ME, Erasmus J, Gupta S, Alden CM, Liu S, Tang X, Khuri FR, Tran HT, Johnson BE, Heymach JV, Mao L, Fossella F, Kies MS, Papadimitrakopoulou, David SE, Lippman SM, Hong WK (2011). The BATTLE Trial: Personalizing Therapy for Lung Cancer. *Cancer Discovery*, Vol. 1, No. 1, pp. 43.

Kim, H., et al. Integrative genome analysis reveals an oncomir/oncogene cluster regulating glioblastoma survivorship. *Proc Natl Acad Sci U S A*, Vol. 107, No. 5, (Feb 2) pp. 2183-2188.

Kim, H. P., et al. (2008). Combined lapatinib and cetuximab enhance cytotoxicity against gefitinib-resistant lung cancer cells. *Mol Cancer Ther*, Vol. 7, No. 3, (Mar) pp. 607-615.

Koch, D., et al. (2007). Local intracerebral administration of O(6)-benzylguanine combined with systemic chemotherapy with temozolomide of a patient suffering from a recurrent glioblastoma. *J Neurooncol*, Vol. 82, No. 1, (Mar) pp. 85-89.

Kurokawa, H., et al. (2000). Inhibition of HER2/neu (erbB-2) and mitogen-activated protein kinases enhances tamoxifen action against HER2-overexpressing, tamoxifen-resistant breast cancer cells. *Cancer Res*, Vol. 60, No. 20, (Oct 15) pp. 5887-5894.

Lai, A., et al. (2011). Phase II study of bevacizumab plus temozolomide during and after radiation therapy for patients with newly diagnosed glioblastoma multiforme. *J Clin Oncol*, Vol. 29, No. 2, (Jan 10) pp. 142-148.

Laigle-Donadey, F., et al. (2005). [Molecular biology of oligodendroglial tumors]. *Neurochirurgie*, Vol. 51, No. 3-4 Pt 2, (Sep) pp. 260-268.

Layfield, L. J., et al. (2006). Epidermal growth factor receptor gene amplification and protein expression in glioblastoma multiforme: prognostic significance and relationship to other prognostic factors. *Appl Immunohistochem Mol Morphol*, Vol. 14, No. 1, (Mar) pp. 91-96.

Li, Y., et al. (2009). MicroRNA-21 targets LRRFIP1 and contributes to VM-26 resistance in glioblastoma multiforme. *Brain Res*, Vol. 1286, No., (Aug 25) pp. 13-18.

Liu, Q., et al. (2009). Molecular properties of CD133+ glioblastoma stem cells derived from treatment-refractory recurrent brain tumors. *J Neurooncol*, Vol. 94, No. 1, (Aug) pp. 1-19.

Macdonald, D. R., et al. (1990). Response criteria for phase II studies of supratentorial malignant glioma. *J Clin Oncol*, Vol. 8, No. 7, (Jul) pp. 1277-1280.

Mao, X. G., et al. (2011). Overexpression of ZNF217 in glioblastoma contributes to the maintenance of glioma stem cells regulated by hypoxia-inducible factors. *Lab Invest*, Vol., No., (Apr 11).

Mellai, M., et al. (2009). MGMT promoter hypermethylation in a series of 104 glioblastomas. *Cancer Genomics Proteomics*, Vol. 6, No. 4, (Jul-Aug) pp. 219-227.

Mellinghoff, I. K., et al. (2005). Molecular determinants of the response of glioblastomas to EGFR kinase inhibitors. *N Engl J Med*, Vol. 353, No. 19, (Nov 10) pp. 2012-2024.

Mikkelsen, T., et al. (2009). Temozolomide single-agent chemotherapy for newly diagnosed anaplastic oligodendroglioma. *Journal of neuro-oncology*, Vol. 92, No. 1, pp. 57-63.

Mokhtari, K., et al. (2011). Alpha-internexin expression predicts outcome in anaplastic oligodendroglial tumors and may positively impact the efficacy of chemotherapy: European organization for research and treatment of cancer trial 26951. *Cancer*, Vol., No., (Jan 18).

Mukasa, A., et al. (2004). Selective expression of a subset of neuronal genes in oligodendroglioma with chromosome 1p loss. *Brain Pathol*, Vol. 14, No. 1, (Jan) pp. 34-42.

Mukasa, A., et al. (2002). Distinction in gene expression profiles of oligodendrogliomas with and without allelic loss of 1p. *Oncogene*, Vol. 21, No. 25, (Jun 6) pp. 3961-3968.

Nakamura, M., et al. (2001). Promoter methylation of the DNA repair gene MGMT in astrocytomas is frequently associated with G:C --> A:T mutations of the TP53 tumor suppressor gene. *Carcinogenesis*, Vol. 22, No. 10, (Oct) pp. 1715-1719.

Newlands, E. S., et al. (2003). Phase I study of temozolamide (TMZ) combined with procarbazine (PCB) in patients with gliomas. *Br J Cancer*, Vol. 89, No. 2, (Jul 21) pp. 248-251.

Noushmehr, H., et al. (2010). Identification of a CpG island methylator phenotype that defines a distinct subgroup of glioma. *Cancer Cell*, Vol. 17, No. 5, (May 18) pp. 510-522.

Nutt, C. L., et al. (2003). Gene expression-based classification of malignant gliomas correlates better with survival than histological classification. *Cancer Res*, Vol. 63, No. 7, (Apr 1) pp. 1602-1607.

Parsa, A. T., et al. (2007). Loss of tumor suppressor PTEN function increases B7-H1 expression and immunoresistance in glioma. *Nat Med*, Vol. 13, No. 1, (Jan) pp. 84-88.

Parsons, D. W., et al. (2008). An integrated genomic analysis of human glioblastoma multiforme. *Science*, Vol. 321, No. 5897, (Sep 26) pp. 1807-1812.

Paz-Ares, L., et al. (2010). Clinical outcomes in non-small-cell lung cancer patients with EGFR mutations: pooled analysis. *J Cell Mol Med*, Vol. 14, No. 1-2, (Jan) pp. 51-69.

Paz, M. F., et al. (2004). CpG island hypermethylation of the DNA repair enzyme methyltransferase predicts response to temozolomide in primary gliomas. *Clin Cancer Res*, Vol. 10, No. 15, (Aug 1) pp. 4933-4938.

Pegg, A. E. (1990). Mammalian O6-alkylguanine-DNA alkyltransferase: regulation and importance in response to alkylating carcinogenic and therapeutic agents. *Cancer Res*, Vol. 50, No. 19, (Oct 1) pp. 6119-6129.

Pelloski, C. E., et al. (2007). Epidermal growth factor receptor variant III status defines clinically distinct subtypes of glioblastoma. *J Clin Oncol*, Vol. 25, No. 16, (Jun 1) pp. 2288-2294.

Perry, J. R., et al. (2010). Phase II trial of continuous dose-intense temozolomide in recurrent malignant glioma: RESCUE study. *J Clin Oncol*, Vol. 28, No. 12, (Apr 20) pp. 2051-2057.

Perry, J. R., et al. (2008). Temozolomide rechallenge in recurrent malignant glioma by using a continuous temozolomide schedule: the "rescue" approach. *Cancer*, Vol. 113, No. 8, (Oct 15) pp. 2152-2157.

Phillips, H. S., et al. (2006). Molecular subclasses of high-grade glioma predict prognosis, delineate a pattern of disease progression, and resemble stages in neurogenesis. *Cancer Cell*, Vol. 9, No. 3, (Mar) pp. 157-173.

Pierson, J., et al. (2008). Regulation of cyclin dependent kinase 6 by microRNA 124 in medulloblastoma. *J Neurooncol*, Vol. 90, No. 1, (Oct) pp. 1-7.

Pillai, R. S., et al. (2005). Inhibition of translational initiation by Let-7 MicroRNA in human cells. *Science*, Vol. 309, No. 5740, (Sep 2) pp. 1573-1576.

Prados, M., et al. (2011). Response as a predictor of survival in patients with recurrent glioblastoma treated with bevacizumab. *Neuro Oncol*, Vol. 13, No. 1, (Jan) pp. 143-151.

Prados, M. D., et al. (2009). Phase II study of erlotinib plus temozolomide during and after radiation therapy in patients with newly diagnosed glioblastoma multiforme or gliosarcoma. *J Clin Oncol*, Vol. 27, No. 4, (Feb 1) pp. 579-584.

Prasad, G., et al. (2011). Inhibition of PI3K/mTOR pathways in glioblastoma and implications for combination therapy with temozolomide. *Neuro Oncol*, Vol. 13, No. 4, (Apr) pp. 384-392.

Preusser, M., et al. (2008). Anti-O6-methylguanine-methyltransferase (MGMT) immunohistochemistry in glioblastoma multiforme: observer variability and lack of association with patient survival impede its use as clinical biomarker. *Brain Pathol*, Vol. 18, No. 4, (Oct) pp. 520-532.

Puzanov, I., et al. (2011). Biological challenges of BRAF inhibitor therapy. *Mol Oncol*, Vol. 5, No. 2, (Apr) pp. 116-123.

Quinn, J. A., et al. (2005). Phase I trial of temozolomide plus O6-benzylguanine for patients with recurrent or progressive malignant glioma. *J Clin Oncol*, Vol. 23, No. 28, (Oct 1) pp. 7178-7187.

Quinn, J. A., et al. (2002). Phase II trial of carmustine plus O(6)-benzylguanine for patients with nitrosourea-resistant recurrent or progressive malignant glioma. *J Clin Oncol*, Vol. 20, No. 9, (May 1) pp. 2277-2283.

Ramirez, C., et al. (2010). Loss of 1p, 19q, and 10q heterozygosity prospectively predicts prognosis of oligodendroglial tumors--towards individualized tumor treatment? *Neuro-oncology*, Vol. 12, No. 5, pp. 490-499.

Reardon, D. A., et al. (2010). Phase 2 trial of erlotinib plus sirolimus in adults with recurrent glioblastoma. *J Neurooncol*, Vol. 96, No. 2, (Jan) pp. 219-230.

Reardon, D. A., et al. (2011). Cilengitide: an RGD pentapeptide alphanubeta3 and alphanubeta5 integrin inhibitor in development for glioblastoma and other malignancies. *Future Oncol*, Vol. 7, No. 3, (Mar) pp. 339-354.

Reitman, Z. J., et al. (2011). Profiling the effects of isocitrate dehydrogenase 1 and 2 mutations on the cellular metabolome. *Proc Natl Acad Sci U S A*, Vol. 108, No. 8, (Feb 22) pp. 3270-3275.

Reitman, Z. J., et al. (2010). IDH1 and IDH2: not your typical oncogenes. *Cancer Cell*, Vol. 17, No. 3, (Mar 16) pp. 215-216.

Reitman, Z. J. and H. Yan (2010). Isocitrate dehydrogenase 1 and 2 mutations in cancer: alterations at a crossroads of cellular metabolism. *J Natl Cancer Inst*, Vol. 102, No. 13, (Jul 7) pp. 932-941.

Ruano, Y., et al. (2009). Worse outcome in primary glioblastoma multiforme with concurrent epidermal growth factor receptor and p53 alteration. *Am J Clin Pathol*, Vol. 131, No. 2, (Feb) pp. 257-263.

Saidi, A., et al. (2009). Combined targeting of interleukin-6 and vascular endothelial growth factor potently inhibits glioma growth and invasiveness. *Int J Cancer*, Vol. 125, No. 5, (Sep 1) pp. 1054-1064.

Salter, K. H., et al. (2008). An integrated approach to the prediction of chemotherapeutic response in patients with breast cancer. *PLoS One*, Vol. 3, No. 4, pp. e1908.

Sampson, J. H., et al. (2011). Greater chemotherapy-induced lymphopenia enhances tumor-specific immune responses that eliminate EGFRvIII-expressing tumor cells in patients with glioblastoma. *Neuro Oncol*, Vol. 13, No. 3, (Mar) pp. 324-333.

Sasayama, T., et al. (2009). MicroRNA-10b is overexpressed in malignant glioma and associated with tumor invasive factors, uPAR and RhoC. *Int J Cancer*, Vol. 125, No. 6, (Sep 15) pp. 1407-1413.

Sawlani, R. N., et al. (2011). Glioblastoma: a method for predicting response to antiangiogenic chemotherapy by using MR perfusion imaging--pilot study. *Radiology*, Vol. 255, No. 2, (May) pp. 622-628.

Server, A., et al. (2011). Diagnostic examination performance by using microvascular leakage, cerebral blood volume, and blood flow derived from 3-T dynamic susceptibility-weighted contrast-enhanced perfusion MR imaging in the differentiation of glioblastoma multiforme and brain metastasis. *Neuroradiology*, Vol. 53, No. 5, (May) pp. 319-330.

Settle, S. H. and E. P. Sulman (2011). Tumor profiling: development of prognostic and predictive factors to guide brain tumor treatment. *Curr Oncol Rep*, Vol. 13, No. 1, (Feb) pp. 26-36.

Shi, L., et al. (2008). hsa-mir-181a and hsa-mir-181b function as tumor suppressors in human glioma cells. *Brain Res*, Vol. 1236, No., (Oct 21) pp. 185-193.

Shinojima, N., et al. (2003). Prognostic value of epidermal growth factor receptor in patients with glioblastoma multiforme. *Cancer Res*, Vol. 63, No. 20, (Oct 15) pp. 6962-6970.

Shiraishi, S., et al. (2002). Influence of p53 mutations on prognosis of patients with glioblastoma. *Cancer*, Vol. 95, No. 2, (Jul 15) pp. 249-257.

Silber, J., et al. (2008). miR-124 and miR-137 inhibit proliferation of glioblastoma multiforme cells and induce differentiation of brain tumor stem cells. *BMC Med*, Vol. 6, No., pp. 14.

Silber, J. R., et al. (1998). O6-methylguanine-DNA methyltransferase activity in adult gliomas: relation to patient and tumor characteristics. *Cancer Res*, Vol. 58, No. 5, (Mar 1) pp. 1068-1073.

Sorensen, A. G., et al. (2009). A "vascular normalization index" as potential mechanistic biomarker to predict survival after a single dose of cediranib in recurrent glioblastoma patients. *Cancer Res*, Vol. 69, No. 13, (Jul 1) pp. 5296-5300.

Sreekanthreddy, P., et al. (2010). Identification of potential serum biomarkers of glioblastoma: serum osteopontin levels correlate with poor prognosis. *Cancer Epidemiol Biomarkers Prev*, Vol. 19, No. 6, (Jun) pp. 1409-1422.

Stingl, J. C., et al. (2010). Impact of CYP2D6*4 genotype on progression free survival in tamoxifen breast cancer treatment. *Curr Med Res Opin*, Vol. 26, No. 11, (Nov) pp. 2535-2542.

Stupp, R., et al. (2009). Effects of radiotherapy with concomitant and adjuvant temozolomide versus radiotherapy alone on survival in glioblastoma in a randomised phase III study: 5-year analysis of the EORTC-NCIC trial. *Lancet Oncol*, Vol. 10, No. 5, (May) pp. 459-466.

Stupp, R., et al. (2010). Phase I/IIa study of cilengitide and temozolomide with concomitant radiotherapy followed by cilengitide and temozolomide maintenance therapy in patients with newly diagnosed glioblastoma. *J Clin Oncol*, Vol. 28, No. 16, (Jun 1) pp. 2712-2718.

Stupp, R., et al. (2005). Radiotherapy plus concomitant and adjuvant temozolomide for glioblastoma. *N Engl J Med*, Vol. 352, No. 10, (Mar 10) pp. 987-996.

Tews, B., et al. (2006). Identification of novel oligodendroglioma-associated candidate tumor suppressor genes in 1p36 and 19q13 using microarray-based expression profiling. *Int J Cancer*, Vol. 119, No. 4, (Aug 15) pp. 792-800.

Tews, B., et al. (2007). Hypermethylation and transcriptional downregulation of the CITED4 gene at 1p34.2 in oligodendroglial tumours with allelic losses on 1p and 19q. *Oncogene*, Vol. 26, No. 34, (Jul 26) pp. 5010-5016.

Thiessen, B., et al. (2010). A phase I/II trial of GW572016 (lapatinib) in recurrent glioblastoma multiforme: clinical outcomes, pharmacokinetics and molecular correlation. *Cancer Chemother Pharmacol*, Vol. 65, No. 2, (Jan) pp. 353-361.

Tolcher, A. W., et al. (2003). Marked inactivation of O-6-alkylguanine-DNA alkyltransferase activity with protracted temozolomide schedules. *British Journal Of Cancer*, Vol. 88, No. 7, (Apr 7) pp. 1004-1011.

Tsien, C., et al. (2011). Parametric response map as an imaging biomarker to distinguish progression from pseudoprogression in high-grade glioma. *J Clin Oncol*, Vol. 28, No. 13, (May 1) pp. 2293-2299.

Uhm, J. H., et al. (2010). Phase II Evaluation of Gefitinib in Patients with Newly Diagnosed Grade 4 Astrocytoma: Mayo/North Central Cancer Treatment Group Study N0074. *Int J Radiat Oncol Biol Phys*, Vol., No., (May 24).

van den Bent, M. J., et al. (2009). Randomized phase II trial of erlotinib versus temozolomide or carmustine in recurrent glioblastoma: EORTC brain tumor group study 26034. *J Clin Oncol*, Vol. 27, No. 8, (Mar 10) pp. 1268-1274.

van den Bent, M. J., et al. (2006). Adjuvant procarbazine, lomustine, and vincristine improves progression-free survival but not overall survival in newly diagnosed anaplastic oligodendrogliomas and oligoastrocytomas: a randomized European Organisation for Research and Treatment of Cancer phase III trial. *J Clin Oncol*, Vol. 24, No. 18, (Jun 20) pp. 2715-2722.

Verhaak, R. G., et al. (2010). Integrated genomic analysis identifies clinically relevant subtypes of glioblastoma characterized by abnormalities in PDGFRA, IDH1, EGFR, and NF1. *Cancer Cell*, Vol. 17, No. 1, (Jan 19) pp. 98-110.

Verhaak, R. G. and P. J. Valk (2010). Genes predictive of outcome and novel molecular classification schemes in adult acute myeloid leukemia. *Cancer Treat Res*, Vol. 145, No., pp. 67-83.

Vredenburgh, J. J., et al. (2007). Bevacizumab plus irinotecan in recurrent glioblastoma multiforme. *J Clin Oncol*, Vol. 25, No. 30, (Oct 20) pp. 4722-4729.

Vredenburgh, J. J., et al. (2011). The Addition of Bevacizumab to Standard Radiation Therapy and Temozolomide Followed by Bevacizumab, Temozolomide and Irinotecan for Newly Diagnosed Glioblastoma. *Clin Cancer Res*, Vol., No., (Apr 29).

Walker, C., et al. (2006). Clinical use of genotype to predict chemosensitivity in oligodendroglial tumors. *Neurology*, Vol. 66, No. 11, (Jun 13) pp. 1661-1667.

Wang, R., et al. (2011). Glioblastoma stem-like cells give rise to tumour endothelium. *Nature*, Vol. 468, No. 7325, (Dec 9) pp. 829-833.

Wang, S. and E. N. Olson (2009). AngiomiRs--key regulators of angiogenesis. *Curr Opin Genet Dev*, Vol. 19, No. 3, (Jun) pp. 205-211.

Webster, R. J., et al. (2009). Regulation of epidermal growth factor receptor signaling in human cancer cells by microRNA-7. *J Biol Chem*, Vol. 284, No. 9, (Feb 27) pp. 5731-5741.

Wen, P. Y., et al. (2010). Updated response assessment criteria for high-grade gliomas: response assessment in neuro-oncology working group. *J Clin Oncol*, Vol. 28, No. 11, (Apr 10) pp. 1963-1972.

Whittaker, S., et al. (2010). Gatekeeper mutations mediate resistance to BRAF-targeted therapies. *Sci Transl Med*, Vol. 2, No. 35, (Jun 9) pp. 35ra41.

Wick, A., et al. (2007). Efficacy and tolerability of temozolomide in an alternating weekly regimen in patients with recurrent glioma. *J Clin Oncol*, Vol. 25, No. 22, (Aug 1) pp. 3357-3361.

Wick, W., et al. (2009). NOA-04 randomized phase III trial of sequential radiochemotherapy of anaplastic glioma with procarbazine, lomustine, and vincristine or temozolomide. *J Clin Oncol*, Vol. 27, No. 35, (Dec 10) pp. 5874-5880.

Wick, W., et al. (2010). Phase III study of enzastaurin compared with lomustine in the treatment of recurrent intracranial glioblastoma. *J Clin Oncol*, Vol. 28, No. 7, (Mar 1) pp. 1168-1174.

Wick, W., et al. (2011). Phase III study of enzastaurin compared with lomustine in the treatment of recurrent intracranial glioblastoma. *J Clin Oncol*, Vol. 28, No. 7, (Mar 1) pp. 1168-1174.

Wick, W., et al. (2004). One week on/one week off regimen of temozolomide for recurrent glioblastoma: A phase III study. *Journal Of Clinical Oncology*, Vol. 22, No. 14, (Jul 15) pp. 116S-116S.

Wick, W. and M. Weller (2005). How lymphotoxic is dose-intensified temozolomide? The glioblastoma experience. *Journal Of Clinical Oncology*, Vol. 23, No. 18, (Jun 20) pp. 4235-4236.

Wu, L. e. a. (2006). MicroRNA direct rapid demethylation of mRNA. *PNAS*, Vol. 103, No., pp. 4034-4039.

Xu, W., et al. (2011). Oncometabolite 2-hydroxyglutarate is a competitive inhibitor of alpha-ketoglutarate-dependent dioxygenases. *Cancer Cell*, Vol. 19, No. 1, (Jan 18) pp. 17-30.

Yan, H., et al. (2009). IDH1 and IDH2 mutations in gliomas. *N Engl J Med*, Vol. 360, No. 8, (Feb 19) pp. 765-773.

Yekta, S. e. a. (2004). MicroRNA-directed cleavage of *HOXB8* mRNA. *Science*, Vol. 304, No., pp. 594-596.

Zhang, Y., et al. (2009). MicroRNA-128 inhibits glioma cells proliferation by targeting transcription factor E2F3a. *J Mol Med*, Vol. 87, No. 1, (Jan) pp. 43-51.

Part 2

Gliomagenesis

5

Genomic Abnormalities in Gliomas

Giovanny Pinto et al.[*]

Federal University of Piauí, Parnaíba,
Brazil

1. Introduction

In general, studies reveal that cancer arises through genetic and epigenetic alterations that affect specific genes within a given cell type. These changes involve a gain of function when the alterations involve oncogenes, a loss of function when the target genes are tumor suppressor genes. Thus, both genetic and epigenetic changes promote the instability of cellular homeostasis (Bello & Rey, 2006; Richardson, 2003; Sugimura & Ushijima, 2000). This lack of stability reflects the complexity of cancer because the loss of controlled cell growth occurs due to changes in one or more genes. These genetic and epigenetic events are followed by the growing accumulation of changes in hundreds, if not thousands, of genes. Over time, this accumulation causes the tumor to reach its highest degree of malignancy, which usually culminates in metastasis (Bartek & Lukas, 2001). However, in recent years, a subpopulation of tumor cells has been found to display a slow rate of cell division, high tumorigenic potential and characteristics similar to those of normal stem cells. This discovery has changed the concept of metastasis to one associated with strictly terminal states (Stiles & Rowitch, 2008).

Hanahan & Weinberg (2000) proposed that all tumor cells must acquire six essential alterations in cell physiology that collectively dictate malignant growth: (1) loss of normal signaling for cell proliferation arrest, (2) loss of signaling for cell differentiation, (3) autocrine signaling for cell division, (4) reduction in apoptosis, (5) ability to enter the basement membrane and other tissues and organs, and (6) induction of angiogenesis. All of these processes involve biochemical pathways that form a complex network of cell signaling. These processes are usually altered in tumors because the genes that compose them are changed, resulting in cell cycle dysregulation. Therefore, the identification and determination of oncogenes and tumor suppressor genes is essential for understanding both cancer biology and clinical applications, such as the identification of therapeutic targets, early detection, and prediction of the disease course. Studies concerning cell cycle control genes have served as a starting point for identifying genes related to tumorigenesis and their biochemical role in various pathways (Paige, 2003).

[*] France Yoshioka[1], Fábio Motta[1], Renata Canalle[1], Rommel Burbano[2], Juan Rey[3],
Aline Custódio[4] and Cacilda Casartelli[4]
[1]*Federal University of Piauí, Parnaíba,Brazil*
[2]*Federal University of Pará, Belém, Brazil*
[3]*University Hospital La Paz, Madrid, Spain*
[4]*University of São Paulo, Ribeirão Preto, Brazil*

Changes in oncogenes can lead to constitutive activation, which involves activation under conditions in which an oncogene would normally be inactive. For this process to occur, a cell needs only one allele of an oncogene to be altered, resulting in a selective growth advantage. In contrast, changes in tumor suppressor genes often reduce the gene product and consequently its activity. For this reason, cells that develop a selective advantage with changes in tumor suppressor genes usually require inactivation of both alleles of the target gene. Conceptually, tumor suppressor genes can be subdivided into two categories: "gatekeepers" that directly inhibit tumor growth and thereby suppress tumor formation and "caretakers" that ensure DNA integrity by repairing damage or preventing genomic instability (Vogelstein & Kinzler, 2004).

Studies of hereditary and sporadic forms of tumors, particularly retinoblastoma, culminated in the formulation of Knudson's "two events" model in 1971. In hereditary tumors, the first mutation occurs in one allele in the germline and results in a predisposition to develop tumors. Throughout development, a second change (mutation or loss of heterozygosity) inactivates the other allele and silences the altered gene. In contrast, sporadic tumors acquire the two allelic alterations that lead to gene silencing throughout the organism's development (Knudson, 1971). Over time, the neoplastic transformation and metabolic-phenotype of the cell can evolve. Ultimately, these changes result in a cancer in which clonal expansion of modified somatic cells destroys the adjacent normal tissue (Bartek & Lukas, 2001).

For many years, research in cancer genetics has prioritized understanding the role of genetic alterations in carcinogenesis. Studies revealed that base deletions, insertions, recombination and amplification in oncogenes and tumor suppressor genes were related to metastasis and invasion. These changes were also closely related to tumorigenesis and tumor progression. For this reason, the scientific community accepted that genetic changes almost exclusively explained the process of carcinogenesis (Sugimura & Ushijima, 2000). However, studies also indicated that embryogenesis and differentiation, which are characterized by specific patterns of gene expression in tissues and organs, can occur without changes in the DNA sequence. This notion has interested the scientific community in potential epigenetic mechanisms of carcinogenesis (Jones & Buckley, 1990; Rush & Plass, 2002).

An epigenetic phenomenon is defined as a change in gene function that is heritable through mitosis or meiosis but cannot be explained by changes in the DNA sequence. Aberrant epigenetic mechanisms, such as promoter hypermethylation, histone modifications, or non-coding RNA expression, are known to be important for tumor formation and comprise the "third pathway" in Knudson's model. These mechanisms result in transcriptional repression equivalent to that observed with the mutations and deletions proposed in Knudson's model (Jones & Baylin, 2007).

DNA methylation, the main epigenetic modification studied, occurs at cytosine residues in the cytosine-guanine sequences (CpG) of DNA through the action of an enzyme family called DNA methyltransferases (DNMT). In humans, approximately 70% of CpG sites, which are generally located in repetitive DNA sequences, are methylated. Clusters of unmethylated CpG sites are present in the genome as well, and these clusters are referred to as CpG islands. Approximately 60% of genes have CpG islands in the promoter regions and in the first exon. CpG islands are often dimethylated when associated with housekeeping genes. Moreover, CpG islands are tissue specific and are generally methylated except in those tissues where the associated gene is expressed (Cross & Bird, 1995; Gonzalez-Gomez et al., 2003). A recent genome-wide analysis revealed that CpG islands are also found in non-promoter regions. In addition, epigenetic abnormalities causing loss of gene function are more frequent than genetic abnormalities in cancer cells (Schuebel et al., 2007). Thus, cellular epigenetic inheritance mediated by aberrant DNA methylation resulting in gene silencing, gene imprinting, and/or activation of cancer-associated genes is now accepted as an important factor defining the transformed phenotype (Natsume et al., 2010)

2. Tumors of the central nervous system

Tumors of the central nervous system (CNS) are relatively rare and represent approximately 5-9% of all cancers, with an estimated incidence of 4.2 to 5.4 per 100,000 people/year. Moreover, tumors of the CNS carry a very poor prognosis and are associated with considerable morbidity and mortality. They are a leading cause of childhood cancer deaths, the second leading cause of cancer-related death in men aged 20–39, and the fifth leading cause of cancer-related death in women aged 20–39 (Ohgaki & Kleihues, 2005).

Although the incidence of CNS tumors is small compared with the incidence of other cancers, CNS tumors are among the most serious human malignancies because they affect the organ responsible for the coordination and integration of all biological activities. Moreover, as each region of the brain has a vital function, therapies used to treat other cancers (e.g., total surgical removal of an organ or tumor with a generous margin of normal tissue) cannot be applied to brain tumors. The inability to use these therapies hinders quality of life and patient survival (Louis et al., 2002).

In CNS tumors, the histopathological classifications are extensive and based primarily on descriptive morphology. Because the histogenesis of these tumors is unique and heterogeneous, it is difficult to characterize several of the tumor subtypes, which is reflected in the difficulties encountered in tumor diagnosis (Gilbertson, 2002).

In contrast with the first World Health Organization (WHO) classifications for CNS tumors (Kleihues et al., 1993; Zülch, 1979), the third edition by Kleihues & Cavenee (2000) incorporated genetic profiles as additional aids in defining brain tumors. The fourth edition of the WHO classifications for CNS tumors, which was published in 2007, lists several new characteristics. The fourth edition is based on consensus from an international working group of 25 pathologists and geneticists, as well as contributions from more than 70 international experts. Currently, this edition is the standard for defining brain tumors for clinical oncology and cancer research communities world-wide (Louis et al., 2007).

3. Gliomas

Gliomas are the most common tumors of the CNS. However, in spite of marked progress in characterizing the molecular pathogenesis of gliomas, these tumors remain incurable. In most cases, gliomas are also refractory to treatment because of their molecular heterogeneity. Gliomas rarely metastasize outside of the brain but instead infiltrate extensively into the surrounding normal brain. Therefore, surgery is not curative but can establish the diagnosis and relieve symptoms by decompressing the brain, which is located in the rigid intracranial cavity. Radiation therapy and chemotherapy increase survival; however, disease recurrence is frequently inevitable (Park & Rich, 2009).

The following four degrees of malignancy are recognized by the WHO: grades I and II (low-grade), which are biologically less aggressive and grades III and IV (high-grade), which are the most aggressive. The histological criteria for grading malignances are not uniform for all subtypes of gliomas. Thus, all tumors should be classified before the degree of malignancy is determined. This classification is made according to the cell type thought to be responsible for the tumor and based on the characteristics exhibited by astrocytes, oligodendrocytes, ependymal cells, or their neuronal progenitors (Louis et al., 2007). Table 1 shows the heterogeneous WHO classification for gliomas according to the degree of malignancy.

Astrocytic tumors	WHO Grade					Ependymal tumors	WHO Grade			
	I	II	III	IV			I	II	III	IV
Subependymal giant cell astrocytoma	●					Subependymoma	●			
Pilocytic astrocytoma	●					Myxopapillary ependymoma	●			
Pilomyxoid astrocytoma		●				Ependymoma		●		
Diffuse astrocytoma		●				Anaplastic ependymoma			●	
Pleomorphic xanthoastrocytoma		●								
Anaplastic astrocytoma			●			**Choroid plexus tumors**				
Glioblastoma				●		Choroid plexus papilloma	●			
Giant cell glioblastoma				●		Atypical choroid plexus papilloma		●		
Gliosarcoma				●		Choroid plexus carcinoma			●	
Oligodendroglial tumors						**Other neuroepithelial tumors**				
Oligodendroglioma		●				Angiocentric glioma	●			
Anaplastic oligodendroglioma			●			Chordoid glioma of the third ventricle		●		
Oligoastrocytic tumors										
Oligoastrocytoma		●								
Anaplastic oligoastrocytoma			●							

Table 1. WHO grading of gliomas (Louis et al., 2007).

Gliomas of astrocytic, oligodendroglial, and ependymal origin account for 80% of CNS tumors. For this reason, some morphological and genetic characteristics of these tumors are discussed below.

3.1 Astrocytomas

Astrocytomas represent the vast majority of gliomas and account for 70% of the total gliomas seen in patients. Astrocytomas can be further characterized as pilocytic astrocytomas (WHO grade I) or diffuse astrocytomas, including low-grade astrocytomas (WHO grade II), anaplastic astrocytomas (WHO grade III) and glioblastomas (WHO grade IV) (Kleihues et al., 2002).

Pilocytic astrocytomas are more commonly seen in children and carry a good prognosis because of their biology. Patients with neurofibromatosis type 1, a familial syndrome caused by germline mutations in the gene NF1 (neurofibromin 1), have an increased incidence of pilocytic astrocytomas. These tumors are usually not aggressive and stand out among astrocytomas because they have maintained their WHO grade I status for years and even decades, in contrast to diffuse astrocytic tumors (WHO grades II-IV). However, some cases can progress to a higher degree of malignancy, though such a progression is rare (Listernick et al., 1999).

More than 100 cases of pilocytic astrocytomas were analyzed by cytogenetics and many others were used for comparative genomic hybridization (CGH); however, the vast majority of the results indicated normal patterns (Bigner et al., 1997; Sanoudou et al., 2000; Zattara-Cannoni et al., 1998). In adults, genetic changes were more frequent but were still rare. The few molecular genetics studies on these tumors indicated allelic loss of both gene loci TP53 (tumor protein p53) and NF1 in regions 17p and 17q, respectively. In sporadic tumors, few mutations were reported in the TP53 locus and none in NF1 (Gutmann et al., 2000; Kluwe et al., 2001).

The relevance of a malignancy-grading scheme based on histopathology is indicated by the correlation with patient survival. Patients with low-grade astrocytomas (WHO grade II) have a median survival of approximately seven years, whereas patients with anaplastic astrocytomas (WHO grade III) have a mean survival of half that time (McCormack et al., 1992). Patients with glioblastomas have a median survival time of 9 to 11 months (Simpson et al., 1993).

Unlike pilocytic astrocytomas, diffuse astrocytic tumors are often seen in adults. Low-grade astrocytomas have a peak incidence between 25 and 50 years of age, whereas glioblastomas have a peak incidence between 45 and 50 years (Colins, 2004).

Ng & Lam (1998) suggested dividing glioblastomas into two distinct molecular and clinical entities: primary or de novo glioblastomas, which occur in elderly patients and are clinically very aggressive and secondary glioblastomas, which develop from low-grade astrocytomas and have a more prolonged clinical course.

Many mechanisms are involved in the initiation and progression of secondary glioblastomas, including the loss of NF1 and TP53 genes and the activation of signal transduction pathways, such as PDGF (platelet-derived growth factor) and its receptor PDGFR (PDGF receptor). These pathways are involved in the induction of low-grade tumors (e.g., pilocytic astrocytomas), which can progress to high-grade tumors (e.g., anaplastic astrocytomas and secondary glioblastoma). This progression is associated with the lack of a functional RB1 (retinoblastoma 1) because of the loss of RB1 or gene amplification/overexpression of CDK4 (cyclin-dependent kinase 4) (Fig. 1a). In primary glioblastomas, the same genetic pathways are disrupted but by different mechanisms. For example, reduction of the *TP53* pathway generally occurs through the loss of the gene *ARF4* (ADP-ribosylation factor 4) or less frequently through amplification of the gene *MDM2* (transformed 3T3 cell double minute 2). The lack of *RB1* also occurs via a loss of the gene *CDKN2A* (cyclin-dependent kinase inhibitor 2A). In primary glioblastomas, amplification and/or mutation of *EGFR* (epidermal growth factor receptor) and loss of *PTEN* (phosphatase and tensin homolog) are the most frequently observed genetic defects (Fig. 1b) (Zu & Parada, 2002).

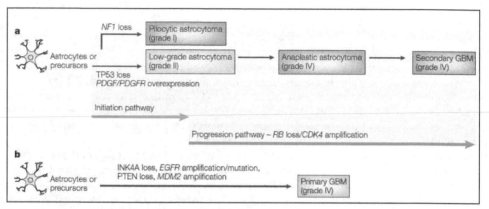

Fig. 1. Genetic pathways involved in the development of (a) primary and (b) secondary glioblastomas (Zhu & Parada, 2000).

Sequencing of the genome recently identified mutations in the *IDH1/IDH2* genes (isocitrate dehydrogenase 1 and 2 genes) that occur in the majority of WHO grade II–III gliomas and secondary glioblastomas (Hartmann et al., 2009; Yan et al., 2009), all of which harbor a better prognosis compared with the wild-type cases (Sanson et al., 2009). However, pilocytic astrocytomas (WHO grade I) that are potentially curable by complete resection rarely harbor *IDH* mutations. *IDH* appears to function as a tumor suppressor when inactivated through mutation, rendering the IDH enzyme unable to catalyze conversion of isocitrate to alphaketoglutarate. This process also induces HIF1-alpha (hypoxia-inducible factor), which triggers the angiogenic process. However, the precise mechanism of its effect on tumor biology remains unclear (Dang et al., 2009).

Aberrant activation of the *BRAF* proto-oncogene (v-raf murine sarcoma viral oncogene homolog B1) at 7q34, which is most commonly caused by gene duplication and fusion or less frequently by point mutation, has only recently been identified as the characteristic genetic aberration in pilocytic astrocytomas. *BRAF* abnormalities occur in 60–80% of pilocytic astrocytomas but almost never in diffuse, infiltrating astrocytomas (Jones et al., 2009). Thus, testing for *BRAF* gene alterations might be helpful for differentiating during diagnosis between pilocytic astrocytomas and low-grade, diffuse astrocytomas (Korshunov et al., 2009).

The importance of silencing DNA repair pathways, especially the DNA-repair enzyme AGAT (O6-alkylguanine DNA alkyltransferase), which is encoded by the gene *MGMT* (O6-methylguanine-DNA-methyltransferase), has been the subject of substantial debate in recent years (Hofer & Lassman, 2010). The *MGMT* gene is frequently silenced by promoter hypermethylation in diffuse gliomas, and this hypermethylation has been pinpointed as an epigenetic mechanism that reduces *MGMT* expression levels. There are 97 CpG islands in the *MGMT* promoter, and these CpG islands are further divided into two hypermethylated regions (Nakagawachi et al., 2003). Because of its critical role in DNA repair, the epigenetic silencing of *MGMT* is associated with an increased number of mutations and with a poorer outcome in glioblastomas. Thus, *MGMT* silencing is considered to be a biomarker for poor prognosis (Komine et al., 2003). However, an association between *MGMT* promoter methylation and the response of malignant gliomas to alkylating chemotherapy using nitrosourea compounds, temozolomide, or a combination of both has been observed (Esteller et al., 2000; Herrlinger et al., 2006). Furthermore, Hegi et al. (2005) reported that patients treated with radiotherapy and temozolomide, and whose tumors had a methylated *MGMT* promoter (which is seen in approximately 40% of primary glioblastomas), survived significantly longer than did patients whose tumors lacked *MGMT* promoter methylation. Rivera et al. (2010) recently reported that *MGMT* promoter methylation in anaplastic gliomas (WHO grade III) is also predictive of the response to radiotherapy and linked to longer survival in the absence of adjuvant chemotherapy. The use of temozolomide based on *MGMT* methylation status highlights the importance of understanding epigenetic changes in glioblastomas for the discovery of novel therapies and prognostic factors for the treatment of this deadly cancer (Komine et al., 2003; Nakagawachi et al., 2003)

3.2 Oligodendrogliomas

Oligodendrogliomas represent approximately 10-15% of gliomas, are more common in adults, and can be divided into two histological subtypes: low-grade (WHO grade II) and anaplastic (WHO grade III) (Kleihues et al., 2002).

Low-grade oligodendrogliomas are less biologically aggressive than are astrocytic tumors. Therefore, the prognosis is quite favorable and survival beyond 15 years is achieved in up to 90% of cases that receive a complete surgical resection. There is potential for malignancy, but even the aggressive tumors respond well to additional treatments (e.g., radiation and chemotherapy). Anaplastic oligodendrogliomas have a more aggressive course; however, survival is still five to eight years longer than that observed with anaplastic astrocytomas (Reifenberger & Louis, 2003).

In 1990, the PCV chemotherapy regimen (procarbazine, carmustine, and vincristine) was shown to result in a dramatic tumor response in oligodendrogliomas. Since that time, the identification of all forms of gliomas with oligodendroglial components became crucial (Macdonald et al., 1990). Importantly, these studies indicated that the prognostic power of oligodendroglial components was independent of whether radiotherapy, chemotherapy or combined radio-chemotherapy was used (Wick et al., 2009). This phenomenon is likely due to oligodendrogliomas exhibiting specific genetic abnormalities that distinguish them from other gliomas. Reifenberger et al. (1994), after a thorough analysis of the genome, reported a loss of genetic information in the 1p and 19q loci in oligodendrogliomas, the so-called chromosome 1p/19q co-deletion. This loss was later linked with a good response to PCV and provided the first molecular indicator of treatment response in brain tumors (Cairncross et al., 1998; Reifenberger et al., 2003). Further studies corroborated these findings, and it is now known that the chromosomal loss results from an unbalanced translocation (Franco-Hernandez et al., 2009; Jenkins et al., 2006). Approximately 85% of low-grade oligodendrogliomas and 65% of anaplastic oligodendrogliomas present with 1p/19q co-deletions (Smith et al., 2000).

Low-grade oligodendrogliomas and astrocytomas present a loss of *ARF4* expression and overexpression of *EGFR* and PDGF signaling. Malignant progression is associated with additional genetic abnormalities that are similar to those described above for astrocytomas, including a lack of the *RB1* pathway, loss of *RB1*, or gene amplification/overexpression of the *CDK4* gene (Franco-Hernandez et al., 2007; Reifenberger & Louis, 2003).

3.3 Ependymomas

Ependymomas arise in or near the ependymal surface, and these tumors can occur anywhere in the ventricular system, spinal cord and even occasionally at extraneural sites. The most common location is in the fourth ventricle, followed by the spinal cord, the lateral ventricles and the third ventricle. These tumors are more common in children but can also occur in adults (Ebert et al., 1999).

WHO classification identifies four major subtypes of ependymomas: subependymomas (WHO grade I), myxopapillary ependymomas (WHO grade I), low-grade ependymomas (WHO grade II) and anaplastic ependymomas (WHO grade III). Subependymomas are intraventricular in location, while myxopapillary ependymomas are commonly found in the cauda equina. The low-grade ependymomas can be differentiated from their anaplastic counterparts based on the low rate of mitosis and the low level of nuclear polymorphism; however, the distinction between the two tumors remains poorly defined (Kleihues et al., 2002).

In ependymomas, chromosomal abnormalities detected by classic cytogenetics and CGH involve chromosomes 1, 6, 7, 9, 10, 13, 17, 19 and 22. Deletions are the most commonly observed changes, and chromosome 22 losses are common in adults (50%) but rare in pediatric ependymomas (Kraus et al., 2001; Lamszus et al., 2001; von Haken et al., 1996). The target genes, located in regions of chromosomal gain or loss, are unknown, with the exception of cases in which both copies of the wild-type *NF2* gene (neurofibromin 2) are lost in intramedullary ependymomas (Alonso et al., 2002). Isolated cases of *MEN1* gene (multiple endocrine neoplasia I) loss have also been reported (Urioste et al., 2002). Germline mutations in *TP53* are uncommon, in contrast with those seen in diffuse astrocytomas (Nozaki et al., 1998).

When reviewed together, the data on genetic and epigenetic abnormalities presented above allow us to define four molecular biomarkers: *MGMT* hypermethylation in glioblastomas and anaplastic gliomas, *IDH1* and *IDH2* mutations in diffuse gliomas, *BRAF* aberrations in pilocytic astrocytomas, and combined deletions of chromosome arms 1p and 19q in oligodendroglial tumors. These biomarkers and their clinical significance are summarized in Table 2.

4. Single nucleotide polymorphisms and gliomas

A single nucleotide polymorphism (SNP) is generally defined as a stable replacement of only one DNA base, with a frequency greater than 1% in at least one population (Taylor et al., 2001). In human genetics studies, SNPs are simply referred to as bi-allelic markers because tri-and tetra-allelic markers are rare (Brookes, 1999).

Initially, only a few thousand SNPs were thought to exist in the entire genome. However, since 2000, that number has increased about one thousand-fold. In 2001, an international consortium on mapping SNPs described 1.42 million polymorphic loci. More important than this large number is the precision of their placement in the genome; there is approximately one polymorphism every 1.91 Kb. Therefore, 90% of sequences greater than 20 Kb in length have at least one SNP, and this density can be higher in genic regions. Of the known genes, 93% contain SNPs and 98% are at least 5 Kb away from a SNP. Soon, almost all genes or gene regions will be marked by one of these variable sequences (Sachidanandam et al., 2001).

Molecular marker	Clinical significance
IDH1/IDH2 mutation	• Diagnostic marker for diffuse WHO grade II and III gliomas, as well as secondary glioblastomas, and associated with a better prognosis in these tumors • Rare in primary glioblastomas, but when present, it is associated with a more favorable outcome • Not predictive for response to a particular type of therapy
BRAF duplication/fusion	• Diagnostic marker for pilocytic astrocytomas and helpful in distinguishing these tumors from diffuse astrocytomas • Prognostic significance within the group of pilocytic astrocytoma patients is unknown
MGMT promoter methylation	• Predictive for response of glioblastomas to alkylating chemotherapy • Associated with longer survival in glioblastoma patients treated with radiotherapy combined with concurrent and adjuvant temozolomide • Prognostic in anaplastic glioma patients treated with radiotherapy and/or alkylating chemotherapy
1p/19q co-deletion	• Associated with improved prognosis in oligodendroglial tumor patients receiving adjuvant radiotherapy and/or chemotherapy • Not predictive for response to a particular type of therapy

Table 2. The four most relevant markers for the molecular diagnosis of gliomas (Hofer & Lassman, 2010; Riemenschneider et al., 2010).

Because they are found throughout the genome, some alleles containing SNPs produce functional or physiologically relevant gene products. For example, SNPs in a coding region can affect the coded protein. When located in an intron, SNPs can influence the splicing mechanism, and when located in the promoter, SNPs can alter gene transcription (Krawczak et al., 1992). For this reason, SNPs are recognized as important tools in human genetics and medicine and have been widely used in genetic association studies of various complex diseases, including cancer. In humans, several reviews of SNPs have been carried out in an attempt to determine the patterns of SNP haplotypes in different populations (Conrad et al., 2006; Gonzalez-Neira et al., 2006; Jakobsson et al., 2008; Nothnagel & Rohde, 2005; Salisbury et al., 2003). Data from these tests are extremely useful for studying the genetic basis of cancer. For this reason, several research groups have focused on elucidating the role of SNPs in different genes related to the initiation and progression of gliomas in different populations. We performed association studies between SNPs, the risk of developing gliomas, and the prognosis for gliomas in a Brazilian population. Brazilians form one of the most heterogeneous populations in the world, which is the result of five centuries of interethnic crosses of peoples from three continents: the European colonizers who are mainly represented by the Portuguese, the African slaves, and the autochthonous Amerindians (Parra et al., 2003).

Until recently, we were the only laboratory investigating the association between *WRN* Cys1367Arg, the risk for brain tumor development, and the prognosis of brain tumors, especially with regard to gliomas (Pinto et al., 2008a). Werner syndrome (WS) is a premature aging disorder characterized by early onset of symptoms related to normal aging and is caused by inherited, recessive mutations in the *WRN* gene. The *WRN* gene encodes a member of the RecQ family of helicases involved in DNA replication and in maintaining the integrity of the genome (Harrigan et al., 2006). The cells of WS patients exhibit a high level of chromosomal translocations and deletions, and these patients present an increased predisposition to various types of cancer, including CNS tumors (Kobayashi et al., 1980). However, despite its putative tumor suppressor function, little is known about the contribution of the WRN protein to sporadic human malignancies. Taking into account that almost all cancers occur in the elderly and that mutations in the *WRN* gene lead to accelerated aging, it has been suggested that polymorphisms of the *WRN* gene, similar to Cys1367Arg, might be associated with age-related pathologies and cancer predisposition. However, our data indicate that neither glioma risk (OR = 1.38; 95% CI, 0.78-2.43; P = 0.334) nor patient survival (overall and disease-free survival, P = 0.396 and P = 0.843, respectively) was associated with variant alleles.

Similar results were found when we evaluated the genotype distribution of *TP53* Pro47Ser and Arg72Pro SNPs for their involvement in susceptibility to gliomas and in determining the oncologic prognosis of patients (Pinto et al., 2008b). A critical site in the TP53 protein for apoptosis signaling is a proline-rich region located between codons 64 and 92. Dumont et al. (2003) reported that the homozygous Arg72 allele induces apoptosis at a rate that is 15-fold higher than the Pro72 allele. According to Leu et al. (2004), the apoptosis-inducing ability of the Arg72 allele is in part due to its mitochondrial location, which makes it possible for TP53 to directly interact with the pro-apoptotic protein, BAK. However, the *TP53* Pro47Ser SNP resulted in a significantly decreased ability of the TP53 protein to induce apoptosis. A critical event in TP53-induced apoptosis is phosphorylation of the serine residue at codon 46. This region is where allele Pro47 acts as a substrate for proline-directed kinases such as the MAPK1 protein. Li et al. (2005) reported that the Ser47 allele, which is a poor substrate for MAPK1, has an apoptosis-inducing ability that is 5-fold lower than that of the wild-type Pro47 allele. However, our data again indicated that neither glioma susceptibility nor patient survival was associated with the *TP53* Arg72Pro or Pro47Ser alleles in the Brazilian population.

In 2009, we investigated the role of *EGF* +61 A>G as a potential risk factor and/or prognostic marker for gliomas in the Brazilian population. The *EGF* gene encodes a ligand for EGFR that activates a cascade of events responsible for promoting cell proliferation, inhibition of apoptosis, and differentiation. Alterations in the EGF/EGFR signaling pathway are associated with tumor progression in a variety of human cancers. Therefore, high expression of EGF may play a key role in glioma development and progression (Salomon et al., 1995). Shahbazi et al. (2002) first reported that the +61 A>G SNP in the 5′-UTR region of *EGF* is associated with increased EGF production and risk of malignant melanoma. Since that discovery, other research groups have obtained conflicting findings regarding the relationship of this functional SNP with different human cancers, including gliomas (Bao et al., 2010; Bhowmick et al., 2004; Costa et al., 2007; Liu et al., 2009; Vauleon et al., 2007; Wang et al., 2010). In our results, the genotype and allele frequencies between cases and controls were similar, indicating no significant association with glioma risk (P = 0.94 and P = 0.887, respectively) and suggesting that *EGF* +61 A>G may not significantly contribute to the susceptibility to gliomas in the Brazilian population. This result is consistent with that of Vauleon et al. (2007) and Liu et al. (2009) in French and Chinese populations, respectively. However, we found that the major +61G allele (frequency among controls, 0.51) was associated with a shorter overall survival in patients (P = 0.023). Thus, with regard to patient survival, our results corroborate those of Bhowmick et al. (2004) in a population of North American patients.

We have also studied the *GSTP1* gene, which encodes a protein accounting for approximately 90% of the enzymatic activity of the glutathione S-transferase (GST) family (Custodio et al., 2010). GSTs constitute a superfamily of ubiquitous, multifunctional enzymes that are involved in cellular detoxification of a large number of endogenous and exogenous chemical agents that possess electrophilic functional groups (Ryberg et al., 1997). The GSTP1 protein is a pi-class enzyme and *GSTP1* structure has been extensively examined in association with the risk of cancer (White et al., 2008). The influence of the *GSTP1* Ile105Val SNP on cancer has been reported with inconsistent results from different parts of the world (Syamala et al., 2008). Our results demonstrate that the Val105 allele was more frequent in a population of cancer patients than in a healthy population (0.29 and 0.06, respectively; P < 0.001) and that the presence of this genotype may increase the risk of developing astrocytomas and glioblastomas (OR = 8.60; 95% CI, 4.14-17.87; P < 0.001). However, we did not find an association between the *GSTP1* Ile105Val SNP and patient survival.

Recently, we began studying SNPs in DNA repair genes and we performed association analysis of SNPs in genes for the *XRCC* (X-ray cross-complementing) family, *XRCC1* and *XRCC3*, in a series of gliomas (unpublished data). Human tumors may develop through alterations to the DNA repair system, which is crucially important for cellular life (Kawabata et al., 2005). To ensure the integrity of the genome, a complex system of DNA repair was developed. Base excision repair is the first defense mechanism of cells against DNA damage and a major means for preventing mutagenesis (Hu et al., 2005). Repair genes may play an important role in maintaining genomic stability through different pathways mediating base excision repair (Sreeja et al., 2008). For this reason, much attention has been given to the study of SNPs in *XRCCs* and their involvement in different types of cancer, including gliomas. We performed analysis of the Arg194Trp and Arg399Gln SNPs in *XRCC1* and the Thr241Met SNP in *XRCC3* to assess their roles in the risk and prognosis for gliomas in Brazilians. Our results provide evidence that the *XRCC1* Arg194Trp SNP may contribute to the etiology of human gliomas because the Trp194 allele was strongly associated with risk and the Gln399 allele revealed a small, increased risk for tumor development. In regard to the *XRCC3* Thr241Met SNP, we also found evidence that *XRRC3* Thr241Met may contribute to the etiology of human gliomas. However, when the Arg194Trp and Arg399Gln SNPs in *XRCC1* and the Thr241Met SNP in *XRCC3* were considered together, we did not find statistical difference between genotypes and patient survival.

Around the globe, other groups have analyzed the association between SNPs found in *XRCCs* genes and the risk of developing gliomas. Kiuru et al. (2003) evaluated the association between the *XRCC1* Arg194Trp, Arg280His, and Arg399Gln SNPS, the *XRCC3*

Thr241Met SNP, and glioma risk in a prospective, population-based, case-control study conducted in Denmark, Finland, Sweden, and the UK. They found no significant association with gliomas for any of the SNPs when examined individually. However, the results indicated possible associations between combinations of *XRCC1* and *XRCC3* SNPs and the risk of glioma development, as carriers of both homozygous variant genotypes, i.e., *XRCC1* Gln399Gln and *XRCC3* Met241Met were associated with a three-fold increased risk of glioma (OR = 3.18; 95% CI, 1.26-8.04). In a haplotype-based approach in a Chinese population, Liu et al. (2007) investigated the role of 22 tagging SNPs (tSNPs) of *XRCC5*, *XRCC6* and *XRCC7*. They found that glioma risk was significantly associated with three of the *XRCC5* tSNPs (rs828704, rs3770502 and rs9288516, P = 0.005, 0.042 and 0.003, respectively), one *XRCC6* tSNP (rs6519265, P = 0.044), and none of the *XPCC7* tSNPs in a single-locus analysis. Haplotype-based association analysis revealed that glioma risk was significantly associated with one protective *XRCC5* haplotype "CAGTT," which accounted for a 40% reduction (OR = 0.60, 95% CI, 0.43-0.85) in glioma risk. In a study of North Americans, Wang et al. (2004) found that the variant XRCC7T allele of the *XRCC7* G6721T SNP was significantly more common in the glioma cases than in the controls (P = 0.045). The *XRCC7* genotype frequency was also significant when comparing the cases and controls (P = 0.040). Likewise, the difference in distribution of the combined T-variant genotype (GT + TT) between the cases and controls was also statistically significant (P = 0.012), suggesting that the T allele may be a risk factor for glioma.

In addition to the studies mentioned above, several others were published indicating the results of associations, positive or negative, of genomic variations with the risk of developing gliomas. However, the ethnic variations, methodological variations, and the presence of responsible, functionally unknown SNPs in linkage disequilibrium with those SNPs analyzed have contributed to the dissemination of conflicting results in different parts of the world. Gu et al. (2009) presented a review including a list of eight literature-defined, putative, functional, SNPs associated with gliomas in at least two populations from case-control studies. A summary of this list is presented in Table 3.

Gene selection for association studies has previously been based on studies reporting the role of genes and their SNPs in the regulation of cellular functions. However, after the completion of the human genome project and the development of analytical platforms capable of parallel genotype processing, which resulted in new selection strategies for identifying susceptibility genes in many complex genetic disorders, gene selection is currently based on genome-wide association (GWA) studies.

The two glioma GWA studies performed so far were published in 2010 in the same issue of Nature Genetics. In the first pages, Shete et al. (2009) presented the results of a meta-analysis of two GWA studies that involved the genotyping of 454,576 tSNPs in a total of 1,878 glioma cases and 3,670 controls, with posterior validation in three additional independent series totaling 2,545 cases and 2,953 controls. The authors identified five risk loci for glioma at 5p15.33 (*TERT* rs2736100), 8q24.21 (*CCDC26* rs4295627), 9p21.3 (*CDKN2A-CDKN2B* rs4977756), 11q23.3 (*PHLDB1* rs498872), and 20q13.33 (*RTEL1* rs6010620). In the second study, Wrensch et al. (2009) analyzed 275,895 SNPs in 692 adult patients with high-grade glioma and 3,992 controls, with a replication series of 176 high-grade glioma cases and 174 controls. That analysis provided further evidence to implicate 9p21 (*CDKN2B* rs1412829) and 20q13.3 (*RTEL1* rs6010620) in glioma risk.

Main paths, genes	Associated SNPs	Effect	OR (95% CI)
DNA repair			
XRCC7	G6721T	Risk	GG vs. TT, 1.82 (1.13–2.93)[1]
			GG vs. TT, 1.44 (1.13–1.84)[2]
XRCC1	Arg399Gln	Risk	AA vs. GG, 1.23 (0.96–1.57)[2]
			AA vs. GG, 1.32 (0.97–1.81)[3]
			GA/AA vs. GG, 1.44 (1.05–1.92)[4]
PARP1	Val762ala	Protective	CT/CC vs. TT, 0.80 (0.67–0.95)[2]
			CT/CC vs. TT, 0.71 (0.52–0.97)[4]
ERCC1	A8092C	Risk	AA/AC vs. CC, 4.41 (1.6–12.2)[5]
			AA/AC vs. CC, 1.67 (0.93–3.02)[6]
ERCC2	Gln751Lys	Risk	CC vs. AA, 1.19 (0.93–1.52)[2]
			AA vs. AC/CC, 1.66 (1.01–2.72)[6]
MGMT	Phe84Leu	Protective or risk?	CT/TT vs. CC, 0.66 (0.45–0.94)[4]
			CT/TT vs. CC, 1.26 (0.90–1.75)[7]
Cell cycle, EGF	+61 A>G	Risk	$P = 0.032$[8]
			AG/GG vs. AA, 1.52 (1.03–2.23)[9]
Inflammation: IL13	Arg130Gln	Protective	AG vs. GG, 0.75 (0.48–1.17)[10]
			TT vs. CC/CT, 0.39 (0.16–0.93)[11]

Table 3. Selected glioma susceptibility genes and SNPs observed in at least two studies.
[1]Wang et al. (2004); [2]McKean-Cowdin et al. (2009); [3]Kiuru et al. (2008); [4]Liu et al. (2009);
[5]Chen et al. (2000); [6]Wrensch et al. (2005); [7]Felini et al. (2007); [8]Bhowmick et al. (2004); [9]Costa
et al. (2007); [10]Schwartzbaum et al. (2005); [11]Amirian et al. (2010).

5. Cancer stem cells

Both the invasive nature of the tumor and its heterogeneity probably contribute to the poor
response to the treatment regimens available today. Tumor heterogeneity is traditionally
attributed to the accumulation of regional variations in the tumor microenvironment and
the diversity of subpopulations of cancer cells, which result from random genetic changes
(Reya et al., 2001).
The majority tumors consist of a heterogeneous population of cells with different
proliferative potential, as well as the ability to re-form the tumor upon transplantation into
immunodeficient mice (Visvader & Lindeman, 2008). Recently, evidence has accumulated
that tumors contain a population with characteristics similar to normal stem cells called

cancer stem cells, which are also multipotent cells. This subpopulation has the ability to repair itself and is believed to control tumor initiation, a process that is responsible for tumor recurrence and the resistance to therapy observed in different tumor types, including gliomas (Bao et al., 2006). The observation that normal stem cells and cancer stem cells share common features (e.g., undifferentiated state and unlimited capacity for self-regeneration) led to the hypothesis of cancer stem cells (Park & Rich, 2009).

A practical component of the cancer stem cell hypothesis is directed to the matter of intrinsic resistance to radiation and chemotherapy. Cancer stem cells are predicted to be difficult targets for tumor therapy because they exhibit a slowed cell cycle and high levels of drug export. Furthermore, these cells may not express or may not be dependent on the oncoproteins that are targeted by the most recent generation of cancer drugs (Cheng et al., 2010).

Cancer stem cells, similar to normal stem cells, are dependent on the microenvironment in which they are located. This microenvironment, formed by cells and extracellular matrix, controls the maintenance of organ functions. Therefore, disturbance of the local microenvironment in neoplastic processes can trigger tumor development (Barcellos-Hoff et al., 2009). In glioma, for example, studies have shown that the microenvironment is surrounded by blood vessels, which provide access to signaling molecules, nutrition, and possibly to the use of the nascent vasculature for migration, which provides direct cell contact and secreted factors that are responsible for maintaining the state of quiescence of cancer stem cells, regulating their self-renewal and multipotency (Gilbertson & Rich, 2007; Jandial et al., 2008). Thus, one can say that cancer stem cells and the microenvironment are parts of the tumor. Therefore, knowledge of the associated characteristics will lead to a new understanding of tumor biology and the development of new therapeutic strategies against these cells. For this reason, it is extremely important to characterize the different subpopulations of cancer stem cells that contribute to tumor formation (Denysenko et al., 2010).

6. Conclusion

The development and progression of gliomas may likely be due to a multistep process that involves the functional inactivation of tumor suppressor genes and DNA repair genes, as well as the activation of oncogenes. Given the limitations of current therapies, understanding the pathways that lead to tumor progression should remain a high priority in cancer research. If the mechanisms that culminate in metastasis are fully understood, the development of new diagnostic and therapeutic methods may allow for a substantial improvement in the quality of life of affected patients and a better means of predicting patient prognosis. Genetic and epigenetic studies involving large cohorts of glioma patients in different populations have provided important information for understanding the role of key genes in the development and risk of gliomas. Because it is considered a work in progress, the WHO classification for brain tumors may soon incorporate molecular data to refine the classification of these diseases, which are complex from a therapeutic standpoint.

SNPs have become increasingly popular in the genetic study of gliomas because of the quick, inexpensive and accurate analysis of SNPs. The identification of SNPs as risk factors for different glioma subtypes can be important for prevention, diagnosis and prognosis. Variations in the genomic sequence contribute to phenotypic diversity and susceptibility to or protection against many complex diseases. Thus, it is estimated that the risk of gliomas may be strongly influenced by the patterns of SNPs in certain key susceptibility genes; these SNPs are still being identified. The same reasoning can be applied to inter-individual variations in genetic responses to medications, which is a field of great interest to the pharmaceutical industry. The benefit of having a SNP map of different populations is that it allows for coverage of the entire genome so that researchers can compare the patterns and frequencies of SNPs in their patients and associate these patterns with the disease concerned. The GWA studies with significant numbers and carefully matched controls have become a powerful tool in identifying genes involved in common genetic diseases, including gliomas. The identification of susceptibility alleles provides a greater understanding of gliomagenesis and provides target genes for potential therapeutic intervention. Unlike environmental exposure, SNPs do not change during the process of tumorigenesis. Therefore, SNPs may be useful as indicators of risk.

The main features of normal stem cells are the capacity for self-regeneration and differentiation to different cell types. These characteristics are heavily regulated by the local microenvironment. Because studies have shown that cancer stem cells behave like normal stem cells, understanding the regulatory mechanisms of cancer stem cells and their microenvironment has changed our understanding of the biology of gliomas and has precipitated a reassessment of current therapies. The cure of glioma will require the elimination of all tumor cells, including cancer stem cells. Therefore, further studies to provide a better understanding of the origin of cancer stem cells and their interactions with the microenvironment are needed. These findings hold great promise for the development of new therapies that can help us improve the results achieved with current therapies and thereby prolong patient survival.

7. References

Alonso, M.E., Bello, M.J., Arjona, D., Gonzalez-Gomez, P., Lomas, J., de Campos, J.M., Kusak, M.E., Isla, A. & Rey, J.A. (2002). Analysis of the NF2 gene in oligodendrogliomas and ependymomas. *Cancer Genet Cytogenet*, Vol.134, No.1, pp. 1-5

Amirian, E., Liu, Y., Scheurer, M.E., El-Zein, R., Gilbert, M.R. & Bondy, M.L. (2010). Genetic variants in inflammation pathway genes and asthma in glioma susceptibility. *Neuro Oncol*, Vol.12, No.5, pp. 444-452

Bao, G., Wang, M., Guo, S., Han, Y. & Xu, G. (2010). Association between epidermal growth factor +61 G/A polymorphism and glioma risk in a Chinese Han population. *J Int Med Res*, Vol.38, No.5, pp. 1645-1652

Bao, S., Wu, Q., McLendon, R.E., Hao, Y., Shi, Q., Hjelmeland, A.B., Dewhirst, M.W., Bigner, D.D. & Rich, J.N. (2006). Glioma stem cells promote radioresistance by preferential activation of the DNA damage response. *Nature*, Vol.444, No.7120, pp. 756-760

Barcellos-Hoff, M.H., Newcomb, E.W., Zagzag, D. & Narayana, A. (2009). Therapeutic targets in malignant glioblastoma microenvironment. *Semin Radiat Oncol*, Vol.19, No.3, pp. 163-170

Bartek, J. & Lukas, J. (2001). Are all cancer genes equal? *Nature*, Vol.411, No.6841, pp. 1001-1002

Bello, M.J. & Rey, J.A. (2006). The p53/Mdm2/p14ARF cell cycle control pathway genes may be inactivated by genetic and epigenetic mechanisms in gliomas. *Cancer Genet Cytogenet*, Vol.164, No.2, pp. 172-173

Bhowmick, D.A., Zhuang, Z., Wait, S.D. & Weil, R.J. (2004). A functional polymorphism in the EGF gene is found with increased frequency in glioblastoma multiforme patients and is associated with more aggressive disease. *Cancer Res*, Vol.64, No.4, pp. 1220-1223

Bigner, S.H., McLendon, R.E., Fuchs, H., McKeever, P.E. & Friedman, H.S. (1997). Chromosomal characteristics of childhood brain tumors. *Cancer Genet Cytogenet*, Vol.97, No.2, pp. 125-134

Brookes, A.J. (1999). The essence of SNPs. *Gene*, Vol.234, No.2, pp. 177-186

Cairncross, J.G., Ueki, K., Zlatescu, M.C., Lisle, D.K., Finkelstein, D.M., Hammond, R.R., Silver, J.S., Stark, P.C., Macdonald, D.R., Ino, Y., Ramsay, D.A. & Louis, D.N. (1998). Specific genetic predictors of chemotherapeutic response and survival in patients with anaplastic oligodendrogliomas. *J Natl Cancer Inst*, Vol.90, No.19, pp. 1473-1479

Chen, P., Wiencke, J., Aldape, K., Kesler-Diaz, A., Miike, R., Kelsey, K., Lee, M., Liu, J. & Wrensch, M. (2000). Association of an ERCC1 polymorphism with adult-onset glioma. *Cancer Epidemiol Biomarkers Prev*, Vol.9, No.8, pp. 843-847

Cheng, L., Bao, S. & Rich, J.N. (2010). Potential therapeutic implications of cancer stem cells in glioblastoma. *Biochem Pharmacol*, Vol.80, No.5, pp. 654-665

Collins, V.P. (2004). Brain tumours: classification and genes. *J Neurol Neurosurg Psychiatry*, Vol.75 Suppl 2, pp. ii2-11

Conrad, D.F., Jakobsson, M., Coop, G., Wen, X., Wall, J.D., Rosenberg, N.A. & Pritchard, J.K. (2006). A worldwide survey of haplotype variation and linkage disequilibrium in the human genome. *Nat Genet*, Vol.38, No.11, pp. 1251-1260

Costa, B.M., Ferreira, P., Costa, S., Canedo, P., Oliveira, P., Silva, A., Pardal, F., Suriano, G., Machado, J.C., Lopes, J.M. & Reis, R.M. (2007). Association between functional EGF+61 polymorphism and glioma risk. *Clin Cancer Res*, Vol.13, No.9, pp. 2621-2626

Cross, S.H. & Bird, A.P. (1995). CpG islands and genes. *Curr Opin Genet Dev*, Vol.5, No.3, pp. 309-314

Custodio, A.C., Almeida, L.O., Pinto, G.R., Santos, M.J., Almeida, J.R., Clara, C.A., Rey, J.A. & Casartelli, C. (2010). GSTP1 Ile105Val polymorphism in astrocytomas and glioblastomas. *Genet Mol Res*, Vol.9, No.4, pp. 2328-2334

Dang, L., White, D.W., Gross, S., Bennett, B.D., Bittinger, M.A., Driggers, E.M., Fantin, V.R., Jang, H.G., Jin, S., Keenan, M.C., Marks, K.M., Prins, R.M., Ward, P.S., Yen, K.E., Liau, L.M., Rabinowitz, J.D., Cantley, L.C., Thompson, C.B., Vander Heiden, M.G. & Su, S.M. (2009). Cancer-associated IDH1 mutations produce 2-hydroxyglutarate. *Nature*, Vol.462, No.7274, pp. 739-744

Denysenko, T., Gennero, L., Roos, M.A., Melcarne, A., Juenemann, C., Faccani, G., Morra, I., Cavallo, G., Reguzzi, S., Pescarmona, G. & Ponzetto, A. (2010). Glioblastoma cancer stem cells: heterogeneity, microenvironment and related therapeutic strategies. *Cell Biochem Funct*, Vol.28, No.5, pp. 343-351

Dumont, P., Leu, J.I., Della Pietra, A.C., 3rd, George, D.L. & Murphy, M. (2003). The codon 72 polymorphic variants of p53 have markedly different apoptotic potential. *Nat Genet*, Vol.33, No.3, pp. 357-365

Ebert, C., von Haken, M., Meyer-Puttlitz, B., Wiestler, O.D., Reifenberger, G., Pietsch, T. & von Deimling, A. (1999). Molecular genetic analysis of ependymal tumors. NF2 mutations and chromosome 22q loss occur preferentially in intramedullary spinal ependymomas. *Am J Pathol*, Vol.155, No.2, pp. 627-632

Esteller, M., Garcia-Foncillas, J., Andion, E., Goodman, S.N., Hidalgo, O.F., Vanaclocha, V., Baylin, S.B. & Herman, J.G. (2000). Inactivation of the DNA-repair gene MGMT and the clinical response of gliomas to alkylating agents. *N Engl J Med*, Vol.343, No.19, pp. 1350-1354

Franco-Hernandez, C., Martinez-Glez, V., Alonso, M.E., De Campos, J.M., Isla, A., Vaquero, J., Gutierrez, M. & Rey, J.A. (2007). Gene dosage and mutational analyses of EGFR in oligodendrogliomas. *Int J Oncol*, Vol.30, No.1, pp. 209-215

Franco-Hernandez, C., Martinez-Glez, V., de Campos, J.M., Isla, A., Vaquero, J., Gutierrez, M., Casartelli, C. & Rey, J.A. (2009). Allelic status of 1p and 19q in oligodendrogliomas and glioblastomas: multiplex ligation-dependent probe amplification versus loss of heterozygosity. *Cancer Genet Cytogenet*, Vol.190, No.2, pp. 93-96

Felini, M.J., Olshan, A.F., Schroeder, J.C., North, K.E., Carozza, S.E., Kelsey, K.T., Liu, M., Rice, T., Wiencke, J.K. & Wrensch, M.R. (2007). DNA repair polymorphisms XRCC1 and MGMT and risk of adult gliomas. *Neuroepidemiology*, Vol.29, No.1-2, pp. 55-58

Gilbertson, R. (2002). Paediatric embryonic brain tumours. biological and clinical relevance of molecular genetic abnormalities. *Eur J Cancer*, Vol.38, No.5, pp. 675-685

Gilbertson, R.J. & Rich, J.N. (2007). Making a tumour's bed: glioblastoma stem cells and the vascular niche. Nat Rev Cancer, Vol.7, No.10, pp. 733-736

Gonzalez-Gomez, P., Bello, M.J., Arjona, D., Lomas, J., Alonso, M.E., De Campos, J.M., Vaquero, J., Isla, A., Gutierrez, M. & Rey, J.A. (2003). Promoter hypermethylation of multiple genes in astrocytic gliomas. Int J Oncol, Vol.22, No.3, pp. 601-608

Gonzalez-Neira, A., Ke, X., Lao, O., Calafell, F., Navarro, A., Comas, D., Cann, H., Bumpstead, S., Ghori, J., Hunt, S., Deloukas, P., Dunham, I., Cardon, L.R. & Bertranpetit, J. (2006). The portability of tagSNPs across populations: a worldwide survey. *Genome Res*, Vol.16, No.3, pp. 323-330

Gu, J., Liu, Y., Kyritsis, A.P. & Bondy, M.L. (2009). Molecular epidemiology of primary brain tumors. *Neurotherapeutics*, Vol.6, No.3, pp. 427-435

Gutmann, D.H., Donahoe, J., Brown, T., James, C.D. & Perry, A. (2000). Loss of neurofibromatosis 1 (NF1) gene expression in NF1-associated pilocytic astrocytomas. *Neuropathol Appl Neurobiol*, Vol.26, No.4, pp. 361-367

Hanahan, D. & Weinberg, R.A. (2000). The hallmarks of cancer. *Cell*, Vol.100, No.1, pp. 57-70

Harrigan, J.A., Wilson, D.M., 3rd, Prasad, R., Opresko, P.L., Beck, G., May, A., Wilson, S.H. & Bohr, V.A. (2006). The Werner syndrome protein operates in base excision repair and cooperates with DNA polymerase beta. *Nucleic Acids Res*, Vol.34, No.2, pp. 745-754

Hartmann, C., Meyer, J., Balss, J., Capper, D., Mueller, W., Christians, A., Felsberg, J., Wolter, M., Mawrin, C., Wick, W., Weller, M., Herold-Mende, C., Unterberg, A.,

Jeuken, J.W., Wesseling, P., Reifenberger, G. & von Deimling, A. (2009). Type and frequency of IDH1 and IDH2 mutations are related to astrocytic and oligodendroglial differentiation and age: a study of 1,010 diffuse gliomas. *Acta Neuropathol*, Vol.118, No.4, pp. 469-474

Hegi, M.E., Diserens, A.C., Gorlia, T., Hamou, M.F., de Tribolet, N., Weller, M., Kros, J.M., Hainfellner, J.A., Mason, W., Mariani, L., Bromberg, J.E., Hau, P., Mirimanoff, R.O., Cairncross, J.G., Janzer, R.C. & Stupp, R. (2005). MGMT gene silencing and benefit from temozolomide in glioblastoma. *N Engl J Med*, Vol.352, No.10, pp. 997-1003

Herrlinger, U., Rieger, J., Koch, D., Loeser, S., Blaschke, B., Kortmann, R.D., Steinbach, J.P., Hundsberger, T., Wick, W., Meyermann, R., Tan, T.C., Sommer, C., Bamberg, M., Reifenberger, G. & Weller, M. (2006). Phase II trial of lomustine plus temozolomide chemotherapy in addition to radiotherapy in newly diagnosed glioblastoma: UKT-03. *J Clin Oncol*, Vol.24, No.27, pp. 4412-4417

Hofer, S. & Lassman, A.B. (2010). Molecular markers in gliomas: impact for the clinician. *Target Oncol*, Vol.5, No.3, pp. 201-210

Hu, Z., Ma, H., Chen, F., Wei, Q. & Shen, H. (2005). XRCC1 polymorphisms and cancer risk: a meta-analysis of 38 case-control studies. *Cancer Epidemiol Biomarkers Prev*, Vol.14, No.7, pp. 1810-1818

Jakobsson, M., Scholz, S.W., Scheet, P., Gibbs, J.R., VanLiere, J.M., Fung, H.C., Szpiech, Z.A., Degnan, J.H., Wang, K., Guerreiro, R., Bras, J.M., Schymick, J.C., Hernandez, D.G., Traynor, B.J., Simon-Sanchez, J., Matarin, M., Britton, A., van de Leemput, J., Rafferty, I., Bucan, M., Cann, H.M., Hardy, J.A., Rosenberg, N.A. & Singleton, A.B. (2008). Genotype, haplotype and copy-number variation in worldwide human populations. *Nature*, Vol.451, No.7181, pp. 998-1003

Jandial, R., U, H., Levy, M.L. & Snyder, E.Y. (2008). Brain tumor stem cells and the tumor microenvironmen. *Neurosurg Focus*, Vol.24, No.3-4, pp. E27

Jenkins, R.B., Blair, H., Ballman, K.V., Giannini, C., Arusell, R.M., Law, M., Flynn, H., Passe, S., Felten, S., Brown, P.D., Shaw, E.G. & Buckner, J.C. (2006). A t(1;19)(q10;p10) mediates the combined deletions of 1p and 19q and predicts a better prognosis of patients with oligodendroglioma. *Cancer Res*, Vol.66, No.20, pp. 9852-9861

Jones, D.T., Kocialkowski, S., Liu, L., Pearson, D.M., Ichimura, K. & Collins, V.P. (2009). Oncogenic RAF1 rearrangement and a novel BRAF mutation as alternatives to KIAA1549:BRAF fusion in activating the MAPK pathway in pilocytic astrocytoma. *Oncogene*, Vol.28, No.20, pp. 2119-2123

Jones, P.A. & Baylin, S.B. (2007). The epigenomics of cancer. *Cell*, Vol.128, No.4, pp. 683-692

Jones, P.A. & Buckley, J.D. (1990). The role of DNA methylation in cancer. *Adv Cancer Res*, Vol.54, pp. 1-23

Kawabata, M., Kawabata, T. & Nishibori, M. (2005). Role of recA/RAD51 family proteins in mammals. *Acta Med Okayama*, Vol.59, No.1, pp. 1-9

Kiuru, A., Lindholm, C., Heinavaara, S., Ilus, T., Jokinen, P., Haapasalo, H., Salminen, T., Christensen, H.C., Feychting, M., Johansen, C., Lonn, S., Malmer, B., Schoemaker, M.J., Swerdlow, A.J. & Auvinen, A. (2008). XRCC1 and XRCC3 variants and risk of glioma and meningioma. *J Neurooncol*, Vol.88, No.2, pp. 135-142

Kleihues, P. & Cavenee, W.K. (2000). World Health Organisation classification of tumours: Pathology and genetics of tumours of the nervous system. IARC Press, Lyon, France

Kleihues, P., Louis, D.N., Scheithauer, B.W., Rorke, L.B., Reifenberger, G., Burger, P.C. & Cavenee, W.K. (2002). The WHO classification of tumors of the nervous system. *J Neuropathol Exp Neurol*, Vol.61, No.3, pp. 215-225; discussion 226-219

Kleihues, P.; Burger, P.C. & Scheithauer, B.W. (1993). Histological typing of tumours of the central nervous system. World Health Organization international histological classification of tumours. Springer Verlag, Berlin, Heidelberg

Kluwe, L., Hagel, C., Tatagiba, M., Thomas, S., Stavrou, D., Ostertag, H., von Deimling, A. & Mautner, V.F. (2001). Loss of NF1 alleles distinguish sporadic from NF1-associated pilocytic astrocytomas. *J Neuropathol Exp Neurol*, Vol.60, No.9, pp. 917-920

Knudson, A.G., Jr. (1971). Mutation and cancer: statistical study of retinoblastoma. *Proc Natl Acad Sci U S A*, Vol.68, No.4, pp. 820-823

Kobayashi, S., Gibo, H., Sugita, K., Komiya, I. & Yamada, T. (1980). Werner's syndrome associated with meningioma. *Neurosurgery*, Vol.7, No.5, pp. 517-520

Komine, C., Watanabe, T., Katayama, Y., Yoshino, A., Yokoyama, T. & Fukushima, T. (2003). Promoter hypermethylation of the DNA repair gene O6 methylguanine-DNA methyltransferase is an independent predictor of shortened progression free survival in patients with low-grade diffuse astrocytomas. *Brain Pathol*, Vol.13, No.2, pp. 176-184

Korshunov, A., Meyer, J., Capper, D., Christians, A., Remke, M., Witt, H., Pfister, S., von Deimling, A. & Hartmann, C. (2009). Combined molecular analysis of BRAF and IDH1 distinguishes pilocytic astrocytoma from diffuse astrocytoma. *Acta Neuropathol*, Vol.118, No.3, pp. 401-405

Kraus, J.A., de Millas, W., Sorensen, N., Herbold, C., Schichor, C., Tonn, J.C., Wiestler, O.D., von Deimling, A. & Pietsch, T. (2001). Indications for a tumor suppressor gene at 22q11 involved in the pathogenesis of ependymal tumors and distinct from hSNF5/INI1. *Acta Neuropathol*, Vol.102, No.1, pp. 69-74

Krawczak, M., Reiss, J. & Cooper, D.N. (1992). The mutational spectrum of single base-pair substitutions in mRNA splice junctions of human genes: causes and consequences. *Hum Genet*, Vol.90, No.1-2, pp. 41-54

Lamszus, K., Lachenmayer, L., Heinemann, U., Kluwe, L., Finckh, U., Hoppner, W., Stavrou, D., Fillbrandt, R. & Westphal, M. (2001). Molecular genetic alterations on chromosomes 11 and 22 in ependymomas. *Int J Cancer*, Vol.91, No.6, pp. 803-808

Leu, J.I., Dumont, P., Hafey, M., Murphy, M.E. & George, D.L. (2004). Mitochondrial p53 activates Bak and causes disruption of a Bak-Mcl1 complex. *Nat Cell Biol*, Vol.6, No.5, pp. 443-450

Li, X., Dumont, P., Della Pietra, A., Shetler, C. & Murphy, M.E. (2005). The codon 47 polymorphism in p53 is functionally significant. *J Biol Chem*, Vol.280, No.25, pp. 24245-24251

Listernick, R., Charrow, J. & Gutmann, D.H. (1999). Intracranial gliomas in neurofibromatosis type 1. *Am J Med Genet*, Vol.89, No.1, pp. 38-44

Liu, Y., Scheurer, M.E., El-Zein, R., Cao, Y., Do, K.A., Gilbert, M., Aldape, K.D., Wei, Q., Etzel, C. & Bondy, M.L. (2009). Association and interactions between DNA repair gene polymorphisms and adult glioma. *Cancer Epidemiol Biomarkers Prev*, Vol.18, No.1, pp. 204-214

Liu, Y., Zhang, H., Zhou, K., Chen, L., Xu, Z., Zhong, Y., Liu, H., Li, R., Shugart, Y.Y., Wei, Q., Jin, L., Huang, F., Lu, D. & Zhou, L. (2007). Tagging SNPs in non-homologous end-joining pathway genes and risk of glioma. *Carcinogenesis*, Vol.28, No.9, pp. 1906-1913

Louis, D.N., Ohgaki, H., Wiestler, O.D., Cavenee, W.K., Burger, P.C., Jouvet, A., Scheithauer, B.W. & Kleihues, P. (2007). The 2007 WHO classification of tumours of the central nervous system. *Acta Neuropathol*, Vol.114, No.2, pp. 97-109

Louis, D.N., Pomeroy, S.L. & Cairncross, J.G. (2002). Focus on central nervous system neoplasia. *Cancer Cell*, Vol.1, No.2, pp. 125-128

Macdonald, D.R., Gaspar, L.E. & Cairncross, J.G. (1990). Successful chemotherapy for newly diagnosed aggressive oligodendroglioma. *Ann Neurol*, Vol.27, No.5, pp. 573-574

McCormack, B.M., Miller, D.C., Budzilovich, G.N., Voorhees, G.J. & Ransohoff, J. (1992). Treatment and survival of low-grade astrocytoma in adults--1977-1988. *Neurosurgery*, Vol.31, No.4, pp. 636-642; discussion 642

McKean-Cowdin, R., Barnholtz-Sloan, J., Inskip, P.D., Ruder, A.M., Butler, M., Rajaraman, P., Razavi, P., Patoka, J., Wiencke, J.K., Bondy, M.L. & Wrensch, M. (2009). Associations between polymorphisms in DNA repair genes and glioblastoma. *Cancer Epidemiol Biomarkers Prev*, Vol.18, No.4, pp. 1118-1126

Nakagawachi, T., Soejima, H., Urano, T., Zhao, W., Higashimoto, K., Satoh, Y., Matsukura, S., Kudo, S., Kitajima, Y., Harada, H., Furukawa, K., Matsuzaki, H., Emi, M., Nakabeppu, Y., Miyazaki, K., Sekiguchi, M. & Mukai, T. (2003). Silencing effect of CpG island hypermethylation and histone modifications on O6-methylguanine-DNA methyltransferase (MGMT) gene expression in human cancer. *Oncogene*, Vol.22, No.55, pp. 8835-8844

Natsume, A., Kondo, Y., Ito, M., Motomura, K., Wakabayashi, T. & Yoshida, J. (2010). Epigenetic aberrations and therapeutic implications in gliomas. *Cancer Sci*, Vol.101, No.6, pp. 1331-1336

Ng, H.K. & Lam, P.Y. (1998). The molecular genetics of central nervous system tumors. *Pathology*, Vol.30, No.2, pp. 196-202

Nothnagel, M. & Rohde, K. (2005). The effect of single-nucleotide polymorphism marker selection on patterns of haplotype blocks and haplotype frequency estimates. *Am J Hum Genet*, Vol.77, No.6, pp. 988-998

Nozaki, M., Tada, M., Matsumoto, R., Sawamura, Y., Abe, H. & Iggo, R.D. (1998). Rare occurrence of inactivating p53 gene mutations in primary non-astrocytic tumors of the central nervous system: reappraisal by yeast functional assay. *Acta Neuropathol*, Vol.95, No.3, pp. 291-296

Ohgaki, H. & Kleihues, P. (2005). Epidemiology and etiology of gliomas. *Acta Neuropathol*, Vol.109, No.1, pp. 93-108

Paige, A.J. (2003). Redefining tumour suppressor genes: exceptions to the two-hit hypothesis. *Cell Mol Life Sci*, Vol.60, No.10, pp. 2147-2163

Park, D.M. & Rich, J.N. (2009). Biology of glioma cancer stem cells. *Mol Cells*, Vol.28, No.1, pp. 7-12

Parra, F.C., Amado, R.C., Lambertucci, J.R., Rocha, J., Antunes, C.M. & Pena, S.D. (2003). Color and genomic ancestry in Brazilians. *Proc Natl Acad Sci U S A*, Vol.100, No.1, pp. 177-182

Pinto, G.R., Yoshioka, F.K., Clara, C.A., Santos, M.J., Almeida, J.R., Burbano, R.R., Rey, J.A. & Casartelli, C. (2008a). WRN Cys1367Arg SNP is not associated with risk and prognosis of gliomas in Southeast Brazil. *J Neurooncol*, Vol.90, No.3, pp. 253-258

Pinto, G.R., Yoshioka, F.K., Silva, R.L., Clara, C.A., Santos, M.J., Almeida, J.R., Burbano, R.R., Rey, J.A. & Casartelli, C. (2008b). Prognostic value of TP53 Pro47Ser and Arg72Pro single nucleotide polymorphisms and the susceptibility to gliomas in individuals from Southeast Brazil. *Genet Mol Res*, Vol.7, No.1, pp. 207-216

Reifenberger, G. & Louis, D.N. (2003). Oligodendroglioma: toward molecular definitions in diagnostic neuro-oncology. *J Neuropathol Exp Neurol*, Vol.62, No.2, pp. 111-126

Reifenberger, J., Reifenberger, G., Liu, L., James, C.D., Wechsler, W. & Collins, V.P. (1994). Molecular genetic analysis of oligodendroglial tumors shows preferential allelic deletions on 19q and 1p. *Am J Pathol*, Vol.145, No.5, pp. 1175-1190

Reya, T., Morrison, S.J., Clarke, M.F. & Weissman, I.L. (2001). Stem cells, cancer, and cancer stem cells. *Nature*, Vol.414, No.6859, pp. 105-111

Richardson, B. (2003). Impact of aging on DNA methylation. *Ageing Res Rev*, Vol.2, No.3, pp. 245-261

Riemenschneider, M.J., Jeuken, J.W., Wesseling, P. & Reifenberger, G. (2010). Molecular diagnostics of gliomas: state of the art. *Acta Neuropathol*, Vol.120, No.5, pp. 567-584

Rivera, A.L., Pelloski, C.E., Gilbert, M.R., Colman, H., De La Cruz, C., Sulman, E.P., Bekele, B.N. & Aldape, K.D. (2010). MGMT promoter methylation is predictive of response to radiotherapy and prognosis in the absence of adjuvant alkylating chemotherapy for glioblastoma. *Neuro Oncol*, Vol.12, No.2, pp. 116-121

Rush, L.J. & Plass, C. (2002). Alterations of DNA methylation in hematologic malignancies. *Cancer Lett*, Vol.185, No.1, pp. 1-12

Ryberg, D., Skaug, V., Hewer, A., Phillips, D.H., Harries, L.W., Wolf, C.R., Ogreid, D., Ulvik, A., Vu, P. & Haugen, A. (1997). Genotypes of glutathione transferase M1 and P1 and their significance for lung DNA adduct levels and cancer risk. *Carcinogenesis*, Vol.18, No.7, pp. 1285-1289

Sachidanandam, R., Weissman, D., Schmidt, S.C., Kakol, J.M., Stein, L.D., Marth, G., Sherry, S., Mullikin, J.C., Mortimore, B.J., Willey, D.L., Hunt, S.E., Cole, C.G., Coggill, P.C., Rice, C.M., Ning, Z., Rogers, J., Bentley, D.R., Kwok, P.Y., Mardis, E.R., Yeh, R.T., Schultz, B., Cook, L., Davenport, R., Dante, M., Fulton, L., Hillier, L., Waterston, R.H., McPherson, J.D., Gilman, B., Schaffner, S., Van Etten, W.J., Reich, D., Higgins, J., Daly, M.J., Blumenstiel, B., Baldwin, J., Stange-Thomann, N., Zody, M.C., Linton, L., Lander, E.S. & Altshuler, D. (2001). A map of human genome sequence variation containing 1.42 million single nucleotide polymorphisms. *Nature*, Vol.409, No.6822, pp. 928-933

Salisbury, B.A., Pungliya, M., Choi, J.Y., Jiang, R., Sun, X.J. & Stephens, J.C. (2003). SNP and haplotype variation in the human genome. *Mutat Res*, Vol.526, No.1-2, pp. 53-61

Salomon, D.S., Brandt, R., Ciardiello, F. & Normanno, N. (1995). Epidermal growth factor-related peptides and their receptors in human malignancies. *Crit Rev Oncol Hematol*, Vol.19, No.3, pp. 183-232

Sanoudou, D., Tingby, O., Ferguson-Smith, M.A., Collins, V.P. & Coleman, N. (2000). Analysis of pilocytic astrocytoma by comparative genomic hybridization. *Br J Cancer*, Vol.82, No.6, pp. 1218-1222

Sanson, M., Marie, Y., Paris, S., Idbaih, A., Laffaire, J., Ducray, F., El Hallani, S., Boisselier, B., Mokhtari, K., Hoang-Xuan, K. & Delattre, J.Y. (2009). Isocitrate dehydrogenase 1 codon 132 mutation is an important prognostic biomarker in gliomas. *J Clin Oncol*, Vol.27, No.25, pp. 4150-4154

Schuebel, K.E., Chen, W., Cope, L., Glockner, S.C., Suzuki, H., Yi, J.M., Chan, T.A., Van Neste, L., Van Criekinge, W., van den Bosch, S., van Engeland, M., Ting, A.H., Jair, K., Yu, W., Toyota, M., Imai, K., Ahuja, N., Herman, J.G. & Baylin, S.B. (2007). Comparing the DNA hypermethylome with gene mutations in human colorectal cancer. *PLoS Genet*, Vol.3, No.9, pp. 1709-1723

Schwartzbaum, J., Ahlbom, A., Malmer, B., Lonn, S., Brookes, A.J., Doss, H., Debinski, W., Henriksson, R. & Feychting, M. (2005). Polymorphisms associated with asthma are inversely related to glioblastoma multiforme. *Cancer Res*, Vol.65, No.14, pp. 6459-6465

Shahbazi, M., Pravica, V., Nasreen, N., Fakhoury, H., Fryer, A.A., Strange, R.C., Hutchinson, P.E., Osborne, J.E., Lear, J.T., Smith, A.G. & Hutchinson, I.V. (2002). Association between functional polymorphism in EGF gene and malignant melanoma. *Lancet*, Vol.359, No.9304, pp. 397-401

Shete, S., Hosking, F.J., Robertson, L.B., Dobbins, S.E., Sanson, M., Malmer, B., Simon, M., Marie, Y., Boisselier, B., Delattre, J.Y., Hoang-Xuan, K., El Hallani, S., Idbaih, A., Zelenika, D., Andersson, U., Henriksson, R., Bergenheim, A.T., Feychting, M., Lonn, S., Ahlbom, A., Schramm, J., Linnebank, M., Hemminki, K., Kumar, R., Hepworth, S.J., Price, A., Armstrong, G., Liu, Y., Gu, X., Yu, R., Lau, C., Schoemaker, M., Muir, K., Swerdlow, A., Lathrop, M., Bondy, M. & Houlston, R.S. (2009). Genome-wide association study identifies five susceptibility loci for glioma. *Nat Genet*, Vol.41, No.8, pp. 899-904

Simpson, J.R., Horton, J., Scott, C., Curran, W.J., Rubin, P., Fischbach, J., Isaacson, S., Rotman, M., Asbell, S.O., Nelson, J.S. & et al. (1993). Influence of location and extent of surgical resection on survival of patients with glioblastoma multiforme: results of three consecutive Radiation Therapy Oncology Group (RTOG) clinical trials. *Int J Radiat Oncol Biol Phys*, Vol.26, No.2, pp. 239-244

Smith, J.S., Perry, A., Borell, T.J., Lee, H.K., O'Fallon, J., Hosek, S.M., Kimmel, D., Yates, A., Burger, P.C., Scheithauer, B.W. & Jenkins, R.B. (2000). Alterations of chromosome arms 1p and 19q as predictors of survival in oligodendrogliomas, astrocytomas, and mixed oligoastrocytomas. *J Clin Oncol*, Vol.18, No.3, pp. 636-645

Sreeja, L., Syamala, V.S., Syamala, V., Hariharan, S., Raveendran, P.B., Vijayalekshmi, R.V., Madhavan, J. & Ankathil, R. (2008). Prognostic importance of DNA repair gene polymorphisms of XRCC1 Arg399Gln and XPD Lys751Gln in lung cancer patients from India. *J Cancer Res Clin Oncol*, Vol.134, No.6, pp. 645-652

Stiles, C.D. & Rowitch, D.H. (2008). Glioma stem cells: a midterm exam. *Neuron*, Vol.58, No.6, pp. 832-846

Sugimura, T. & Ushijima, T. (2000). Genetic and epigenetic alterations in carcinogenesis. *Mutat Res*, Vol.462, No.2-3, pp. 235-246

Syamala, V.S., Sreeja, L., Syamala, V., Raveendran, P.B., Balakrishnan, R., Kuttan, R. & Ankathil, R. (2008). Influence of germline polymorphisms of GSTT1, GSTM1, and GSTP1 in familial versus sporadic breast cancer susceptibility and survival. *Fam Cancer*, Vol.7, No.3, pp. 213-220

Taylor, J.G., Choi, E.H., Foster, C.B. & Chanock, S.J. (2001). Using genetic variation to study human disease. *Trends Mol Med*, Vol.7, No.11, pp. 507-512

Urioste, M., Martinez-Ramirez, A., Cigudosa, J.C., Colmenero, I., Madero, L., Robledo, M., Martinez-Delgado, B. & Benitez, J. (2002). Complex cytogenetic abnormalities including telomeric associations and MEN1 mutation in a pediatric ependymoma. *Cancer Genet Cytogenet*, Vol.138, No.2, pp. 107-110

Vauleon, E., Auger, N., Benouaich-Amiel, A., Laigle-Donadey, F., Kaloshi, G., Lejeune, J., Delattre, J.Y., Thillet, J. & Sanson, M. (2007). The 61 A/G EGF polymorphism is functional but is neither a prognostic marker nor a risk factor for glioblastoma. *Cancer Genet Cytogenet*, Vol.172, No.1, pp. 33-37

Visvader, J.E. & Lindeman, G.J. (2008). Cancer stem cells in solid tumours: accumulating evidence and unresolved questions. *Nat Rev Cancer*, Vol.8, No.10, pp. 755-768

Vogelstein, B. & Kinzler, K.W. (2004). Cancer genes and the pathways they control. *Nat Med*, Vol.10, No.8, pp. 789-799

von Haken, M.S., White, E.C., Daneshvar-Shyesther, L., Sih, S., Choi, E., Kalra, R. & Cogen, P.H. (1996). Molecular genetic analysis of chromosome arm 17p and chromosome arm 22q DNA sequences in sporadic pediatric ependymomas. *Genes Chromosomes Cancer*, Vol.17, No.1, pp. 37-44

Wang, L.E., Bondy, M.L., Shen, H., El-Zein, R., Aldape, K., Cao, Y., Pudavalli, V., Levin, V.A., Yung, W.K. & Wei, Q. (2004). Polymorphisms of DNA repair genes and risk of glioma. *Cancer Res*, Vol.64, No.16, pp. 5560-5563

Wang, S., Zhao, Y., Ruan, Z., Chen, H., Fan, W., Chen, J., Wu, Q., Qian, J., Zhang, T., Huang, Y. & Lu, D. (2010). Association between EGF +61 G/A and glioma risk in a Chinese population. *BMC Cancer*, Vol.10, pp. 221

White, D.L., Li, D., Nurgalieva, Z. & El-Serag, H.B. (2008). Genetic variants of glutathione S-transferase as possible risk factors for hepatocellular carcinoma: a HuGE systematic review and meta-analysis. *Am J Epidemiol*, Vol.167, No.4, pp. 377-389

Wick, W., Hartmann, C., Engel, C., Stoffels, M., Felsberg, J., Stockhammer, F., Sabel, M.C., Koeppen, S., Ketter, R., Meyermann, R., Rapp, M., Meisner, C., Kortmann, R.D., Pietsch, T., Wiestler, O.D., Ernemann, U., Bamberg, M., Reifenberger, G., von Deimling, A. & Weller, M. (2009). NOA-04 randomized phase III trial of sequential radiochemotherapy of anaplastic glioma with procarbazine, lomustine, and vincristine or temozolomide. *J Clin Oncol*, Vol.27, No.35, pp. 5874-5880

Wrensch, M., Jenkins, R.B., Chang, J.S., Yeh, R.F., Xiao, Y., Decker, P.A., Ballman, K.V., Berger, M., Buckner, J.C., Chang, S., Giannini, C., Halder, C., Kollmeyer, T.M., Kosel, M.L., LaChance, D.H., McCoy, L., O'Neill, B.P., Patoka, J., Pico, A.R., Prados, M., Quesenberry, C., Rice, T., Rynearson, A.L., Smirnov, I., Tihan, T., Wiemels, J., Yang, P. & Wiencke, J.K. (2009). Variants in the CDKN2B and RTEL1 regions are associated with high-grade glioma susceptibility. *Nat Genet*, Vol.41, No.8, pp. 905-908

Wrensch, M., Kelsey, K.T., Liu, M., Miike, R., Moghadassi, M., Sison, J.D., Aldape, K., McMillan, A., Wiemels, J. & Wiencke, J.K. (2005). ERCC1 and ERCC2 polymorphisms and adult glioma. *Neuro Oncol*, Vol.7, No.4, pp. 495-507

Yan, H., Parsons, D.W., Jin, G., McLendon, R., Rasheed, B.A., Yuan, W., Kos, I., Batinic-Haberle, I., Jones, S., Riggins, G.J., Friedman, H., Friedman, A., Reardon, D., Herndon, J., Kinzler, K.W., Velculescu, V.E., Vogelstein, B. & Bigner, D.D. (2009). IDH1 and IDH2 mutations in gliomas. *N Engl J Med*, Vol.360, No.8, pp. 765-773

Zattara-Cannoni, H., Gambarelli, D., Lena, G., Dufour, H., Choux, M., Grisoli, F. & Vagner-Capodano, A.M. (1998). Are juvenile pilocytic astrocytomas benign tumors? A cytogenetic study in 24 cases. *Cancer Genet Cytogenet*, Vol.104, No.2, pp. 157-160

Zhu, Y. & Parada, L.F. (2002). The molecular and genetic basis of neurological tumours. *Nat Rev Cancer*, Vol.2, No.8, pp. 616-626

Zülch, K.J. (1979). Histologic typing of tumours of the central nervous system. World Health Organization, Geneva, Switzerland

6

Genetic Diversity of Glioblastoma Multiforme: Impact on Future Therapies

Franz-Josef Klinz[1], Sergej Telentschak[1],
Roland Goldbrunner[2] and Klaus Addicks[1]
[1]*Department of Anatomy I,*
University of Cologne,
[2]*Department of Neurosurgery,*
University of Cologne,
Germany

1. Introduction

Glioblastoma multiforme (GBM; WHO grade IV) is the most malignant type of glioma and in addition the most abundant malignant cancer of the adult human brain. Despite progress in diagnosis, surgery and chemotherapy, the median survival time of patients suffering from GBM is approximately 15 months (Stupp et al., 2005). The five years survival time is less than 5% (CBTRUS, 2010). Because glioblastoma cells show a highly infiltrating growth into the brain tissue, a total resection is not possible. In addition, glioblastoma cells are remarkably resistant to chemotherapy and ionizing radiation. In addition, the association of a portion of these cells with hypoxic and necrotic areas within the tumor increases their resistance.

Gliobastoma multiforme tumors can be classified:

1. by histopathology (WHO) in conventional glioblastomas (93%), giant cell glioblastoma (5%) and gliosarcoma (2%);
2. by pathogenesis in primary GBM (90%) and secondary GBM (10%);
3. by gene expression analysis in (I) classical, (II) mesenchymal, (III) proneural or (IV) neural type of GBM;
4. by genomic analysis in subgroups harboring specific mutations and/or altered gene dosage/chromosome number.

Conventional glioblastomas constitute approximately 93% of all glioblastomas and can be divided into primary or secondary tumors: primary glioblastomas represent approximately 90% and develop de novo, whereas the incidence of secondary glioblastomas that arise from astroyctomas WHO grade II and III is in the range of 5 to 10%. Primary and secondary glioblastomas differ in their genetic defects: for example 39% of primary glioblastomas harbor an amplification of the EGF receptor (EGFR) locus, whereas in secondary glioblastomas no amplification was detected. Mutations within the p53 gene are more abundant in secondary glioblastomas. Unconventional glioblastomas include giant cell glioblastomas, gliosarcomas and other rare types (for details see section 4).

	Conventional Glioblastoma		Giant cell glioblastoma	Gliosarcoma
	Primary glioblastoma	Secondary glioblastoma		
Frequency	93%		5%	2%
	90%	10%		
Clinical onset	de novo	secondary	de novo	de novo
Preoperative history (mo)	1,7	>25	1,6	2
Age at diagnosis (yr)	55	39	42	56

Table 1. Clinical profile of the common histopathological glioblastoma subtypes according to WHO. Modified from Kleihues et al., 2007; Peraud et al., 1997; Peraud et al., 1999 and Reis et al., 2000.

2. Genetics of glioblastoma multiforme

2.1 Genetic defects in human cancer

For an introduction into the history of this field the reader is referred to the review of Bignold et al. (2006). Abnormalities of mitoses and chromosomes in cancer cells were described in late 1880s and Hansemann (1890) suggested that cancer cells develop from normal cells due to a tendency to maldistribute chromosomes during mitosis. The term somatic mutation was introduced into tumor biology by Tyzzer (1916). To explain the complexity of cancer phenomena "multi-hit" models (Knudson, 1971) increased in popularity over "single-hit" models of somatic mutation. In the multistep progression model of sporadic colorectal carcinoma five to ten genetic alterations seemed to be necessary for generation of the malignant phenotype (for review see: Fearon and Vogelstein, 1990). The onset and extent of genetic alterations in progression of sporadic colorectal tumors was studied in detail by Stoler et al. (1999). Their observation of about 10,000 genomic alterations occurring per cancer cell has brought into attention the issue of genetic instability in human cancer. Genetic and phenotypic instability are hallmarks of cancer cells and appear early in tumor progression; most cancers are of clonal origin, but individual cancer cells are highly heterogenous. There are three major forms of genetic instability in cancer: (1) aneuploidy, in which entire chromosomes are lost or gained; (2) intrachromosomal instability, distinguished by insertions, deletions, translocations or amplifications and (3) point mutations, which accumulate in certain forms of hereditary cancer as well as in a small portion of sporadic cancers. Stanbridge et al. (1981) reported that specific chromosome loss is associated with the expression of tumorigenicity in human cell hybrids. It was published by Duesberg et al. (1998) that genetic instability of cancer cells is proportional to their degree of aneuploidy. Aneuploidy, an abnormal number of chromosomes, is the result of asymmetrical segregation of chromosomes to daughter cells during mitosis. Once aneuploid, cells will continue to segregate chromosomes asymmetrically during subsequent rounds of mitosis, a process that has been termed "chromosome error propagation" (for review see: Holliday, 1989).

Unlike oncogenes, tumor suppressor genes generally follow the "two hit" model, which implies that both alleles of a particular tumor suppressor gene have to be inactivated before an effect is manifested. If only one allele is inactivated, the second correct allele can still produce the correct protein. Whereas mutant oncogene alleles are typically dominant, mutant tumor suppressor genes are usually recessive.

The mutational activation of oncogenes induces loss of heterozygosity and genomic instability in mammalian cells. These results have used to formulate the oncogene-induced replication stress model (for review see: Halazonetis et al., 2008). In precancerous lesions with intact p53 gene, the oncogene-induced DNA damage leads to p53-dependent apoptosis and/or senescence. After the function of p53 is lost, cells are able to escape its apoptotic and/or senescence effects, and the precancerous lesion is predestinated to become cancerous (Gorgoulis et al., 2005; Bartkova et al., 2005; Bartkova et al., 2006; Di Micco et al., 2006). DNA damage has an important role in promoting polyploidization. If cells with altered DNA enter mitosis, defects in chromosomal segregation and cytokinesis occur (for review see: Chow and Poon, 2010).

The gene for the tumor suppressor protein p53 is mutated in about half of human cancers. It was shown recently by several groups, that eliminating p53 function by mutation leads to dramatically increased reprogramming efficiency of differentiated cells into induced pluripotent stem cells. Important for the field of cancer biology is the report of Mizuno et al. (2010), demonstrating that breast and lung cancers harboring TP53 mutations exhibit stem cell-like transcriptional signatures. These data suggest a role for active p53 in preventing the emergence of cancerous stem-like cells during tumor progression. Since TP53 mutations often arise in a late stage of tumor progression, when many cancer cells with different genetic alterations coexist, some cancer cells may be susceptible to reprogramming to generate stem-like cancer cells, leading to further tumor progression and cellular heterogeneity.

2.2 Genetic diversity of glioblastoma multiforme

DNA sequencing and gene dosage analysis of GBM revealed a high number of shared as well as individual-specific mutations, deletions and amplifications of DNA sequences. A hallmark of many primary GBMs is the loss of one copy of chromosome 10 harboring the locus for the PTEN tumor suppressor gene and/or amplification of the EGF receptor locus at chromosome 7. As a consequence, the Akt signalling pathway is often overactivated in GBM. Array comparative genomic hybridization (CGH) analyses revealed, that primary glioblastomas can be divided into three major genetic subgroups, i.e. tumors with chromosome 7 gain and chromosome 10 loss, tumors with chromosome 10 loss and tumors without copy number changes in chromosomes 7 or 10 (Misra et al., 2005).

Parsons et al. (2008) sequenced 20661 genes coding for proteins in 22 GBM samples and 1 normal sample. They observed that 685 genes contained at least 1 non-silent somatic mutation. 94% of these alterations were single base substitutions that were uniformly distributed among the 21 GBM samples, resulting in an average of 47 mutations per GBM. About 15% of the missense mutations were predicted to have a significant effect on protein function. The same 22 GBM samples were analysed for copy number alterations through hybridization of DNA samples to single nucleotide polymorphism (SNP) arrays, leading to the identification of 147 amplifications and 134 homozygous deletions.

Parsons et al. (2008) next studied the probabilities that the mutations were either "driver" or "passenger". Driver mutations may provide a selective advantage to the cancer cell, whereas passenger mutations arise by the instability of the tumor genome and have no effect on tumor growth. Analysis of all data was used to identify GBM candidate cancer genes that were likely drivers, pointing to alterations in several signaling pathways: CDKN2A (altered in 50% of GBMs); TP53, EGFR, and PTEN (altered in 30 to 40%); NF1, CDK4, and RB1 (altered in 12 to 15%); and PIK3CA and PIK3R1 (altered in 8 to 10%). By analysing additional gene members within signaling pathways affected by these genes, the authors identified alterations of critical genes in the RB1 pathway (RB1, CDK4, and CDKN2A; altered in 68% of GBMs), TP53 pathway (TP53, MDM2, and MDM4; altered in 64%), and the PI3K/PTEN pathway (PIK3CA, PIK3R1, PTEN, and IRS1; altered in 50%). Mutations in the NF1 gene (coding for neurofibromatosis-related protein NF-1 or neurofibromin 1, a stimulator of GTPase activity of ras proteins) were observed in 16 of 105 GBMs (15%). Mutations in the IDH1 gene (coding for the citric acid cycle enzyme isocitrate dehydrogenase 1) were reported in 18 of 149 GBMs (12%).

The Cancer Genome Atlas Research Network (2008) study analysed 91 GBM samples and found 453 non-silent somatic mutations in 223 genes. Affected signaling pathways include TP53, PTEN, NF1, EGFR, ERBB2, RB1, NF1, PIK3R1, and PIK3CA. High-level amplifications were observed frequently for EGFR, CDK4, PDGFR, MDM2, and MDM4 genes, whereas homozygous deletion events were often associated with CDKN2A/B and PTEN genes. In this study, GBMs from patients treated with temozolomide and/or lomustine were analysed for mutations. Treatment with alkylating agents resulted in more than tenfold increase in the number of mutations, that was dependent on the methylation status of the gene for the DNA repair enzyme O^6-methylguanine-DNA methyltransferase (MGMT).

Bredel et al. (2009) published "A Network Model of a Cooperative Genetic Landscape in Brain Tumors". The authors demonstrate that a multigene risk scoring model based on gene dosis and expression of 7 landscape genes (POLD2, CYCS, MYC, AKR1C3, YME1L1, ANXA7, and PDCD4) is associated with the overall length of survival in 189 glioblastoma samples. Yadav et al. (2009) reported that loss of function of ANXA7 (annexin 7) stabilizes the EGFR protein and increases EGFR signaling in glioblastoma cells. ANXA7 haploinsuffiency doubles the tumorigenic potential of glioblastoma cells. The heterozygous loss of ANXA7 in about 75% of GBM in the Cancer Genome Atlas Research Network study (2008) plus the observed infrequent ANXA7 mutation in about 6% of GBM is indicative for its role as a haploinsufficiency gene. A multigene predictor model of outcome in GBM based on expression analysis of 9 genes was published by Colman et al. (2009).

Verhaak et al. (2010) used gene expression analysis to divide GBM into 4 subtypes: I. Classical, II. Mesenchymal, III. Proneural, and IV. Neural. The reproducibility of this classification was demonstrated in an independent validation set. To get insight into the genomic events, the authors used copy number and sequence data from the Cancer Genome Atlas Research Network (2008).

I. Classical subtype of GBM (21% of core samples):

Neural precursor and stem cell markers NES, as well as Notch and Sonic hedgehog signaling pathways were highly expressed in the Classical subtype. Chromosome 7 amplification paired with chromosome 10 loss was seen in 100% of the Classical subtype. High level EGF receptor (EGFR) gene amplification was observed in 97% of the Classical subtype and infrequently in other subtypes. Even though TP53 is the most frequently mutated gene in GBM (Cancer Genome Atlas Research Network, 2008), there was a distinct lack of TP53 mutations in the Classical subtype samples sequenced. Deletion events at 10q23 harboring the PTEN locus were observed in 100% of the Classical subtype. Focal 9p21.3 homozygous deletion targeting CDKN2A (encoding for both p16INK4A and p14 ARF) was frequent and co-occurred with EGFR amplification in 94% of the Classical subtype.

II. Mesenchymal subtype of GBM (32% of core samples):

The Mesenchymal subtype displayed expression of mesenchymal markers as described earlier (Phillips et al. 2006). Genes in the tumor necrosis super family pathway are highly expressed in this subtype. Focal hemizygous deletion of a region at 17q11.2, containing the gene NF1 (coding for neurofibromatosis-related protein NF-1 or neurofibromin 1, a stimulator of GTPase activity of ras proteins) occurred predominantly in the Mesenchymal subtype. NF1 mutations were found in 20 samples, 14 of which were classified as Mesenchymal subtype, resulting in 53% of samples with NF1 abnormalities.

Mutated Gene	Classical Subtype	Mesenchymal Subtype	Proneural Subtype	Neural Subtype	Approximate Overall Frequency
TP53	0%	32%	54%	21%	23%
PTEN	23%	32%	16%	21%	17%
NF1	5%	37%	5%	16%	13%
EGFR	32%	5%	16%	26%	13%
IDH1	0%	0%	30%	5%	8%
PIK3R	5%	0%	19%	11%	6%
RB1	0%	13%	3%	5%	5%
ERBB2	5%	3%	5%	16%	5%
EGFRvIII	23%	3%	3%	0%	5%
PIK3CA	5%	3%	8%	5%	4%
PDGFRA	0%	0%	11%	0%	3%

Table 2. Frequently mutated genes in Glioblastoma multiforme and their distribution among GBM subtypes according to Verhaak et al (2010). Outstanding frequencies are grayed out for comparison between subtypes. Modified from Verhaak et al. (2010).

III. Proneural subtype of GBM (31% of core samples):

The Proneural group showed high expression of oligodendrocytic genes, underlining its status as an atypical GBM subtype. The majority of TP53 mutations and TP53 loss of heterozygosity were found in Proneural samples. The classic GBM signature, chromosome 7 amplification associated with chromosome 10 loss was less prevalent and occurred in only 54% of the Proneural subtype. Focal amplifications of the locus at 4q12 harboring the PDGF Receptor A (PDGFRA) gene were seen in all subtypes of GBM but at a much higher rate

(35%) in Proneural samples. 11 of the 12 observed mutations in the isocitrate dehydrogenase 1 gene (IDH1) were found in this class.

IV. Neural subtype of GBM (16% of core samples):

The Neural subtype was typified by the expression of neuron markers. The two normal brain tissues samples examined in this data set were both classified as Neural subtype. Chomosome 7 amplification associated with chromosome 10 loss was prevalent in the Neural subtype.

		Known Cancer Gene in Region	Classical Subtype	Mesenchymal Subtype	Proneural Subtype	Neural Subtype
Amplification Events	7p11.2	EGFR	100%	95%	54%	96%
	7q21.2	CDK6	92%	89%	46%	96%
	7q31.2	MET	86%	91%	54%	92%
	7q34		86%	91%	52%	92%
	4q12	PDGFRA	5%	9%	35%	13%
Homo- and Hemizygous Deletion Events	17q11.2	NF1	5%	38%	6%	17%
	10q23	PTEN	100%	87%	69%	96%
	9p21.3	CDKN2A/CDKN2B	95%	67%	56%	71%
	13q14	RB1	16%	53%	52%	46%

Table 3. Frequency of copy number alterations in Glioblastoma subtypes according to gene expression. Modified from Verhaak et al. (2010).

2.2.1 Subtypes and clinical correlations

Three of four tumors classified as secondary GBMs were found in the Proneural group. The Proneural subtype was associated with younger age, PDGFRA abnormalities, IDH1 and TP53 mutations, all of which have been associated with secondary GBM in earlier studies (Arjona et al., 2006; Furnari et al., 2007; Kleihues and Ohgaki, 1999; Watanabe et al., 1996; Yan et al., 2009). Verhaak et al. (2010) concluded that tumors did not change class at recurrence, because recurrent tumors were found in all subtypes (Murat et al., 2008). Although statistically not significant, there was a trend towards longer survival for patients with a Proneural signature. Aggressive treatment significantly reduced mortality in Classical and Mesenchymal subtypes, had a less pronounced effect in the Neural subtype and did not alter survival in the Proneural subtype. There was no association of GBM subtype with methylation status of the DNA repair gene MGMT, which has been positively linked to therapy response (all data and conclusions from Verhaak et al., 2010).

Bredel et al. (2010) reported that NFKBIA (nuclear factor of κ-light polypeptide gene enhancer in B-cells inhibitor-α), an inhibitor of EGFR signaling pathway, is often deleted in GBM (Table 4). Most deletions occur in non-classical subtypes of GBM. Deletion and low expression of NFKBIA were reported to be associated with unfavorable outcomes. The authors present a two-gene model based on the expression of NFKBIA and MGMT that is strongly associated with the clinical course of GBM (Table 5).

Genetic Alteration	Classical Subtype	Nonclassical Glioblastomas		
		Mesenchymal Subtype	Proneural Subtype	Neural Subtype
NFKBIA deletion	6%	30%	39%	22%
EGFR amplification	80%	20%	11%	46%

Table 4. Relationship of four molecular subtypes of glioblastoma to gene-dosage profiles for NFKBIA and EGFR across 188 glioblastomas. NFKBIA deletions are rare in classical (6%) and more common in non-classical (32%) glioblastomas.

Irrespective of subtype a degree of mutual exclusivity between NFKBIA deletion and EGFR amplification was suggested: NFKBIA deletion or EGFR amplification were observed in 53%, whereas concomitant occurrence (NFKBIA deletion together with EGFR amplification) was observed only in 5%. All data and conclusions are from Bredel et al. (2010). Glioblastoma subtypes were classified according to Verhaak et al. (2010).

Risk Groups	NFKBIA and MGMT Expression	Median Survival	NFKBIA Expression and MGMT Promoter Methylation Status	Media Survival (Weeks)	With Radiotherapie and Temozolomide	
					NFKBIA Expression and MGMT Promoter Methylation Status	Median Survival (Weeks)
High-risk	Low NFKBIA, High MGMT	44	Low NFKBIA, Unmeth. MGMT	45	Low NFKBIA, Unmeth. MGMT	35
Inter-mediate-risk	Low NFKBIA, Low MGMT or High NFKBIA, High MGMT	59	Low NFKBIA, Meth. MGMT or High NFKBIA, Unmeth. MGMT	63	Low NFKBIA, Meth. MGMT or High NFKBIA, Unmeth. MGMT	71
Low-risk	High NFKBIA, Low MGMT	92	High NFKBIA, Meth. MGMT	91	High NFKBIA, Meth. MGMT	122

Table 5. The strong association of the clinical course of GBM with expression of NFKBIA and expression/methylation status of the promoter of O^6-methylguanine-DNA methyltransferase (MGMT). All data and conclusions are from Bredel et al. (2010).

To add an additional level of complexity, gene dosage analysis of separate tumor areas derived from one GBM revealed area-specific genomic imbalances (see chapter 5).

2.3 Correlation between genetic and histopathologic diversity in GBM

Glioblastomas are morphologically highly heterogeneous and in addition the histological features often vary in different areas of one tumor. Currently three distinct common histopathological variants of GBM are recognized by the actual World Health Organization classification scheme, including conventional glioblastoma, giant cell glioblastoma, and gliosarcoma.

Despite of lack of any histopathological difference, *primary* (de novo) and *secondary* (with an evidence of a lower-grade precursor) *conventional glioblastomas* harbor distinct molecular genetic abnormalities: Primary glioblastomas are characterized by relatively high frequencies of EGFR amplification, PTEN deletion, and CDKN2A (p16) loss, whereas secondary glioblastomas often contain TP53 mutations, especially those involving codons 248 and 273 or G:C->A:T mutations at CpG sites (Ohgaki et al., 2004).

Even within the conventional glioblastoma category, the cellular composition is heterogeneous and may include small or fibrillary, gemistocytic, granular, lipidized and occasional giant cells or oligodendroglial components. According to the predomination of one of these cell types indicating patterns of differentiation, the WHO distinguishes respective subtypes of glioblastoma such as small cell glioblastoma, glioblastoma with granular cell astrocytoma features, glioblastoma with lipidized cells; whereas giant cell glioblastoma is recognized as a distinct clinicopathologic entity (Kleihues et al., 2007; Miller and Perry, 2007).

Small cell astrocytoma is an aggressive histologic variant being often misdiagnosed as anaplastic oligodendroglioma because of considerable morphologic similarities. Despite of histological overlap clinicopathologic and genetic features are distinct: there are no small cell astrocytomas harboring 1p/19q codeletions, whereas vIII mutant form of EGFR, EGFR amplification and 10q deletions are present in 50%, 69% and 97% of small cell astrocytomas, respectively (Perry et al., 2004).

Once thought to represent a reactive component, *gemistocytes* have been found to harbor TP53 mutations and cytogenetic abnormalities (chromosome 7p gains and 10q losses); therefore, they are now thought to represent a true neoplastic component (Kros et al., 2000).

In rare cases *granular cells* may predominate and create the impression of a granular cell tumor. Similar to astrocytomas with non-granular cytology, these tumors may also harbor TP53 mutations, high-frequency loss of heterozygosity at 9p, 10q, and 17p, and less frequent loss of heterozygosity at 1p and 19q (Castellano-Sanchez et al., 2003). Brat et al. (2002) reported the largest series of such tumors to date (22 cases, including 4 grade II, 7 grade III, and 11 grade IV tumors) and found that these tumors were more aggressive than non-granular cell astrocytomas of the same grade.

Glioblastoma with oligodendroglioma component is an astrocytoma WHO-grade IV containing oligodendroglial areas varying in size and frequency (Kleihues et al., 2007). Despite of oligodendroglial component and in contrast to rather frequent codeletions in WHO grade III anaplastic oligodendroglioma (approximately 85%), deletion of either 1p (24%), 19q (43%), or combined 1p/19q (22%) is relatively infrequent in glioblastoma with oligodendroglioma component (Miller and Perry, 2007).

Giant cell glioblastoma is a rare variant that constitutes up to 5% of glioblastoma and is recognized as a distinct clinicopathologic entity in the WHO 2007 classification. Although occasional giant cells may be found in conventional glioblastoma, these cells are a predominating cytologic component in giant cell glioblastoma. As the name implies, the tumor cells are markedly enlarged and bizarre, often appear often multi-nucleated and tumor masses are typically well-circumscribed. It occurs in younger patients (fifth decade) (Kleihues et al., 2007).

The molecular genetic features include relatively high frequencies of TP53 mutations (59% to 90%) and PTEN deletion (up to 33%), whereas EGFR amplification/overexpression and homozygous p16 deletion (p16^{INK4a} gene at the CDKN2A locus, 9p21) are lacking in comparison to conventional glioblastoma (Meyer-Puttlitz et al., 1997; Peraud et al., 1997; Peraud et al. 1999; Temme et al. 2010). Therefore, giant cell glioblastomas contain clinical and molecular genetic features of both primary and secondary glioblastomas. Giant cell glioblastomas have an increased expression of Aurora Kinase B; combined with TP53 mutations this may be responsible in induce cytokinesis defects and the development of multinucleated cells (Temme et al., 2010).

	Gliosarcoma	Primary glioblastoma	Giant cell glioblastoma	Secondary glioblastoma
PTEN mutation	38%	32%	33%	4%
EGFR amplification	0%	39%	5%	0%
TP53 mutation	23%	11%	84%	67%
p16^{INK4a} deletion	37%	36%	0%	4%
MDM2 amplification	5%	8%	0%	0%

Table 6. Genetic profile of the common histopathological glioblastoma subtypes. Similar tendencies are indicated by grayscale. Modified from Kleihues et al., 2007; Peraud et al., 1997; Peraud et al., 1999 and Reis et al., 2000.

Despite showing a very poor prognosis giant cell glioblastoma appears to carry a slightly better prognosis than conventional glioblastoma (Burger and Vollmer, 1980; Margetts and Kalyan-Raman, 1989; Shinojima et al., 2004), perhaps because of a less infiltrative behaviour. Gliosarcoma constitutes roughly 2% of GBMs and is also recognized as a distinct clinico-pathologic entity in the WHO 2007 classification. These tumors are characterized by their well-circumscribed, biphasic tissue pattern with clearly distinguishable areas of glial and mesenchymal differentiation. The glial component of gliosarcoma may display any of the aforementioned cytologic attributes and is typically immunoreactive for GFAP. The mesenchymal component is GFAP-negative and may also carry a wide variety of morphologic appearances, with evidence of differentiation along fibroblastic, cartilaginous, osseous, smooth and striated muscle, and adipose lines (Kleihues et al., 2007). There is a cytogenetic and molecular evidence for a monoclonal origin of both components (Actor et al., 2002; Paulus et al., 1994; Reis et al., 2000).

Exept for the infrequent EGFR amplification, gliosarcomas are genetically similar to primary glioblastomas: they harbor likewise low frequency of TP53 mutations (up to 24%) and similar rates of PTEN deletions (38%) as well as deletions of p16^{INK4a} gene (at the CDKN2A locus, 9p21) in roughly 37% (Actor et al., 2002; Reis et al., 2000).

Comparative genomic hybridization analysis in 20 gliosarcomas by Actor et al. (2002) revealed such common chromosomal imbalances as gains on chromosomes 7 (75%), X (20%), 9q and 20q (15% each) as well as losses on chromosomes 13q (15%), 10 and 9p (35% each).

2.4 Area-specific genomic Imbalances in glioblastoma multiforme

Using flow cytometry data analysis Hoshino et al. (1978) reported that different tumor regions of one glioblastoma showed a highly variable distribution of ploidy. By use of a DNA fingerprinting technique Misra et al. (2000) analysed genetic alterations within two or three tumor areas from seven glioblastomas. In all cases except one, different areas of one tumor displayed different fingerprints, indicating a striking extent of intratumoral genetic heterogeneity. Conventional comparative genomic hybridization (CGH) was used to study the intratumoral patterns of genomic imbalance in Glioblastoma multiforme (Harada et al., 1998; Jung et al., 1999). Array comparative genomic hybridization was utilized by Nobusawa et al. (2010) to study in detail tumor area-specific genomic imbalances. Genetic alterations common to all the areas analyzed within a single tumor included gains at chromosomes 1q32.1 (PIK3C2B, MDM4), 4q11-q12 (KIT, PDGFRA), 7p12.1-11.2 (EGFR), 12q13.3-12q14.1 (GLI1, CDK4), and 12q15 (MDM2), and loss of chromosomes at 9p21.1-24.3 (p16[INK4a]/p14[ARF] = CDKN2a), 10p15.3-q26.3 (PTEN, etc.), and 13q12.11-q34 (SPRY2, RB1). These alterations are likely to be causative in the pathogenesis of glioblastomas (driver mutations). Additionally, the authors reported numerous tumor area-specific genomic imbalances, which may be either nonfunctional (passenger mutations) or functional, but constitute secondary events reflecting clonal selection and/or progressive genomic instability, a hallmark of glioblastomas. Area specific-evolution of genomic imbalances in GBM may be comparable to the genetic evolution and genomic instability of metastatic pancreas cancer that has been studied in detail recently (Campbell et al., 2010; Yachida et al., 2010).

Loeper et al. (2001) reported that frequent mitotic errors occur in genetically micro-heterogenous glioblastomas. The authors used fluorescent in situ hybridization (FISH) to study chromosome numbers in a series of 24 glioblastomas. All examined chromosomes showed mitotic instability indicated by numerical aberrations within significant amounts of tumor cells.   For chromosomes 10 and 17 only monosomy was observed, whereas chromosome 7 showed trisomy/polysomy. In contrast to other chromosomes displaying monosomy as well as trisomy, copy number changes of chromosomes 7, 10 and 17 seem to be the result of selection in favor of the respective aberration (Loeper et al., 2001). In this context it is interesting to note that neural stem and progenitor cells in the subventricular zone of mouse postnatal brain are frequently aneuploid (Kaushal et al., 2003) and that chromosome segregation defects contribute to aneuploidy in normal neural progenitor cells of the mouse cerebral cortex (Yang et al., 2003). Studies in mice and human demonstrate that chromosomal mosaicism is a prominent feature of neural stem cells, whereas interchromosomal translocations or partial chromosomal deletions or insertions are extremely rare (for review see: Peterson et al., 2008). Glioblastoma stem cells share several properties with neural stem cells, i.e. the growth in floating spheres under serum-free conditions, the expression of the stem cell marker nestin and the differentiation into neural cells like astrocytes or neurons. This similarity in marker expression and behaviour has led to the hypothesis that glioblastoma stem cells may be derived from NSCs (Berger et al., 2004; Sanai et al., 2005).

Recent research makes clear that GBMs do not behave as a whole; local heterogeneity may arise because the tumor regionally adapts to the microenvironment. The influence of microenvironment-induced stimuli may be the force behind clonal selection and acquisition of area specific genomic imbalances in GBM. In addition, regional genomic alterations may be associated with the development of resistance to irradiation and/or chemotherapy, resulting in tumor recurrence and/or progression.

2.5 Mechanisms leading to genetic alterations in glioblastoma multiforme

Analysis of copy number alterations showed an average of 7 amplifications and 6 homozygous deletions per GBM. In addition, an average of 47 mutations was reported (Parsons et al., 2008).

A characteristic feature of GBM is a chromosomal instability (CIN) phenotype distinguished by the loss or gain of complete chromosomes, for example by the gain of chromosome 7 and/or loss of chromosome 10. These chromosome copy number changes can be explained by merotelic spindle attachment that is associated with bipolar but more often with multipolar mitosis. Multipolar spindle pole coalescence in cells with supernumerary centrosomes has been reported as a major source of chromosomal misattachment and chromosome missegregation in colorectal cancer cell lines (Silkworth et al., 2009). Obviously, specific chromosome aberrations may be associated with growth advantage for clonal populations of cancer cells (for example by the loss of tumor suppressor genes).

In addition to its well-defined role in signal transduction at the plasma membrane, recent results have identified PTEN as a new guardian of the genome (for review see: Yin and Shen, 2008). Pten-deficient mouse embryo fibroblasts revealed an increased frequency of mitotic centromere-associated chromosomal instability as well as spontaneous DNA double-strand breaks (Shen et al., 2007). Li Li et al. (2008) developed a mouse model by infecting PTEN-/- neural precursor cells with an EGFRvIII expressing retrovirus and found that EGFRvIII expression and PTEN loss synergistically induced chromosomal instability and glial tumors.

Interestingly, polyploidization of mammalian hepatocytes occurs through failed cytokinesis and is followed by a process that was called reductive mitoses (Duncan et al. 2010). The authors postulate a dynamic model of hepatocyte polyploidization, ploidy reversal and aneuploidy (ploidy conveyor) and propose that this mechanism evolved to generate genetic diversity and permits adaptation of hepatocytes to xenobiotic and nutritional injury.

Several studies point to a link between centrosome amplification, chromosomal instability and the development of cancer (for review see: D´Assoro et al., 2002). Cells in resected high grade gliomas and cultured glioblastoma cells have been reported to exhibit often centrosome amplifications (Loh et al., 2010) and the centrosomal protein γ-tubulin is over-expressed and shows altered subcellular localization in GBM (Katsetos et al., 2006; Loh et al., 2010). Multipolar mitoses were occasionally observed in time lapse recordings of cultured glioblastoma cells (Hegedüs et al., 2000). Our laboratory used long term life cell imaging to study mitoses in a newly established glioblastoma cell line and found that cytokinesis defects followed by multipolar mitosis may be an important mechanism that is used by glioblastoma cells to reduce ploidy and generate viable daughter cells (our unpublished results).

2.6 Epigenetics in glioblastoma multiforme

To add another level of complexity, many types of cancer cells carry aberrant epigenetic modifications. Changes in epigenetic marks (caused or not caused by genetic alterations) may have an fundamental impact on tumor development and/or tumor progression. Epigenetic markers in human gliomas have been reviewed by Hesson et al. (2008). Two groups have studied in detail DNA methylation profiles in GBM (Etcheverry et al. 2010; Nousmehr et al., 2010). Hypermethylation at a large number of genetic loci occurred in a subgroup (proneural group) of glioblastoma patients and was associated with improved outcome (Nousmehr et al., 2010).

Epigenetic mechanisms like methylation of DNA have already an impact on chemotheraypy of GBM. Temozolomide (TMZ, Temodal®) is an orally administered alkylating drug that is often used for chemotherapy of GBM. O^6-Methylguanine-DNA methyltransferase (MGMT) is a DNA repair enzyme that specifically removes promutagenic alkyl DNA adducts from the O^6 position of guanine residues in DNA which are induced by alkylating agents like temozolomide (Goth and Rajewsky, 1974; Margison and Kleihues, 1975). Loss of MGMT expression may be caused by transcriptional silencing through hypermethylation of its CpG islands (Esteller et al., 1999; Qian & Brent, 1997), is frequently (45% to 75%) present in glioblastomas (Bello et al., 2004; Kamiryo et al., 2004; Nakamura et al., 2001) and results in improved survival of glioblastoma patients treated with the alkylating agent temozolomide (Fukushima et al., 2009; Hegi et al, 2005; Hegi et al., 2008). On the other hand not all glioblastoma patients with MGMT promoter methylation respond to alkylating agents and in addition responding GBMs cannot avoid eventual recurrence (Fukushima et al., 2009; Hegi et al., 2008). MGMT promoter methylation appears to occur with a higher frequency in secondary than in primary glioblastoma (Bello et al., 2004; Nakamura et al., 2001) but there is no evidence about its correlation with other histopathologic subtypes.

However, prospective randomized studies of EORTC (European Organisation for Research and Treatment of Cancer) and NCIC (National Cancer Institute of Canada) trial have revealed a significant prolongation of progression free and overall survival for patients with newly diagnosed glioblastoma treated by the concomitant and adjuvant temozolomide and irradiation. By this means median survival has been increased over one year (Stupp et al., 2005, 2009).

The methylation status of the MGMT gene promoter is being used as a biomarker for the potential benefit of the addition of temozolomide to the therapy because its epigenetic silencing has been identified as a strong and independent predictive factor of treatment response for anaplastic glioma patients undergoing chemotherapy with alkylating agents (Hegi et al., 2005; Wick et al., 2009). 3 to 5% of the GBM patients survive for more than 3 years. MGMT hypermethylation was reported to be significantly more frequent in the long-term survivor group (Krex et al., 2007).

The assumption that DNA methylation of CpG island on the MGMT promoter represses consecutively transcriptional activity of the MGMT gene and expression of MGMT protein has been used to explain the correlation between the positive promoter methylation status and favorable treatment response after chemotherapy with temozolomide (Kaina et al., 2007).

However, studies that were performed to validate a relationship between MGMT promoter methylation and protein expression have yielded contradictory results in brain tumors as well as in other neoplasms (Brell et al., 2011). While some studies report a significant correlation between MGMT protein expression analyzed by immunohistochemistry (IHC) and MGMT promoter status measured by methylation-specific polymerase chain reaction (MSP) in glioblastoma and brain metastases of various origin (Ingold et al., 2009; Spiegl-Kreinecker et al., 2009; Tang et al., 2011), other studies failed to detect correlations between both parameters (Brell et al., 2005, 2011; Christmann et al., 2010; Preusser et al., 2008).

In addition, there is increasing evidence that MGMT mRNA expression, unlike MGMT protein expression, could be a better predictor for tumor sensitivity to alkylating agents than MGMT methylation status (Everhard et al., 2009; Kreth et al., 2011). Kreth et al. (2011) provide not only evidence that the degree of MGMT mRNA expression is highly correlated with the MGMT promoter methylation status, but also that low MGMT mRNA expression is strongly predictive for prolonged time to progression, treatment response, and length of survival. Furthermore, the authors found that in case of discordance the patients with methylated tumors combined with high MGMT mRNA expression did significantly worse than those with low transcriptional activity or unmethylated tumors with low MGMT mRNA expression. Finally Kreth et al. (2011) assume methylation-independent pathways of MGMT expression regulation; however, the exact role of DNA-methyltransferases DNMT1 and DNMT3b that are likely to be involved in methylation of CpG islands of MGMT gene promoter remains unclear.

In the Cancer Genome Atlas Research Network (2008) study, GBMs from patients treated with temozolomide and/or lomustine were analysed for mutations. Treatment with alkylating agents resulted in a more than tenfold increase in the number of mutations that was dependent on the methylation status of the MGMT gene. This phenotype seems to be caused by mutations in the MSH6 gene (Cahill et al., 2007; Hunter et al., 2006; Yip et al., 2009) and other genes of the DNA mismatch repair pathway (Cancer Genome Atlas Research Network, 2008). The loss of the mismatch repair protein MSH6 in GBM is associated with tumor progression during temozolomide treatment (Cahill et al., 2007; Hunter et al., 2006; Yip et al., 2009).

2.7 Stem cells in glioblastoma multiforme

The cancer stem cell concept that is of importance for the genesis of many types of cancer receives increasing credit also in the field of GBM. A minor population of GBM cancer stem cells, which may be derived from genetically altered neural stem cells, is presumed to generate transit amplifying cells with high mitotic activity. Because these stem cells appear to have a low mitotic activity, they are difficult to target by radiotherapy and conventional chemotherapy.

For recent reviews on glioblastoma stem cells the reader is referred to Huang et al. (2010) and McLendon and Rich (2010). Ignatova et al. (2002) firstly described cells with stem-like properties in human cortical glial tumors. Singh et al. (2003) used the cell surface marker CD133 to isolate a clonogenic population of cells showing stem-like features in medullo-blastomas and pilocytic astrocytomas. These cells were declared as tumor stem cells based on their capabilities of self-renewal and multilineage differentiation. Galli et al. (2004) and Yuan et al. (2004) confirmed these findings for glioblastomas. Bao et al. (2006a) selected CD133+ cells from glioblastoma biopsies that were capable of forming tumorspheres in vitro, demonstrated self-renewal and multilineage differentiation and resulted in tumours after transplantation into nude mice. In contrast, CD133- cells did not form tumorspheres in vitro und were not tumorigenic in nude mice. CD133+ cells proved to be a minor population of cells in GBM biopsies. Clinical studies suggested that the percentage of CD133+ cells (Zhang et al., 2008; Zeppernick et al., 2008) or the rate of tumorsphere formation in vitro (Laks et al., 2009; Panosyan et al., 2010) can be used to predict overall survival time of patients. However, it should be noted, that contrary results also exist (Phi et al., 2009; Kim et al., 2011). In recurrent glioblastomas the percentage of CD133+ cells is increased strongly when compared with primary glioblastomas (Pallini et al., 2010). Surprisingly, the increase in expression of CD133 after tumor recurrence was associated significantly with longer survival. Thon et al. (2008) described a correlation between the amount of CD133+ cells within the tumor mass and the WHO grade of glioma (WHO grade II, III and IV). Bao et al. (2006a) demonstrated that CD133+ cells constitutively expressed DNA repair genes at much higher levels that CD133- cells, mediating resistance to X-irradiation in CD133+ cells.

Brain tumor stem cells seem to be localized in a perivascular niche (Bao et al., 2006b; Calabrese et al., 2007; Shen et al., 2008) and low oxygen tension (hypoxia) is associated with its undifferentiated state. In glioblastomas, cancer stem cells express much higher levels of VEGF than non-stem cancer cells and show increased angiogenic potential in vivo (Bao et al., 2006b; Li et al., 2009). Because VEGF expression is under control of transcription factors of the hypoxia inducible factor (HIF) family, one should note that expression of HIF2α is unique to glioma stem cells and correlated with poor patient survival, whereas HIF1α is found in all malignant cells (Li et al., 2009). It has been reported that different human cancers (GBM, colorectal carcinoma, and NSCL carcinoma) converge at the HIF2α oncogenic axis (Franovic et al., 2009). The authors propose that inhibition of HIF2α may be of broad clinical interest in the treatment of cancers with different genetic signatures. Hjelmeland et al. (2010) published recently that acidic stress promotes a glioma stem cell phenotype by induction of HIF2α and other glioma stem cell markers. The authors suggest that an increase in intratumoral pH may be of benefit for targeting the stem cell phenotype.

Three recent papers demonstrate that stem-like cells in GBM are able to differentiate into endothelial cells and may give rise to tumor endothelium (Ricci-Vitiani et al., 2010; Thon et al., 2008; Wang et al., 2010). These results define a novel mechanism for cancer vasculogenesis and may help to explain the failure of currently used inhibitors of angiogenesis. Glioma stem cells as targets for novel strategies of treatment have been recently reviewed (Dietrich et al., 2010; Gilbert & Ross, 2011).

2.8 Promising targets for chemotherapy of glioblastoma multiforme

GBMs are highly infiltrative tumors that show resistance to conventional chemotherapy. Many chemotherapeutic agents are not able to reach the tumor in sufficient doses, because the blood brain barrier is at least partially intact in these tumors.

Most mitotic inhibitors used in clinic impair the function of mitotic spindles by targeting tubulins that are basic components of microtubules. Because microtubules in non-mitotic cells are also affected, these compounds often exhibit significant side effects (for example neurotoxicity). Future therapies of GBM may involve small molecules that inhibit the activity of aurora kinases A or B, polo kinases or the mitotic kinesin Eg5, all proteins that have specific functions in different phases of mitosis (for review see: Kaestner and Bastians, 2010; Sudakin and Yen, 2007). Pharmaceutical companies are on the way to develop selective inhibitors that target these proteins. Phase I and II studies on different forms of solid cancers are currently underway to study newly developed mitosis inhibitors and may also open the way for a more efficient therapy of GBM. Interestingly, it has been reported that in glioblastoma expression of aurora kinases A (Barton et al., 2010) and B (Zeng et al., 2007) were both associated with poor prognosis and may be targets for therapy. Among several other proteins also histone deacetylases (HDACs) may be promising targets for future therapy of GBM (Argyriou and Kalofonos, 2009). ABC transporters play an important role in the development of multidrug resistance. The role of ABC transporters in the resistance network of glioblastoma was reviewed by Bleau et al. (2009).

The humanized monoclonal antibody against vascular endothelial growth factor (Bevacizumab, Avastin®) has been approved by the FDA for treatment of GBM. Although targeting the tumor vasculature with Bevacizumab reduced the number of cancer-like stem cells in orthotopic brain tumor xenografts (Calabrese et al., 2007), a recent phase II study indicates that bevacizumab does not affect median survival of patients with recurrent GBM (Pope et al, 2011).

Potential targets for directed therapy of GBM may include extracellular matrix proteins of the perivascular niche that influence proliferation and/or migration of cancer stem cells. Targeting integrin α6 has recently been shown to inhibit self-renewal, proliferation, and tumor formation capacity of glioblastoma stem cells (Lathia et al., 2010). Cilengitide (Impetreve®) is a cyclic pentapeptide harboring a RGD sequence. RGD sequences present on extracellular matrix proteins mediate the binding to integrins, a class of cell surface receptors. Cilengitide is a selective inhibitor of αvβ3/5 integrins and currently under study as an inhibitor of angiogenesis in several types of solid cancer. Cilengitide monotherapy was well tolerated and exhibited modest antitumor activity among patients with recurrent GBM in a randomized phase II study (Reardon et al., 2008). Also targeting glioma stem cells through the neural cell adhesion molecule L1CAM has been reported to suppress glioma growth (Bao et al., 2008). Glioblastoma cells display complex surface structures with numerous microvilli and filopodia that resist the actions of cytolytic effector lymphocytes (Hoa et al., 2010). It should also be noted that gliomas are accompanied by numerous microglia/macrophages. As was recently reported, inhibition of microglia/macrophage activation may represent a new and effective strategy to suppress proliferation of glioma cells (Zhai et al., 2011).

Subtypes of breast cancer or leukemia can be efficiently treated by inhibiting the one excessively activated signal transduction pathway that is linked to malignancy. For GBM a monocausal therapy by inhibition of a single overactivated signaling pathway seems to be less promising, because cells or even regions with different genetic defects coexist in one tumor. A personalized therapy based on analysis of the individual genetic defects is not yet in sight for GBM.

3. Summary and perspective

Many types of cancer cells evolve through a multistep process in which genetic aberrations accumulate and finally lead to cells exhibiting aberrant gene expression programs. GBM has been considered as a system/network disease (Fathallah-Shaykh, 2010), because its phenotypes appear to be generated by several interconnected aberrant signal transduction pathways as well as numerous molecular abnormalities, thereby resulting in uncontrolled mitosis and migration of GBM cancer cells. In GBM local heterogeneity arises as the tumor regionally adapts to microenvironmental cues. Future molecular therapies of GBM should target its Achilles' heels: the elimination of the small intratumoral subpopulation of cells that exert stem cell properties and the inhibition of mitosis within the population of transit amplifying cells, which is responsible for forming the tumor mass.

4. Acknowledgments

We thank the Maria-Pesch Stiftung and the Nolting-Stiftung for support.

5. References

Actor, B.; Cobbers, J.M., Buschges, R., Wolter, M., Knobbe, C.B., Lichter, P., Reifenberger, G. & Weber, R.G. (2002). Comprehensive analysis of genomic alterations in gliosarcoma and its two tissue components. *Genes Chromosomes Cancer*, Vol.34, No.4, (December 2002), pp. 416–427, ISSN 1045-2257

Argyriou, A.A. & Kalofonos, H.P. (2009). Molecularly targeted therapies for malignant gliomas. *Mol Med*. Vol.15, No.3-4, (March-April 2009), pp. 115-22, ISSN 1076-1551

Arjona, D.; Rey, J.A. & Taylor, S.M. (2006). Early genetic changes involved in low-grade astrocytic tumor development. *Curr Mol Med.*, Vol.6, No.6, (September 2006), pp. 645-50, ISSN 1566-5240

Bao, S.; Wu, Q., McLendon, R.E., Hao, Y., Shi, Q., Hjelmeland, A.B., Dewhirst, M.W., Bigner D.D. & Rich, J.N. (2006a). Glioma stem cells promote radioresistance by preferential activation of the DNA damage response. *Nature*, Vol.444, No.7120, (December 2006a), pp. 756-60, ISSN 0028-0836

Bao, S.; Wu, Q., Sathornsumetee, S., Hao, Y., Li, Z., Hjelmeland, A.B., Shi, Q., McLendon, R.E., Bigner, D.D. & Rich, J.N. (2006b). Stem cell-like glioma cells promote tumor angiogenesis through vascular endothelial growth factor. *Cancer Res.*, Vol.66, No.16, (August 2006b), pp. 7843-7848, ISSN 0008-5472

Bao, S.; Wu, Q., Li, Z., Sathornsumetee, S., Wang, H., McLendon, R.E., Hjelmeland, A.B. & Rich, J.N. (2008). Targeting cancer stem cells through L1CAM suppresses glioma growth. *Cancer Res.*, Vol.68, No.15, (August 2008), pp. 6043-6048, ISSN 0008-5472

Bartkova, J.; Horejsí, Z., Koed, K., Krämer, A., Tort, F., Zieger, K., Guldberg, P., Sehested, M., Nesland, J.M., Lukas, C., Ørntoft, T., Lukas, J. & Bartek, J. (2005). DNA damage response as a candidate anti-cancer barrier in early human tumorigenesis. *Nature*, Vol.434, No.7035, (April 2005), pp. 864-70, ISSN 0028-0836

Bartkova, J.; Rezaei, N., Liontos, M., Karakaidos, P., Kletsas, D., Issaeva, N., Vassiliou, L.V., Kolettas, E., Niforou, K., Zoumpourlis, V.C., Takaoka, M., Nakagawa, H., Tort, F., Fugger, K., Johansson, F., Sehested, M., Andersen, C.L., Dyrskjot, L., Ørntoft, T., Lukas, J., Kittas, C., Helleday, T., Halazonetis, T.D., Bartek, J. & Gorgoulis, V.G. (2006). Oncogene-induced senescence is part of the tumorigenesis barrier imposed by DNA damage checkpoints. *Nature*, Vol.444, No.7119, (November 2006), pp. 633-637, ISSN: 0028-0836

Barton, V.N.; Foreman, N.K., Donson, A.M., Birks, D.K., Handler, M.H. & Vibhakar, R. (2010). Aurora kinase A as a rational target for therapy in glioblastoma. *J Neurosurg Pediatr.*, Vol.6, No.1, (July 2010), pp. 98-105, ISSN 1933-0707

Bello, M.J.; Alonso, M.E., Amiñoso, C., Anselmo, N.P., Arjona, D., Gonzalez-Gomez, P., Lopez-Marin, I., de Campos, J.M., Gutierrez, M., Isla, A., Kusak, M.E., Lassaletta, L., Sarasa, J.L., Vaquero, J., Casartelli, C. & Rey, J.A. (2004). Hypermethylation of the DNA repair gene MGMT: association with TP53 G:C to A:T transitions in a series of 469 nervous system tumors. *Mutat Res.*, Vol.554, No.1-2, (October 2004), pp. 23-32, ISSN 0027-5107

Berger, F.; Gay, E., Pelletier, L., Tropel, P. & Wion, D. (2004). Development of gliomas: potential role of asymmetrical cell division of neural stem cells. *Lancet Oncol.*, Vol.5, No.8, (August 2004), pp. 511-514, ISSN 1470-2045

Bignold, L.P.; Coghlan, B.L. & Jersmann, H.P. (2006). Cancer morphology, carcinogenesis and genetic instability: a background. *EXS*, Vol.96, (2006), pp. 1-24, ISSN 1023-294X

Bleau, A.M.; Huse, J.T. & Holland, E.C. (2009). The ABCG2 resistance network of glioblastoma. *Cell Cycle*, Vol.8, No.18, (September 2009), pp. 2936-2944, ISSN 1538-4101

Brat, D.J.; Scheithauer, B.W., Medina-Flores, R., Rosenblum, M.K. & Burger, P.C. (2002). Infiltrative astrocytomas with granular cell features (granular cell astrocytomas): a study of histopathologic features, grading, and outcome. *Am J Surg Pathol.*, Vol.26, No.6, (June 2002), pp. 750-757, ISSN 0147-5185

Bredel, M.; Scholtens, D.M., Harsh, G.R., Bredel, C., Chandler, J.P., Renfrow, J.J., Yadav, A.K., Vogel, H., Scheck, A.C., Tibshirani, R. & Sikic, B.I. (2009). A network model of a cooperative genetic landscape in brain tumors. *JAMA*, Vol.302, No.3, (Juli 2009), pp. 261-75, ISSN 0098-7484

Bredel, M.; Scholtens, D.M., Yadav, A.K., Alvarez, A.A., Renfrow, J.J., Chandler, J.P., Yu, I.L., Carro, M.S., Dai, F., Tagge, M.J., Ferrarese, R., Bredel, C., Phillips, H.S., Lukac, P.J., Robe, P.A., Weyerbrock, A., Vogel, H., Dubner, S., Mobley, B., He, X., Scheck, A.C., Sikic, B.I., Aldape, K.D., Chakravarti, A. & Harsh, G.R. 4th. (2010). NFKBIA deletion in glioblastomas. *N Engl J Med.*, Vol.364, No.7, (February 2011), pp. 17627-17637, ISSN 0028-4793

Brell, M.; Ibáñez, J. & Tortosa, A. (2011). O6-Methylguanine-DNA methyltransferase protein expression by immunohistochemistry in brain and non-brain systemic tumours: systematic review and meta-analysis of correlation with methylation-specific polymerase chain reaction. *BMC Cancer*, Vol.11, No.1, (January 2011), pp. 35, ISSN 1471-2407

Brell, M.; Tortosa, A., Verger, E., Gil, J.M., Viñolas, N., Villà, S., Acebes, J.J., Caral Pons, J.J., Pujol, T., Ferrer, I., Ribalta, T. & Graus, F. (2005). Prognostic significance of O6 - Methilguanine DNA methyltransferase determined by promoter methylation and immunohistochemical expression in anaplastic gliomas. *Clin Cancer Res.*, Vol.11, No.14, (July 2005), pp. 5167-5174; ISSN 1078-0432

Burger, P.C. & Vollmer, R.T. (1980). Histologic factors of prognostic significance in the glioblastoma multiforme. *Cancer*, Vol.46, No.5, (September 1980), pp. 1179-1186, ISSN 1837-9664

Cahill, D.P.; Levine, K.K., Betensky, R.A., Codd, P.J., Romany, C.A., Reavie, L.B., Batchelor, T.T., Futreal, P.A., Stratton, M.R., Curry, W.T., Iafrate, A.J. & Louis, D.N. (2007). Loss of the mismatch repair protein MSH6 in human glioblastomas is associated with tumor progression during temozolomide treatment. *Clin Cancer Res.*, Vol.13, No.7, (April 2007), pp. 2038-2045, ISSN 1078-0432

Calabrese, C.; Poppleton, H., Kocak, M., Hogg, T.L., Fuller, C., Hamner, B., Oh, E.Y., Gaber, M.W., Finklestein, D., Allen, M., Frank, A., Bayazitov, I.T., Zakharenko, S.S., Gajjar, A., Davidoff, A. & Gilbertson R.J. (2007). A perivascular niche for brain tumor stem cells. *Cancer Cell*, Vol.11, No.1, (January 2007), pp. 69-82, ISSN 1535-6108

Campbell, P.J.; Yachida, S., Mudie, L.J., Stephens, P.J., Pleasance, E.D., Stebbings, L.A., Morsberger, L.A., Latimer, C., McLaren, S., Lin, M.L., McBride, D.J., Varela, I., Nik-Zainal, S.A., Leroy, C., Jia, M., Menzies, A., Butler, A.P., Teague, J.W., Griffin, C.A., Burton, J., Swerdlow, H., Quail, M.A., Stratton, M.R., Iacobuzio-Donahue, C. & Futreal, P.A. (2010). The patterns and dynamics of genomic instability in metastatic pancreatic cancer. *Nature*, Vol.467, No.7319, (October 2010), pp. 1109-1113, ISSN 0028-0836

Cancer Genome Atlas Research Network (2008). Comprehensive genomic characterization defines human glioblastoma genes and core pathways. *Nature,* Vol.455, No.7216, (October 2008), pp. 1061-1068, ISSN 0028-0836

Castellano-Sanchez, A.A.; Ohgaki, H., Yokoo, H., Scheithauer, B.W., Burger, P.C., Hamilton, R.L., Finkelstein, S.D. & Brat, D.J. (2003). Granular cell astrocytomas show a high frequency of allelic loss but are not a genetically defined subset. *Brain Pathol.,* Vol.13, No.2, (April 2003), pp. 185-194, ISSN 1015-6305

Central Brain Tumor Registry of the United States (2010) . Primary Brain and Central Nervous System Tumors Diagnosed in Unated States 2004-2006, In CBRUS Statistical Report (2010), 15.04.2011, Available from http://www.cbtrus.org/2010-NPCR-SEER/CBTRUS-WEBREPORT-Final-3-2-10.pdf

Chow, J. & Poon, R.Y. (2010). DNA damage and polyploidization. *Adv Exp Med Biol.,* Vol.676, (2010), pp. 57-71, ISSN 0065-2598

Colman, H.; Zhang, L., Sulman, E.P., McDonald, J.M., Shooshtari, N.L., Rivera, A., Popoff, S., Nutt, C.L., Louis, D.N., Cairncross, J.G., Gilbert M.R., Phillips, H.S., Mehta, M.P., Chakravarti, A., Pelloski, C.E., Bhat, K., Feuerstein, B.G., Jenkins, R.B. & Aldape, K. (2009). A multigene predictor of outcome in glioblastoma. *Neuro Oncol.,* Vol.12, No.1, (January 2010), pp. 49-57, ISSN 1522-8517

Christmann, M.; Nagel, G., Horn, S., Krahn, U., Wiewrodt, D., Sommer, C. & Kaina, B. (2010). MGMT activity, promoter methylation and immunohistochemistry of pretreatment and recurrent malignant gliomas: a comparative study on astrocytoma and glioblastoma. *Int J Cancer,* Vol.127, No.9, (November 2010), pp. 2106-2118, ISSN 0898-6924

D'Assoro, A.B.; Lingle, W.L. & Salisbury, J.L. (2002). Centrosome amplification and the development of cancer. *Oncogene,* Vol.21, No.40, (September 2002), pp. 6146-6153, ISSN 0950-9232

Di Micco, R.; Fumagalli, M., Cicalese, A., Piccinin, S., Gasparini, P., Luise, C., Schurra, C., Garre', M., Nuciforo, P.G., Bensimon A., Maestro, R., Pelicci, P.G. & d'Adda di Fagagna F. (2006). Oncogene-induced senescence is a DNA damage response triggered by DNA hyper-replication. *Nature.* Vol.444, No.7119, (November 2006), pp. 638-42, ISSN 0028-0836

Dietrich, J.; Diamond, E.L., & Kesari, S. (2010). Glioma stem cell signaling: therapeutic opportunities and challenges. *Expert Rev Anticancer Ther.,* Vol.10, No.5, (May 2010), pp. 709-22, ISSN 1473-7140

Duesberg, P.; Rausch, C., Rasnick, D. & Hehlmann, R. (1998). Genetic instability of cancer cells is proportional to their degree of aneuploidy. *Proc Natl Acad Sci U S A,* Vol.95, No.23, (November 1998), pp. 13692-13697, ISSN 0027-8424

Duncan, A.W.; Taylor, M.H., Hickey, R.D., Hanlon Newell, A.E., Lenzi, M.L., Olson, S.B., Finegold, M.J. & Grompe, M. (2010). The ploidy conveyor of mature hepatocytes as a source of genetic variation. *Nature,* Vol.467, No.7316, (October 2010), pp. 707-710, ISSN 0028-0836

Etcheverry, A.; Aubry, M., de Tayrac, M., Vauleon, E., Boniface, R., Guenot, F., Saikali, S., Hamlat, A., Riffaud, L., Menei, P., Quillien, V. & Mosser, J. (2010). DNA methylation in glioblastoma: impact on gene expression and clinical outcome. *BMC Genomics,* Vol.11, (December 2010), pp. 701, ISSN 1471-2164

Esteller, M.; Hamilton, S.R., Burger, P.C., Baylin, S.B. & Herman, J.G. (1999). Inactivation of the DNA repair gene O6-methylguanine-DNA methyltransferase by promoter hypermethylation is a common event in primary human neoplasia. *Cancer Res.*, Vol.59, No.4, (February 1999), pp. 793-797, ISSN 0008-5472

Everhard, S.; Tost, J., El Abdalaoui, H., Crinière, E., Busato, F., Marie, Y., Gut, I.G., Sanson, M., Mokhtari, K., Laigle-Donadey, F., Hoang-Xuan, K., Delattre, J.Y. & Thillet, J. (2009). Identification of regions correlating MGMT promoter methylation and gene expression in glioblastomas. *Neuro Oncol.*, Vol.11, (August 2009), pp. 348–356, ISSN 1522-8517

Fathallah-Shaykh, H.M. (2010). Malignant astrocytomas: a system disease. *Arch Neurol.*, Vol.67, No.3, (March 2010), pp. 353-355, ISSN 0003-9942

Fearon, E.R. & Vogelstein, B. (1990). A genetic model for colorectal tumorigenesis. *Cell*, Vol.61, No.5, (June 1990), pp. 759-767

Franovic, A.; Holterman, C.E., Payette, J. & Lee, S. (2009). Human cancers converge at the HIF-2alpha oncogenic axis. *Proc Natl Acad Sci U S A*, Vol.106, No.50, (December 2009), pp. 21306-21311, ISSN 0027-8424

Fukushima, T.; Takeshima, H. & Kataoka, H. (2009). Anti-glioma therapy with temozolomide and status of the DNA-repair gene MGMT. *Anticancer Res.*, Vol.29, No.11, (November 2009), pp. 4845-4854, ISSN 0250-7005

Furnari, F.B.; Fenton, T., Bachoo, R.M., Mukasa, A., Stommel, J.M., Stegh, A., Hahn, W.C., Ligon, K.L., Louis, D.N., Brennan, C., Chin, L., DePinho, R.A. & Cavenee, W.K. (2007). Malignant astrocytic glioma: genetics, biology, and paths to treatment. *Genes Dev.*, Vol.21, No.21, (November 2007), pp. 2683-2710, ISSN 0890-9369

Galli, R.; Binda, E., Orfanelli, U., Cipelletti, B., Gritti, A., De Vitis, S., Fiocco, R., Foroni C., Dimeco, F. & Vescovi, A. (2004). Isolation and characterization of tumorigenic, stem-like neural precursors from human glioblastoma. *Cancer Res.*, Vol.64, No.19, (October 2004), pp. 7011-7021, ISSN 0008-5472

Gilbert, C.A. and Ross A.H. (2011). Glioma Stem Cells: Cell Culture, Markers and Targets for New Combination Therapies, In: *Cancer Stem Cells Theories and Prac*tice, S. Shostak (Ed.), InTech, Retrieved from http://www.intechopen.com/articles /show/title/glioma-stem-cells-cell-culture-markers-and-targets-for-new-combination-therapies

Gorgoulis, V.G.; Vassiliou, L.V., Karakaidos, P., Zacharatos, P., Kotsinas, A., Liloglou, T., Venere, M., Ditullio, R.A.Jr., Kastrinakis, N.G., Levy, B., Kletsas, D., Yoneta, A., Herlyn, M., Kittas, C. & Halazonetis, T.D. (2005). Activation of the DNA damage checkpoint and genomic instability in human precancerous lesions. *Nature*, Vol. 434, No.7035, (April 2005), pp. 907-913, ISSN 0028-0836

Goth, R. & Rajewsky, M.F. (1974). Persistence of O6-ethylguanine in rat-brain DNA: correlation with nervous system-specific carcinogenesis by ethylnitrosourea. *Proc Natl Acad Sci U S A.* Vol.71, No.3, (March 1974), pp. 639-43, ISSN 0027-8424

Halazonetis, T.D.; Gorgoulis, V.G. & Bartek, J. (2008). An oncogene-induced DNA damage model for cancer development. *Science*, Vol.319, No.5868, (March 2008), pp. 1352-5, ISSN 0193-4511

Hansemann, D. (1890). Ueber asymmetrische Zellteilung in Epithelkrebsen und deren biologische Bedeutung [On the asymmetrical cell divisions in epithelial cancers and its biological significance]. *Arch Pathol Anat etc., Berlin (Virchow's Arch)*, Vol.119, (1890), pp. 299-326

Harada, K.; Nishizaki, T., Ozaki, S., Kubota, H., Ito, H. & Sasaki, K. (1998). Intratumoral cytogenetic heterogeneity detected by comparative genomic hybridization and laser scanning cytometry in human gliomas. *Cancer Res.* Vol.58, No.20, (October 1998), pp. 4694-700, ISSN 0008-5472

Hegedüs, B.; Czirók, A., Fazekas, I., B'abel, T., Madar'asz, E. & Vicsek, T. (2000). Locomotion and proliferation of glioblastoma cells in vitro: statistical evaluation of videomicroscopic observations. *J Neurosurg.*, Vol.92, No.3, (March 2000), pp. 428-34, ISSN 0022-3085

Hegi, M.E.; Diserens, A.C., Gorlia, T., Hamou, M.F., de Tribolet, N., Weller, M., Kros, J.M., Hainfellner, J.A., Mason, W., Mariani, L., Bromberg, J.E., Hau, P., Mirimanoff, R.O., Cairncross, J.G., Janzer, R.C. & Stupp, R. (2005). MGMT gene silencing and benefit from temozolomide in glioblastoma. *N Engl J Med.*, Vol.352, No.10, (March 2005),pp. 997-1003, ISSN 0028-4793

Hegi, M.E.; Liu, L., Herman, J.G., Stupp, R., Wick, W., Weller, M., Mehta, M.P. & Gilbert, M.R. (2008). Correlation of O6-methylguanine methyltransferase (MGMT) promoter methylation with clinical outcomes in glioblastoma and clinical strategies to modulate MGMT activity. *J Clin Oncol.*, Vol.26, No.25, (September 2008), pp. 4189-99 ISSN 0732-183X

Hesson, L.B. ; Krex, D. & Latif, F. (2008). Epigenetic markers in human gliomas: prospects for therapeutic intervention. *Expert Rev Neurother.*, Vol.8, No.10, (October 2008), pp. 1475-96, ISSN 1473-7175

Hjelmeland, A.B.; Wu, Q., Heddleston, J.M., Choudhary, G.S., Macswords, J., Lathia, J.D., McLendon, R., Lindner, D., Sloan, A. & Rich, J.N. (2010). Acidic stress promotes a glioma stem cell phenotype. *Cell Death Differ.*, [Epub ahead of print], ISSN 1476-5403

Hoa, N.; Ge, L., Kuznetsov, Y., McPherson, A., Cornforth, A.N., Pham, J.T., Myers, M.P., Ahmed, N., Salsman, V.S., Lamb, L.S.Jr., Bowersock, J.E., Hu, Y., Zhou, Y.H. & Jadus M.R. (2010). Glioma cells display complex cell surface topographies that resist the actions of cytolytic effector lymphocytes. *J Immunol.*, Vol.185, No.8, (October 2010), pp. 4793-803, ISSN 0022-1767

Holliday, R. (1989). Chromosome error propagation and cancer. *Trends Genet.* Vol.5, No.2, (February 1989), pp. 42-5, ISSN 0168-9525

Hoshino, T.; Nomura, K., Wilson, C.B., Knebel, K.D. & Gray, J.W. (1978). The distribution of nuclear DNA from human brain-tumor cells. *J Neurosurg.*, Vol.49, No.1, (July 1978), pp. 13-21, ISSN 0022-3085

Huang, Z.; Cheng, L., Guryanova, O.A., Wu, Q. & Bao, S. (2010). Cancer stem cells in glioblastoma-molecular signaling and therapeutic targeting. *Protein Cell*, Vol.1, No.7, (July 2010), pp. 638-55, ISSN 1674-800X

Hunter,C.; Smith, R., Cahill, D.P., Stephens, P., Stevens, C., Teague, J., Greenman, C., Edkins, S., Bignell, G., Davies, H., O'Meara, S., Parker, A., Avis, T., Barthorpe, S., Brackenbury, L., Buck, G., Butler, A., Clements, J., Cole, J., Dicks, E., Forbes, S., Gorton, M., Gray, K., Halliday, K., Harrison, R., Hills, K., Hinton, J., Jenkinson, A., Jones, D., Kosmidou, V., Laman, R., Lugg, R., Menzies, A., Perry, J., Petty, R., Raine,

K., Richardson, D., Shepherd, R., Small, A., Solomon, H., Tofts, C., Varian, J., West, S., Widaa, S., Yates, A., Easton, D.F., Riggins, G., Roy, J.E., Levine, K.K., Mueller, W., Batchelor, T.T., Louis, D.N., Stratton, M.R., Futreal, P.A. & Wooster R. (2006). A hypermutation phenotype and somatic MSH6 mutations in recurrent human malignant gliomas after alkylator chemotherapy. Cancer Res., Vol.66, No.8, (April 2006), pp. 3987-91, ISSN-0008-5472

Ignatova, T.N.; Kukekov, V.G., Laywell, E.D., Suslov, O.N., Vrionis, F.D. & Steindler, D.A. (2002). Human cortical glial tumors contain neural stem-like cells expressing astroglial and neuronal markers in vitro. Glia, Vol.39, No.3, (September 2002), pp. 193-206, ISSN 0894-1491

Ingold, B.; Schraml, P., Heppner, F.L. & Moch, H. (2009). Homogeneous MGMT immuno-reactivity correlates with an unmethylated MGMT promoter status in brain metastases of various solid tumors. PLoS ONE, Vol.4, No.3, (March 2009), pp. e4775, ISSN 1932-6203

Jung, V.; Romeike, B.F., Henn, W., Feiden, W., Moringlane, J.R., Zang, K.D. & Urbschat, S. (1999). Evidence of focal genetic microheterogeneity in glioblastoma multiforme by area-specific CGH on microdissected tumor cells. J Neuropathol Exp Neurol., Vol. 58, No.9, (September 1999), pp. 993-9, ISSN 0022-3069

Kaestner, P. & Bastians, H. (2010). Mitotic drug targets. J Cell Biochem., Vol.111, No.2, (October 2010), pp. 258-65, ISSN 0730-2312

Kaina, B.; Christmann, M., Naumann, S. & Roos, W.P. (2007). MGMT: key node in the battle against genotoxicity, carcinogenicity and apoptosis induced by alkylating agents. DNA Repair (Amst), Vol.6, No.8, (August 2007), pp. 1079–1099, ISSN 1568-7864

Kamiryo, T.; Tada, K., Shiraishi, S., Shinojima, N., Kochi, M. & Ushio, Y. (2004). Correlation between promoter hypermethylation of the O6-methylguanine-deoxyribonucleic acid methyltransferase gene and prognosis in patients with high-grade astrocytic tumors treated with surgery, radiotherapy, and 1-(4-amino-2-methyl-5-pyrimidinyl)methyl-3-(2-chloroethyl)-3-nitrosourea-based chemotherapy. Neuro-surgery, Vol.54, No.2, (February 2004), pp. 349-57, ISSN 0148-396X

Katsetos, C.D.; Reddy, G., Dráberová, E., Smejkalová, B., Del Valle, L., Ashraf, Q., Tadevosyan, A., Yelin, K., Maraziotis, T., Mishra, O.P., Mörk, S., Legido, A., Nissanov, J., Baas, P.W., de Chadarévian, J.P. & Dráber, P. (2006). Altered cellular distribution and subcellular sorting of gamma-tubulin in diffuse astrocytic gliomas and human glioblastoma cell lines. J Neuropathol Exp Neurol., Vol.65, No.5, (May 2006), pp. 465-77, ISSN 0022-3069

Kaushal, D.; Contos, J.J., Treuner, K., Yang, A.H., Kingsbury, M.A., Rehen, S.K., McConnell M.J., Okabe, M., Barlow, C. & Chun, J. (2003). Alteration of gene expression by chromosome loss in the postnatal mouse brain. J Neurosci., Vol.23, No.13, (July 2003), pp. 5599-606, ISSN 0270-6474

Kim, K.J.; Lee, K.H., Kim, H.S., Moon, K.S., Jung, T.Y., Jung, S. & Lee, M.C. (2011). The presence of stem cell marker-expressing cells is not prognostically significant in glioblastomas. Neuropathology, (January 2011), [Epub ahead of print], ISSN 0919-6544

Kleihues, P.; Burger, P.C., Aldape, K.D., Brat, D.J., Biernat, W., Bigner, D.D., Nakazato, Y., Plate, K.H., Giangaspero, F., von Deimling, A., Ohgaki, H., Cavenee, W.K. (2007).

Glioblastoma. In: *Classification of Tumors of the Central Nervous System*, Louis, D.N., Ohgaki, H., Wiestler, O.D., Cavenee, W.K., pp. 33-49, WHO, ISBN 978-92-832-2430-2, Lyon: IARC

Kleihues, P. & Ohgaki, H.(1999). Primary and secondary glioblastomas: from concept to clinical diagnosis. *Neuro Oncol.*, Vol.1, No.1, (January 1999), pp. 44-51, ISSN 1522-8517

Knudson, A. (1971). Mutation and cancer: statistical study of retinoblastoma. *Proc Natl Acad Sci U S A*, Vol.68, No.4, (April 1971), pp. 820-3, ISSN 0027-8424

Kreth, S.; Thon, N., Eigenbrod, S, Lutz, J., Ledderose, C., Egensperger, R., Tonn, J.C., Kretzschmar, H.A., Hinske, L.C. & Kreth, F.W. (2011). O-Methylguanine-DNA Methyltransferase (MGMT) mRNA Expression Predicts Outcome in Malignant Glioma Independent of MGMT Promoter Methylation. *PLoS One*, Vol.6, No.2, (February 2011), pp. e17156, ISSN 1932-6203

Krex, D.; Klink, B., Hartmann, C., von Deimling, A., Pietsch, T., Simon, M., Sabel, M., Steinbach, J.P., Heese, O., Reifenberger, G., Weller, M. & Schackert, G. (2007). German Glioma Network. Long-term survival with glioblastoma multiforme. *Brain*, Vol.130, No.10, (October 2007), pp. 2596-606, ISSN 0006-8950

Kros, J.M.; Waarsenburg, N., Hayes, D.P., Hop, W.C. & van Dekken, H. (2000). Cytogenetic analysis of gemistocytic cells in gliomas. *J Neuropathol Exp Neurol.*, Vol.59, No.8, (August 2000), pp. 679-686, ISSN 0022-3069

Laks, D.R.; Masterman-Smith, M., Visnyei, K., Angenieux, B., Orozco, N.M., Foran, I., Yong, W.H., Vinters, H.V., Liau, L.M., Lazareff, J.A., Mischel, P.S., Cloughesy, T.F., Horvath, S. & Kornblum, H.I. (2009). Neurosphere formation is an independent predictor of clinical outcome in malignant glioma. *Stem Cells*, Vol.27, No.4, (April 2009), pp. 980-7, ISSN 0250-6793

Lathia, J.D.; Gallagher, J., Heddleston, J.M., Wang, J., Eyler, C.E., Macswords, J., Wu, Q., Vasanji, A., McLendon, R.E., Hjelmeland, A.B. & Rich, J.N. (2010). Integrin alpha 6 regulates glioblastoma stem cells. *Cell Stem Cell*, Vol.6, No.5, (May 2010), pp. 421-32, ISSN 1934-5909

Li, Z.; Bao, S., Wu, Q., Wang, H., Eyler, C., Sathornsumetee, S., Shi, Q., Cao, Y., Lathia, J., McLendon, R.E., Hjelmeland, A.B. & Rich, J.N. (2009). Hypoxia-inducible factors regulate tumorigenic capacity of glioma stem cells. *Cancer Cell*, Vol.15, No.6, (June 2009), pp. 501-13, ISSN 1535-6108

Li, L.; Dutra, A., Pak, E., Labrie, J.E. 3rd, Gerstein, R.M., Pandolfi, P.P., Recht, L.D., Ross, A.H(2008). EGFRvIII expression and PTEN loss synergistically induce chromosomal instability and glial tumors. *Neuro Oncol.* Vol.11, No.1, (February 2009),pp. 9-21, ISSN 1522-8517

Loeper, S.; Romeike, B.F., Heckmann, N., Jung, V., Henn, W., Feiden, W., Zang, K.D. & Urbschat, S. (2001). Frequent mitotic errors in tumor cells of genetically micro-heterogeneous glioblastomas. *Cytogenet Cell Genet.*, Vol.94, No.1-2, (2001), pp. 1-8, ISSN 0301-0171

Loh, J.K.; Lieu, A.S., Chou, C.H., Lin, F.Y., Wu, C.H., Howng, S.L., Chio, C.C. & Hong, Y.R. (2010). Differential expression of centrosomal proteins at different stages of human glioma. *BMC Cancer*, Vol.10, (June 2010); pp. 268, ISSN 1471-2407

Margetts, J.C. & Kalyan-Raman, U.P. (1989). Giant-celled glioblastoma of brain. A clinico-pathological and radiological study of ten cases (including immunohistochemistry and ultrastructure). Cancer, Vol.63, No.3, (Feb 1989), pp. 524-31

Margison, G.P. & Kleihues, P. (1975). Chemical carcinogenesis in the nervous system. Preferential accumulation of O6-methylguanine in rat brain deoxyribonucleic acid during repetitive administration of N-methyl-N-nitrosourea. Biochem J., Vol.148, No.3, (June 1975), pp. 521-5, ISSN 0264-6021

McLendon, R.E. & Rich, J.N. (2010). Glioblastoma Stem Cells: A Neuropathologist's View. J Oncol., Vol.2011, (2011), pp. 397195, ISSN 1687-8450

Meyer-Puttlitz, B.; Hayashi, Y., Waha, A., Rollbrocker, B., Boström, J., Wiestler, O.D., Louis, D.N., Reifenberger, G., von Deimling, A. (1997). Molecular genetic analysis of giant cell glioblastomas. Am J Pathol., Vol.151, No.3, (September 1997), pp. 853–857, ISSN 0002-9440

Miller, C.R. & Perry, A. (2007). Glioblastoma. Morphologic and Molecular Genetic Diversity. Arch Pathol Lab Med., Vol.131, No.3, (March 2007), pp. 397-406, ISSN 0003-9985

Misra, A.; Chattopadhyay, P., Dinda, A.K., Sarkar, C., Mahapatra, A.K., Hasnain, S.E. & Sinha, S. (2000). Extensive intra-tumor heterogeneity in primary human glial tumors as a result of locus non-specific genomic alterations. J Neurooncol. Vol.48, No.1, (May 2000), pp. 1-12, ISSN 0167-594X

Misra, A.; Pellarin, M., Nigro, J., Smirnov, I., Moore, D., Lamborn, K.R., Pinkel, D., Albertson, D.G. & Feuerstein, B.G. (2005). Array comparative genomic hybridization identifies genetic subgroups in grade 4 human astrocytoma. Clin Cancer Res., Vol.11, No.8, (April 2005), pp. 2907-18, ISSN 1078-0432

Mizuno, H.; Spike B.T., Wahl, G.M. & Levine, A.J. (2010). Inactivation of p53 in breast cancers correlates with stem cell transcriptional signatures. Proc Natl Acad Sci U S A, Vol.107, No.52, (December 2010), pp. 22745-50, ISSN 0027-8424

Murat, A.; Migliavacca, E., Gorlia, T., Lambiv, W.L., Shay, T., Hamou, M.F., de Tribolet, N., Regli, L., Wick, W., Kouwenhoven, M.C., Hainfellner, J.A., Heppner, F.L., Dietrich, P.Y., Zimmer, Y., Cairncross, J.G., Janzer, R.C., Domany, E., Delorenzi, M., Stupp, R. & Hegi, M.E. (2008). Stem cell-related "self-renewal" signature and high epidermal growth factor receptor expression associated with resistance to concomitant chemoradiotherapy in glioblastoma. J Clin Oncol., Vol.26, No.18, (June 2008), pp. 3015-24, ISSN 0732-183X

Nakamura, M.; Watanabe, T., Yonekawa, Y., Kleihues, P. & Ohgaki, H. (2001). Promoter methylation of the DNA repair gene MGMT in astrocytomas is frequently associated with G:C --> A:T mutations of the TP53 tumor suppressor gene. Carcinogenesis, Vol.22, No.10, (October 2001), pp. 1715-9, ISSN 0143-3334

Nobusawa, S.; Lachuer, J., Wierinckx, A., Kim, Y.H., Huang, J., Legras, C., Kleihues, P. & Ohgaki, H. (2010). Intratumoral patterns of genomic imbalance in glioblastomas. Brain Pathol., Vol.20, No.5, (September 2010), pp. 936-44, ISSN 1015-6305

Noushmehr, H.; Weisenberger, D.J., Diefes, K., Phillips, H.S., Pujara, K., Berman, B.P., Pan, F., Pelloski, C.E., Sulman, E.P., Bhat, K.P., Verhaak, R.G., Hoadley, K.A., Hayes, D.N., Perou, C.M., Schmidt, H.K., Ding, L., Wilson, R.K., Van Den Berg, D., Shen, H., Bengtsson, H., Neuvial, P., Cope, L.M., Buckley, J., Herman, J.G., Baylin, S.B., Laird, P.W. & Aldape, K. (2010). Cancer Genome Atlas Research Network.

Identification of a CpG island methylator phenotype that defines a distinct subgroup of glioma. *Cancer Cell,* Vol.17, No.5, (May 2010), pp. 510-22, ISSN 1535-6108

Ohgaki, H., Dessen, P., Jourde, B., Horstmann, S., Nishikawa, T., Di Patre, P.L., Burkhard, C., Schüler, D., Probst-Hensch, N.M., Maiorka, P.C., Baeza, N., Pisani, P., Yonekawa, Y., Yasargil, M.G., Lütolf, U.M. & Kleihues, P. (2004). Genetic pathways to glioblastoma: a population-based study. *Cancer Res.,* Vol.64, No.19, (October 2004), pp. 6892-9, ISSN 0008-5472

Pallini, R.; Ricci-Vitiani, L., Montano, N., Mollinari, C., Biffoni, M., Cenci, T., Pierconti, F., Martini, M., De Maria, R. & Larocca, L.M. (2010). Expression of the stem cell marker CD133 in recurrent glioblastoma and its value for prognosis. *Cancer,* Vol.117, No.1, (January 2011), pp. 162-74

Panosyan, E.H.; Laks, D.R., Masterman-Smith, M., Mottahedeh, J., Yong, W.H., Cloughesy, T.F., Lazareff, J.A., Mischel, P.S., Moore, T.B. & Kornblum, H.I. (2010). Clinical outcome in pediatric glial and embryonal brain tumors correlates with in vitro multi-passageable neurosphere formation. *Pediatr Blood Cancer,* Vol.55, No.4, (October 2010), pp. 644-51, ISSN 1545-5009

Parsons, D.W., Jones, S., Zhang, X., Lin, J.C., Leary, R.J., Angenendt, P., Mankoo, P., Carter, H., Siu, I.M., Gallia, G.L., Olivi, A., McLendon, R., Rasheed, B.A., Keir, S., Nikolskaya, T., Nikolsky, Y., Busam, D.A., Tekleab, H., Diaz, L.A.Jr., Hartigan, J., Smith, D.R., Strausberg, R.L., Marie, S.K., Shinjo, S.M., Yan, H., Riggins, G.J., Bigner, D.D., Karchin, R., Papadopoulos, N., Parmigiani, G., Vogelstein, B., Velculescu, V.E. & Kinzler, K.W. (2008). An integrated genomic analysis of human glioblastoma multiforme. *Science,* Vol.321, No.5897, (September 2008), pp. 1807-12, ISSN 0036-8075

Paulus, W.; Bayas, A., Ott, G. & Roggendorf, W. (1994). Interphase cytogenetics of glioblastoma and gliosarcoma. *Acta Neuropathol (Berl),* Vol.88, No.5, (1994), pp. 420-425, ISSN 0001-6322

Peraud, A.; Watanabe, K., Plate, K.H., Yonekawa, Y., Kleihues, P. & Ohgaki, H. (1997). p53 mutations versus EGF receptor expression in giant cell glioblastomas. *J Neuropathol Exp Neurol.,* Vol.56, No.11, (November 1997), pp. 1236-41, ISSN 0022-3069

Peraud, A.; Watanabe, K., Schwechheimer, K., Yonekawa, Y., Kleihues, P. & Ohgaki, H. (1999). Genetic profile of the giant cell glioblastoma. *Lab Invest,* Vol.79, No.2, (February 1999), pp. 123-129, ISSN 0023-6837

Perry, A.; Aldape, K.D., George, D.H. & Burger, P.C. (2004). Small cell astrocytoma: an aggressive variant that is clinicopathologically and genetically distinct from anaplastic oligodendroglioma. *Cancer,* Vol.101, No.10, (November 2004), pp. 2318-26

Peterson, S.E., Westra, J.W., Paczkowski, C.M. & Chun, J. (2008). Chromosomal mosaicism in neural stem cells. *Methods Mol Biol.* Vol.438, (2008), pp. 197-204, ISSN 1064-3745

Phi, J.H.; Park, S.H., Chung, C.K., Wang, K.C., Cho, B.K. & Kim, S.K. (2009). Atypical cell clusters expressing both neuronal and oligodendrocytic markers: novel histological pattern of glioneuronal tumors? *Pathol Int.,* Vol.59, No.10, (October 2009), pp. 735-43, ISSN 1320-5463

Phillips, H.S.; Kharbanda, S., Chen, R., Forrest, W.F., Soriano, R.H., Wu, T.D., Misra, A., Nigro, J.M., Colman, H., Soroceanu, L., Williams, P.M., Modrusan, Z., Feuerstein, B.G. & Aldape, K. (2006). Molecular subclasses of high-grade glioma predict prognosis, delineate a pattern of disease progression, and resemble stages in neurogenesis. *Cancer Cell*, Vol.9, No.3, (March 2006), pp. 157-73, ISSN 1535-6108

Pope, W.B.; Xia, Q., Paton, V.E., Das, A., Hambleton, J., Kim, H.J., Huo, J., Brown, M.S., Goldin, J. & Cloughesy, T. (2011). Patterns of progression in patients with recurrent glioblastoma treated with bevacizumab. *Neurology*, Vol.76, No.5, (February 2011), pp. 432-7, ISSN 028-3878

Preusser, M.; Charles, J.R., Felsberg, J., Reifenberger, G., Hamou, M.F., Diserens, A.C., Stupp, R., Gorlia, T., Marosi, C., Heinzl, H., Hainfellner, J.A. & Hegi, M. (2008). Anti-O6-methylguanine-methyltransferase (MGMT) immunohistochemistry in glioblastoma multiforme: observer variability and lack of association with patient survival impede its use as clinical biomarker. *Brain Pathol.*, Vo.18, No.4, (October 2008), pp. 520–532, ISSN 1015-6305

Qian, X.C. & Brent, T.P. (1997). Methylation hot spots in the 5' flanking region denote silencing of the O6-methylguanine-DNA methyltransferase gene. *Cancer Res.*, Vol.57, No.17, (September 1997), pp. 3672 7, ISSN 0008-5472

Reardon, D.A.; Fink, K.L., Mikkelsen, T., Cloughesy, T.F., O'Neill, A., Plotkin, S., Glantz, M., Ravin, P., Raizer, J.J., Rich, K.M., Schiff, D., Shapiro, W.R., Burdette-Radoux, S., Dropcho, E.J., Wittemer, S.M., Nippgen, J., Picard, M. & Nabors, L.B. (2008). Randomized phase II study of cilengitide, an integrin-targeting arginine-glycine-aspartic acid peptide, in recurrent glioblastoma multiforme. *J Clin Oncol.*, Vol.26, No.34, (December 2008), pp. 5610-7, ISSN 0732-183X

Reis, R.M.; Konu-Lebleblicioglu, D., Lopes, J.M., Kleihues, P. & Ohgaki, H. (2000). Genetic profile of gliosarcomas. *Am J Pathol.*, Vol.156, (2000), pp. 425–432

Ricci-Vitiani, L.; Pallini, R., Biffoni, M., Todaro, M., Invernici, G., Cenci, T., Maira, G., Parati, E.A., Stassi, G., Larocca, L.M. & De Maria, R. (2010). Tumour vascularization via endothelial differentiation of glioblastoma stem-like cells. *Nature*, Vol.468, No.7325, (December 2010), pp. 824-8, ISSN 0028-0836

Sanai, N.; Alvarez-Buylla, A. & Berger, M.S. (2005). Neural stem cells and the origin of gliomas. *N Engl J Med.*, Vol.353, No.8, (August 2005), pp. 811-22, ISSN 0028-4793

Shen, W.H.; Balajee, A.S., Wang, J., Wu, H., Eng, C., Pandolfi, P.P., Yin, Y (2007) Essential role for nuclear PTEN in maintaining chromosomal integrity. *Cell.* Vol.128, No.1, (January 2007), pp. 157-70, ISSN:0092-8674

Shen, Q.; Wang, Y., Kokovay, E., Lin, G., Chuang, SM., Goderie, S.K., Roysam, B. & Temple, S. (2008). Adult SVZ stem cells lie in a vascular niche: a quantitative analysis of niche cell-cell interactions. *Cell Stem Cell*, Vol.3, No.3, (September 2008), pp. 289-300, ISSN 1934-5909

Shinojima, N.; Kochi, M., Hamada, J., Nakamura, H., Yano, S., Makino, K., Tsuiki, H., Tada, K., Kuratsu, J., Ishimaru, Y. & Ushio, Y. (2004). The influence of sex and the presence of giant cells on postoperative long-term survival in adult patients with supratentorial glioblastoma multiforme. *J Neurosurg.*, Vol.101, (2004), pp. 219–226

Silkworth, W.T.; Nardi, I.K., Scholl, L.M. & Cimini, D. (2009). Multipolar spindle pole coalescence is a major source of kinetochore mis-attachment and chromosome mis-segregation in cancer cells. *PLoS One*, Vol.4, No.8, (August 2009), pp. e6564, ISSN 1932-6203

Singh, S.K.; Clarke, I.D., Terasaki, M., Bonn, V.E., Hawkins, C., Squire, J. & Dirks, P.B. (2003). Identification of a cancer stem cell in human brain tumors. *Cancer Res.*, Vol.63, No.18, (September 2003), pp. 5821-8, ISSN 0099-7013

Spiegl-Kreinecker, S.; Pirker, C., Filipits, M., Lötsch, D., Buchroithner, J., Pichler, J., Silye, R., Weis, S., Micksche, M., Fischer, J. & Berger, W. (2009). O6-Methylguanine DNA methyltransferase protein expression in tumor cells predicts outcome of temozolomide therapy in glioblastoma patients. *Neuro Oncol.*, Vol.12, No.1, (January 2010), pp. 28-36, ISSN 1522-8517

Stanbridge, E.J.; Flandermeyer, R.R., Daniels, D.W. & Nelson-Rees, W.A. (1981). Specific chromosome loss associated with the expression of tumorigenicity in human cell hybrids. *Somatic Cell Genet.*, Vol.7, No.6, (November 1981), pp. 699-712, ISSN 0098-0366

Stoler, D.L.; Chen, N., Basik, M., Kahlenberg, M.S., Rodriguez-Bigas, M.A., Petrelli, N.J. & Anderson, G.R. (1999). The onset and extent of genomic instability in sporadic colorectal tumor progression. *Proc Natl Acad Sci U S A*, Vol.96, No.26, (December 1999), pp. 15121-6, ISSN 0027-8424

Stupp, R.; Mason, W.P., van den Bent, M.J., Weller, M., Fisher, B., Taphoorn, M.J., Belanger, K., Brandes, A.A., Marosi, C., Bogdahn, U., Curschmann, J., Janzer, R.C., Ludwin, S.K., Gorlia, T., Allgeier, A., Lacombe, D., Cairncross, J.G., Eisenhauer, E. & Mirimanoff, R.O. (2005). Radiotherapy plus concomitant and adjuvant temozolomide for glioblastoma. *N Engl J Med*, Vol. 352, No.10, (March 2005), pp. 987–996, ISSN 0028-4793

Stupp, R.; Hegi, M.E., Mason, W.P., van den Bent, M.J., Taphoorn, M.J., Janzer R.C., Ludwin, S.K., Allgeier, A., Fisher, B., Belanger, K., Hau, P., Brandes, A.A., Gijtenbeek, J., Marosi, C., Vecht, C.J., Mokhtari, K., Wesseling, P., Villa, S., Eisenhauer, E., Gorlia, T., Weller, M., Lacombe, D., Cairncross, J.G., Mirimanoff, R.O., European Organisation for Research and Treatment of Cancer Brain Tumour and Radiation Oncology Groups & National Cancer Institute of Canada Clinical Trials Group. (2009). Effects of radiotherapy with concomitant and adjuvant temozolomide versus radiotherapy alone on survival in glioblastoma in a randomised phase III study: 5-year analysis of the EORTC-NCIC trial. *Lancet Oncol.*, Vol.10, No.5, (May 2009), pp. 459-66, ISSN 1470-2045

Sudakin, V. & Yen, T.J. (2007). Targeting mitosis for anti-cancer therapy. *BioDrugs*, Vol.21, No.4, (2007), pp. 225-33, ISSN 1173-8804

Tang, K.; Jin, Q., Yan, W., Zhang, W., You, G., Liu, Y. & Jiang, T. (2011). Clinical correlation of MGMT protein expression and promoter methylation in Chinese glioblastoma patients. *Med Oncol.*, (Mar 2011), [Epub ahead of print], ISSN 1357-0560

Temme, A.; Geiger, K.D., Wiedemuth, R., Conseur, K., Pietsch, T., Felsberg, J., Reifenberger, G., Tatsuka, M., Hagel, C., Westphal, M., Berger, H., Simon, M., Weller, M. & Schackert, G. (2010). Giant cell glioblastoma is associated with altered aurora b expression and concomitant p53 mutation. *J Neuropathol Exp Neurol.*, Vol.69, No.6, (June 2010), pp. 632-42, ISSN 0022-3069

Thon, N.; Damianoff, K., Hegermann, J., Grau, S., Krebs, B., Schnell, O., Tonn, J.C. & Goldbrunner, R. (2008). Presence of pluripotent CD133+ cells correlates with malignancy of gliomas. *Mol Cell Neurosci.*, Vol.43, No.1, (January 2010), pp. 51-9, ISSN 1044-7431

Tyzzer, E.E. (1916). Tumor immunity. *J Cancer Res.*, Vol.1, (1916), pp. 125-155

Verhaak, R.G.; Hoadley, K.A., Purdom, E., Wang, V., Qi, Y., Wilkerson, M.D., Miller, C.R., Ding, L., Golub, T., Mesirov, J.P., Alexe, G., Lawrence, M., O'Kelly, M., Tamayo, P., Weir, B.A., Gabriel, S., Winckler, W., Gupta, S., Jakkula, L., Feiler, H.S., Hodgson, J.G., James, C.D., Sarkaria, J.N., Brennan, C., Kahn, A., Spellman, P.T., Wilson, R.K., Speed, T.P., Gray, J.W., Meyerson, M., Getz, G., Perou, C.M., Hayes, D.N., Cancer Genome Atlas Research Network. (2010). Integrated genomic analysis identifies clinically relevant subtypes of glioblastoma characterized by abnormalities in PDGFRA, IDH1, EGFR, and NF1. *Cancer Cell*, Vol.17, No.1, (January 2010), pp. 98-110, ISSN 1535-6108

Wang, R.; Chadalavada, K., Wilshire, J., Kowalik, U., Hovinga, K.E., Geber, A., Fligelman, B., Leversha, M., Brennan, C. & Tabar, V. (2010). Glioblastoma stem-like cells give rise to tumour endothelium. *Nature*, Vol.468, No.7325, (December 2010), pp. 829-33, ISSN 0028-0836

Watanabe, K.; Tachibana, O., Sata, K., Yonekawa, Y., Kleihues, P. & Ohgaki, H. (1996). Overexpression of the EGF receptor and p53 mutations are mutually exclusive in the evolution of primary and secondary glioblastomas. *Brain Pathol.*, Vol.6, No.3, (July 1996), pp. 217-23, ISSN 1015-6305

Wick, W.; Hartmann, C., Engel, C., Stoffels, M., Felsberg, J., Stockhammer, F., Sabel, M.C., Koeppen, S., Ketter, R., Meyermann, R., Rapp, M., Meisner, C., Kortmann, R.D., Pietsch, T., Wiestler, O.D., Ernemann, U., Bamberg, M., Reifenberger, G., von Deimling, A. & Weller, M. (2009). NOA-04 randomized phase III trial of sequential radiochemotherapy of anaplastic glioma with procarbazine, lomustine, and vincristine or temozolomide. *J Clin Oncol*, Vol.27, No.35, (December 2009), pp. 5874-80, ISSN 0732-183X

Yachida, S.; Jones, S., Bozic, I., Antal, T., Leary, R., Fu, B., Kamiyama, M., Hruban, R.H., Eshleman, J.R., Nowak, M.A., Velculescu, V.E., Kinzler, K.W., Vogelstein, B. & Iacobuzio-Donahue, C.A. (2010). Distant metastasis occurs late during the genetic evolution of pancreatic cancer. *Nature*, Vol.467, No.7319, (October 2010), pp. 1114-7, ISSN 0028-0836

Yadav, A.K.; Renfrow, J.J., Scholtens, D.M., Xie, H., Duran, G.E., Bredel, C., Vogel, H., Chandler, J.P., Chakravarti, A., Robe, P.A., Das, S., Scheck, A.C., Kessler, J.A., Soares, M.B., Sikic, B.I., Harsh, G.R. & Bredel, M. (2009). Monosomy of chromosome 10 associated with dysregulation of epidermal growth factor signaling in glioblastomas. *JAMA*, Vol.302, No.3, (July 2009), pp. 276-89, ISSN 0098-7484

Yan, H.; Parsons, D.W., Jin, G., McLendon, R., Rasheed, B.A., Yuan, W., Kos, I., Batinic-Haberle, I., Jones, S., Riggins, G.J., Friedman, H., Friedman, A., Reardon, D., Herndon, J., Kinzler, K.W., Velculescu, V.E., Vogelstein, B. & Bigner, D.D. (2009). IDH1 and IDH2 mutations in gliomas. *N Engl J Med.*, Vol.360, No.8, (February 2009), pp. 765-73, ISSN 0028-4793

Yang, A.H.; Kaushal, D., Rehen, S.K., Kriedt, K., Kingsbury, M.A., McConnell, M.J. & Chun, J. (2003). Chromosome segregation defects contribute to aneuploidy in normal neural progenitor cells. *J Neurosci.*, Vol.23, No.32, (November 2003), pp. 10454-62, ISSN 0270-6474

Yin, Y & Shen, W.H. (2008). PTEN: a new guardian of the genome. Oncogene. Vol.27, No.41, (September 2008), pp. 5443-53, ISSN 0950-9232

Yip, S.; Miao, J., Cahill, D.P., Iafrate, A.J., Aldape, K., Nutt, C.L. & Louis, D.N. (2009). MSH6 mutations arise in glioblastomas during temozolomide therapy and mediate temozolomide resistance. *Clin Cancer Res.*, Vol.15, No.14, (July 2009), pp. 4622-9, ISSN 1078-0432

Yuan, X.; Curtin, J., Xiong, Y., Liu, G., Waschsmann-Hogiu, S., Farkas, D.L., Black, K.L. & Yu, J.S. (2004). Isolation of cancer stem cells from adult glioblastoma multiforme. *Oncogene*, Vol.23, No.58, (December 2004), pp. 9392-400, ISSN 0950-9232

Zeng, W.F.; Navaratne, K., Prayson, R.A. & Weil, R.J. (2007). Aurora B expression correlates with aggressive behaviour in glioblastoma multiforme. *J Clin Pathol.*, Vol.60, No.2, (February 2007), pp. 218-21, ISSN 0021-9746

Zeppernick, F.; Ahmadi, R., Campos, B., Dictus, C., Helmke, B.M., Becker, N., Lichter, P., Unterberg, A., Radlwimmer, B. & Herold-Mende, C.C. (2008). Stem cell marker CD133 affects clinical outcome in glioma patients. *Clin Cancer Res.*, Vol.14, No.1, (January 2008), pp. 123-9, ISSN 1078-0432

Zhai, H.; Heppner, F.L. & Tsirka, S.E. (2011). Microglia/macrophages promote glioma progression. *Glia*, Vol.59, No.3, (March 2011), pp. 472-85, ISSN 0894-1491

Zhang, M.; Song, T., Yang, L., Chen, R., Wu, L., Yang, Z. & Fang, J. (2008). Nestin and CD133: valuable stem cell-specific markers for determining clinical outcome of glioma patients. *J Exp Clin Cancer Res.*, Vol.27, (December 2008), pp. 85, ISSN 0392-9078

7

New Insight on the Role of Transient Receptor Potential (TRP) Channels in Driven Gliomagenesis Pathways

Giorgio Santoni[1], Maria Beatrice Morelli[1,2], Consuelo Amantini[1],
Matteo Santoni[1] and Massimo Nabissi[1]
[1]School of Pharmacy, Section of Experimental Medicine, University of Camerino
[2]Department of Molecular Medicine, Sapienza University, Rome
Italy

1. Role of TRP channels in glioma growth and progression

Gliomas are primary brain tumours believed to arise from glial cells or their progenitors. They account for 78% of malignant brain tumours (Shwartzbaum et al., 2006). The vast majority of gliomas is high-grade glioblastoma multiforme (GBM), and is characterized by almost unrestrained growth. Consequently, the median survival of patients with GBM was approximately 12 months (Huncharek & Muscat, 1998). While research has generated abundant information regarding the growth characteristics of these cancers, clinical care remains palliative and the prognosis dismal (Butowski et al., 2006). Gliomagenesis and progression are complex processes only partly understood. At molecular level, tumor progression and the associated heterogeneity is likely the result of multiple mutations in certain key signaling proteins (Furnari et al., 2007). Among these proteins, the Transient Receptor Potential (TRP) channel family has been identified to profoundly affect a variety of physiological and pathological processes (Kiselyov et al., 2007; Nilius et al., 2007). Members of TRP channels control cellular homeostasis by regulating calcium flux, cell proliferation, differentiation and apoptosis; moreover, in the last years an additional role for TRP ion channel family in malignant cancer growth and progression has been recognized (Xu et al., 2001; Wisnoskey et al., 2003; Xin et al., 2005; Bidaux et al., 2007; Prevarskaya et al., 2007; Gkika & Prevarskaya, 2009). Approximately thirty TRPs have been identified to date, and are classified in seven different families: TRPC (Canonical), TRPV (Vanilloid), TRPM (Melastatin), TRPML (Mucolipin), TRPP (Polycystin), and TRPA (Ankyrin transmembrane protein) and TRPN (NomPC-like) (Montell, 2003) (Fig.1).

The expression levels and activity of members of the TRPC, TRPM, and TRPV families have been correlated with malignant growth and progression (Duncan et al., 1998; Tsavaler et al., 2001; Wissenbach et al., 2001; Thebault et al., 2006; Amantini et al., 2007; Caprodossi et al., 2008; Nabissi et al., 2010). TRP channels may regulate glioma growth and progression at different levels by controlling cell proliferation, inhibiting apoptosis, stimulating angiogenesis and triggering the migration and the invasion during tumor progression (Table 1).

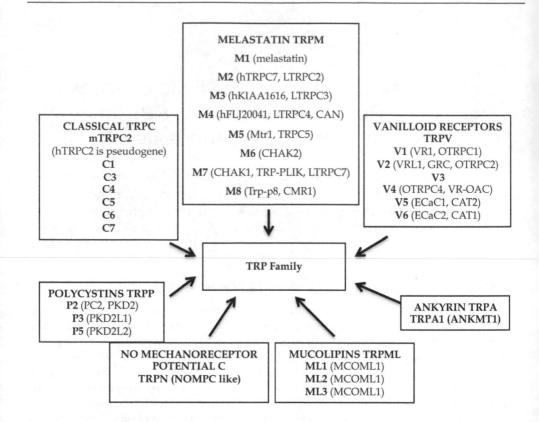

Fig. 1. TRP superfamily. TRP subgroups are represented in square, the members are indicated for each subfamily.

2. Role of TRPC and TRPV channels in cell cycle arrest and cytokinesis in malignant glioma

Growth control of cancer cell populations has been studied extensively over the past decades and research has identified a multitude of transmembrane TRP channels involved in this process (Schönherr, 2005; Santoni et al., 2011) (Fig.2). While our understanding of their exact role in the physiology of cell proliferation remains tentative, many TRP channel agonists or antagonists also stimulate or retard cell population growth, which support the notion that TRP channels are intrinsic component of the cell cycle. In particular, calcium Ca(2+) signaling plays an important role in normal and aberrant cell proliferation, and some members of the Ca(2+)-permeable TRPC family have demonstrated a role in the proliferation of many types of cancer cells (Malarkey et al., 2008). Using a combination of molecular, biochemical and biophysical approaches, it was demonstrated the expression of five TRPC channel proteins (TRPC1, TRPC3, TRPC4, TRPC5 and TRPC6) in patient biopsies and cell lines derived from glioma patients (Tables 1). Activation of TRPC channels typically occurs through the triggering of phospholipase C and this signaling cascade is the target of a number of G-protein-coupled receptors and receptor tyrosine kinases. An important form of

TRP channel	Function/s	References
TRPC1	Chemotaxis in response to EGF stimulation	Sontheimer, 2010
	Calcium signaling during cytokinesis (Multinucleated-giant cells), stimulates proliferation	Bomben & Sontheimer, 2018 Bomben & Sontheimer, 2010
	Up-regulates hypoxia-induced VEGF expression	Wang et al., 2009
	Histamine-induced Ca(2+) entry	Barajas et al., 2008
TRPC3	Ca(2+) influx, PAR-1-mediated astrocytic activation	Nakao et al., 2008
	[Ca(2+)]$_i$ signaling	Grimaldi et al., 2003
TRPC4	Histamine-induced Ca(2+) entry	Barajas et al., 2008
TRPC6	Increase intracellular Ca(2+) induced by PDGF, stimulates G2/M phase transition and clonogenic ability; increases tumor volume in a subcutaneous mouse model of xenografted human tumors and decreases mean survival in mice in an intracranial model	Ding et al., 2010
	Increases [Ca(2+)]$_i$ elevation coupled to NFAT activation; stimulates hypoxia-induced Notch1-driven growth, invasion and angiogenesis	Chigurupati et al., 2010
TRPV1	Ca(2+) influx, p38MAPK-dependent apoptosis	Amantini et al., 2007
TRPV2	Inhibition of cell survival and proliferation, increase sensitivity to Fas-induced apoptosis in an ERK-dependent manner	Nabissi et al., 2010
TRPM2	ROS-induced cell death	Ishii et al., 2007
TRPM8	Increases intracellular Ca(2+), BK channel activity, cell migration	Wondergem et al., 2008 Wondergem & Bartley, 2009

Table 1. Expression and function of TRP channels in human gliomas

TRPC activation has been shown downstream of the epidermal growth factor receptor (EGFR) (Odell et al.,2005) that is the major growth factor receptor activated in malignant gliomas. Indeed, mutated or amplified EGFR is often observed in malignant gliomas and has been associated with the increased cell proliferation seen in them (Bryant et al., 2004). In Cos-7 cells, EGFR activation causes phosphorylation of TRPC4 and results in channel insertion into the plasma membrane (Odell et al., 2005). Additionally, knockdown of TRPC4 in human corneal epithelial cells suppresses epidermal growth factor (EGF)-induced cell proliferation, again linking proliferation to TRPC channels (Yang et al., 2005). Among TRPC channels, TRPC6 and TRPC1 seem to play a major role in the control of cell cycle and glioma cell proliferation. Functional TRPC6 channels were overexpressed in human U251, U87, and T98G glioma cell lines. Moreover, increased TRPC6 expression was found in GBM biopsies compared with normal brain tissue, suggesting a role for TRPC6 in malignant growth of gliomas *in vitro* and *in vivo* (Ding et al., 2010). TRPC6 channels have been implicated in cell proliferation and hypertrophic gene expression through the activation of the calcineurin-nuclear factor of activated T-cell (NFAT) pathway in normal (K. Kuwahara et al., 2006; Onohara et al., 2006) and malignant cells (Bomben & Sontheimer, 2008). Because glioma cells lack the expression of voltage-gated calcium channels (Kunzelmann, 2005) and Ca(2+) signaling promotes G_1/S phase transition and cell cycle progression in a variety of cell types (Lipskaia & Lopré, 2004; M. Kuwahara et al., 2006), the TRPC6-mediated sustained elevation of $[Ca(2+)]_i$ and calcineurin-NFAT pathway activation is vital for the proliferation and malignant growth of gliomas under hypoxia. Consistently, inhibition of hypoxia-induced TRPC6 expression causes a dramatic decrease in NFAT activation (Bucholz & Ellenrieder, 2007). In glioma cells, inhibition of TRPC6 activity or expression by using a dominant-negative mutant TRPC6 (DNC6) or RNA interference, respectively, attenuated the increase in intracellular Ca(2+) induced by platelet-derived growth factor (PDGF), suppressed cell growth and clonogenic ability, induced cell cycle arrest at the G2/M phase, and enhanced the antiproliferative effect of ionizing radiation. Cyclin-dependent kinase 1 (CdK1) activation and cell division cycle 25 homolog C (Cdc25) expression regulated the DNC6-induced cell cycle arrest. Inhibition of TRPC6 activity also significantly reduced tumor volume in a subcutaneous mouse model of xenografted human tumors and increased mean survival in mice in an intracranial model (Ding et al., 2010). In addition to TRPC6 a role for TRPC3 in glioma cell proliferation has been suggested. The TRPC3 channel has been found to cause intracytoplasmic calcium oscillations in rat glial cells (Grimaldi et al., 2003). In rat cortical astrocytes, thrombin via Ca(2+) signal, induces TRPC3 upregulation and enhanced proliferation, and these effects were inhibited by TRPC3 blockers and siTRPC3 RNA (Shirakawa et al., 2010). Ca(2+) mobilization mediated by TRPC3 is associated with thrombin-induced morphological changes in human astrocytoma cells (Nakao et al., 2008). Glioblastoma multiforme proliferates extensively and cells often undergo incomplete cell divisions, resulting in multinucleated cells. Cytokinesis, which begins at the onset of anaphase, is the division of remaining cytoplasmic substances in the cell, aside from the nuclear events of mitosis (Glotzer, 2005; Eggert et al., 2006). Recent evidence (Bomben & Sontheimer, 2010) indicated that the functional loss of TRPC1 channels involved in agonist-induced calcium entry and reloading of intracellular Ca(2+) stores disrupts glioma cytokinesis leading to bizarre and greatly enlarged multinucleated glioma cells (GMGCs) showing slow growth (Palma et al., 1989). Pharmacological inhibition of TRPC1 expression using the continuously administration for up to 4 days of the chronic inhibitor of TRPC channels, SKF96365, or TRPC1 suppression using a doxycycline inducible shRNA knockdown approach, causes loss of functional channels and store-operated calcium entry in glioma cells, and a significant decrease of tumor size, respectively. This effect is associated with reduced cell proliferation and, frequently, with incomplete cell division due to arrest at the G_2/M phase of the cell cycle (Stark & Taylor, 2006). Cytokinesis is typically described with two key components being the central spindle and the contractile ring. RhoA guanosine triphosphatase GTPase is one key player in contractile ring formation, which is important for actin nucleation and myosin activation (Bement et al., 2006). Recently reports have indicated an association between TRPC1 and RhoA (Mehta et al., 2003) and independently of TRPC6 and RhoA in certain cell types (Singh et al., 2007). Finally, receptors belonging to the TRPV channel family have been found to inhibit *in vitro* glioma cell proliferation. In this regard, we have recently reported that TRPV2 mRNA was expressed in benign astrocyte tissues, and its expression progressively declined in high-grade glioma tissues as histological grade increased. TRPV2 negatively controls glioblastoma survival and proliferation. In U87 glioma cells, silencing of TRPV2 by RNA interference (siRNA) affects several genes controlling cell cycle and proliferation (Nabissi et al., 2010). Down-regulation of CD95/Fas and parallel up-regulation of CCNE1, CDK2, E2F1, Raf-1 gene expression was observed in siTRPV2-U87 glioma cells as respect to controls. Moreover, TRPV2 knock-out increased glioblastoma proliferation and survival in an ERK-dependent manner. Inhibition of ERK activation by treatment of siRNA-TRPV2 U87 glioma cells with the specific MEK-1 inhibitor PD98059, promoted Fas expression and restored Akt/PKB pathway activation leading to reduced cell survival and proliferation (Nabissi et al., 2010). Conversely, TRPV2 transfection of primary MZC glioblastoma cells also reduced glioma viability and proliferation (Nabissi et al., 2010).

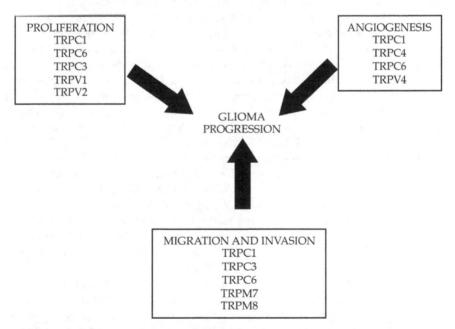

Fig. 2. TRP and glioma progression. In each square are represented the members of the TRP family, that are involved in the main processes driving glioma progression.

3. Role of TRPC and TRPV channels in hypoxia-induced angiogenesis of human gliomas: Role for VEGF and angiopoietin-1

Tumor microvessels are highly tortuous with sluggish flow and diminished gradient for oxygen delivery and increased susceptibility to thrombosis and microhemorrages. The

GBM microvasculature provides little support in oxygen/nutrient delivery, paradoxically contributing to exacerbate a metabolic mismatch between supply and demand leading to progressive hypoxia and eventually necrosis. In addition with the poor vascular architecture, endothelial cells associated with tumor vasculature fail to form tight junctions and have few associated pericytes or astrocytic foot processes leaving the integrity of the brain blood barrier compromised. This process requires that endothelial cells respond to a variety of extracellular signals that activate receptors responsible for growth and differentiation. VEGF (Vascular Endothelial Growth Factor), and Angiopoietin are key molecules in the promotion of angiogenesis via activation of the VEGFR (VEGF Receptor), and Tyrosine kinase with immunoglobulin-like and EGF-like domains 1 (TIE) expressed on vascular endothelial cells (Lutsenko et al., 2003). The Ca(2+) is another important second messenger and its entry through plasma membrane affects the angiogenesis. VEGF causes an increase in intracellular Ca(2+) concentration in cultured endothelial cells (Criscuolo et al., 1989) through both intracellular Ca(2+) release and extracellular Ca(2+) entry (Brock et al., 1991; Faehling et al., 2001; Wu et al., 1999; Cheng et al., 2006) and up-regulates vascular permeability (Criscuolo et al., 1988). Many of its physiological functions are dependent on Ca(2+) influx (Kawasaki et al., 2000; Faehling et al., 2002) through a store-independent mechanism (Pocock et al., 2000). Vascular permeability has been shown to be dependent on calcium influx, possibly through a TRPC-mediated channels. In particular, recent data indicate that TRPC6 represent an obligatory component of cation channels required for the VEGF-mediated increase in cytosolic calcium and subsequent downstream signaling that leads to processes associated with angiogenesis. The TRPC6 channel can be activated by VEGF. Overexpression of a dominant negative TRPC6 construct in human microvascular endothelial cells (HMVECs) inhibited the VEGF-mediated increase in cytosolic calcium, migration, sprouting, and proliferation. In contrast, overexpression of a wild-type TRPC6 construct increased the proliferation and migration of HMVECs (Hamdollah Zadeh et al., 2008). Inhibition of TRPC6 in HUVECs by pharmacological or genetic approaches arrested HUVECs at G2/M phase and suppressed VEGF-induced HUVEC proliferation and tube formation. Furthermore, inhibition of TRPC6 abolished VEGF-, but not FGF-induced angiogenesis in the chick embryo chorioallantoic membrane (Ge et al., 2009). Reduced oxygen availability (hypoxia) in the surrounding brain tissue is a major driving force behind GBM angiogenesis, and the low oxygen environment in the brain is positively related to GBM aggressiveness and poor prognosis (Hockel & Vaupel, 2001). The role of Hif-1α in tumor growth and invasion is well established (Semenza, 2003). Hif-1α protein was undetectable or low in glioma cells under normoxic conditions but increased markedly under hypoxia. Similarly, Notch1 activity was low in glioma cells but was elevated after the hypoxic switch. In addition to Notch1, other components of the Notch pathway were increased in glioma cells after the hypoxic switch. Specifically, the levels of Jagged-1 protein were increased under hypoxia. The molecular signals that link tissue hypoxia, Hif-1α activation to tumor angiogenesis are poorly understood. In glioma cells, the expression of TRPC6 is low or undetectable. Hypoxia by inducing Notch1 activation, increases TRPC6 expression in primary GBM and cell lines derived from GBM. Knockdown of TRPC6 expression inhibits glioma angiogenesis. Moreover, pharmacologic inhibition of Notch blocked the hypoxia-induced upregulation of TRPC6. The induction of TRPC6 expression in gliomas was TRPC subtype specific because other members of TRPC subfamily were unaffected. Although

Notch signaling is critical for TRPC6 upregulation, it remains to be determined whether the Notch pathway directly or indirectly, through cross-talk with other transcription factors (Gustafsson et al., 2005; Song et al., 2008), regulates TRPC6 transcription. TRPC6 activity is increased with EGFR activation (Odell et al., 2005), suggesting a link between growth factor response to tumor growth, and angiogenesis. Functionally, TRPC6 causes a sustained elevation of intracellular calcium that is coupled to the activation of the calcineurin-nuclear factor of activated T-cell (NFAT) pathway. Pharmacologic inhibition of the calcineurin-NFAT pathway substantially reduces hypoxia-induced glioma progression (Mosieniak et al., 1998; Chigurupati et al., 2010). The activation of TRPC6 by Galphaq induces RhoA activation and increased $[Ca(2+)]_i$ that stimulate thrombin-induced increase of actinomyosin-mediated endothelial cell contraction, cell shape change and consequently increased endothelial permeability. Inhibitor of Galphaq or phospholipase C and the Ca(2+) chelator, BAPTA-AM, abrogated thrombin-induced RhoA activation. By contrast, activation of TRPC6 by oleoyl-2-acetyl-sn-glycerol (OAG), the membrane permeable analogue of the Galphaq-phospholipase C product, diacylglycerol, induced RhoA activity. Receptor-operated Ca(2+) activation was mediated by TRPC6. Thus, TRPC6 knockdown significantly reduced Ca(2+) entry and prevented RhoA activation, myosin light chain phosphorylation, and actin stress fiber formation as well as inter-endothelial junctional gap formation in response to either OAG or thrombin (Singh et al., 2007). Lysophosphatidylcholine (lysoPC) has been also found to induce a rapid translocation of TRPC6 in endothelial cells, that triggeres calcium influx resulting in externalization of TRPC5. Activation of this novel TRPC6-TRPC5 channel cascade by lysoPC, inhibits endothelial cell migration. TRPC5 siRNA down-regulates the lysoPC-induced rise in $[Ca(2+)]_i$ and reverts the inhibition of EC migration (Chaudhuri et al., 2008), suggesting a negative role played by this channel in the regulation of EC migration. Finally, the phosphatase and tensin homologue (PTEN), has been found to serves as a scaffold for TRPC6 channel by enabling cell surface expression of the channel. Ca(2+) entry through TRPC6 induces an increase in endothelial permeability and directly promotes angiogenesis (Kini et al., 2010) (Fig 3). PTEN is a dual lipid-protein phosphatase that catalyzes the conversion of phosphoinositol 3,4,5-triphosphate to phosphoinositol 4,5-bisphosphate and thereby inhibits PI3K-Akt-dependent cell proliferation, migration, and tumor vascularization. Recently, a PTEN phosphatase-independent mechanism in regulating Ca(2+) entry through TRPC6 has been reported. PTEN tail-domain residues 394-403 permit PTEN to associate with TRPC6, and thrombin promotes this association. Deletion of PTEN residues 394-403 prevents TRPC6 cell surface expression and Ca(2+) entry (Kini et al., 2010). Other TRPC channels have been found to be involved in glioma angiogenesis. Studies in zebrafish, have demonstrated that the involvement of TRPCs channels in angiogenesis represents a reminiscent of the role of TRPC channels in axon guidance (Yu et al., 2010). Activation of TRPC1 seems to be essential for the angiogenesis *in vivo*. Knockdown of TRPC1 by antisense oligonucleotides severely disrupted angiogenic sprouting of intersegmental vessels (ISVs). *In vivo* time-lapse imaging revealed that the angiogenic defect was attributable to impairment of filopodia extension, migration, and proliferation of ISV tip cells. TRPC1 acts synergistically with VEGFA in controlling ISV growth, and appeared to be downstream to VEGFA in controlling angiogenesis (Yu et al., 2010). Recently a role for TRPC1 in hypoxia-induced VEGF expression in U87 glioma cells has been reported. TRPC1 siRNA markedly inhibits hypoxia-induced up-regulation of

VEGF mRNA and protein levels (Wang et al., 2009). TRPC1-dependent Ca(2+) influx induced by VEGF also increases endothelial permeability. Angiopoietin-1 (Ang1) that exerts a vascular endothelial barrier protective effect by blocking the action of permeability-increasing mediators such as VEGF, inhibited the VEGF-induced Ca(2+) influx and increased the endothelial permeability in a concentration-dependent manner. Ang1 interfered with downstream IP3-dependent plasmalemmal Ca(2+) entry. Anti-TRPC1 antibody (Ab) inhibited the VEGF-induced Ca(2+) entry and the increased endothelial permeability. TRPC1 overexpression in endothelial cells augmented the VEGF-induced Ca(2+) entry, and application of Ang1 opposed this effect. Consistent with the coupling hypothesis of Ca(2+) entry, Ang1 by inhibiting the association of IP3 receptor (IP3R) and TRPC1, abrogates the increase in endothelial permeability (Jho et al., 2005). Although the previously reported study has been focused on Ang1 regulation of TRPC1 activation, we cannot rule out the involvement of other relevant TRPC channels. TRPC4 acts as a functional homologue in mouse endothelia to TRPC1 in humans (Nilius et al., 2003; Tiruppathi et al., 2002). For agonist-induced Ca(2+) entry in mouse aortic endothelial cells, TRPC4 was essential as either a channel-forming subunit or a constituent required for channel activation (Freichel et al., 2001). Because TRPC1 and TRPC4 can oligomerize (Hofmann et al., 2002), it is possible that both may be needed for the VEGF-induced Ca(2+) entry. The importance of TRPC4 in regulation of endothelial permeability in mice has been reinforced by the observations that the effects of Ang1 on VEGF-induced Ca(2+) entry and permeability were mimicked by deletion of the TRPC4 gene in mice (Tiruppathi et al., 2002). Finally, VEGF-induced activation of Ca(2+) entry can also occur via TRPC6 which is activated by PLC-generated DAG (Pocock et al., 2001, 2004). TRPC4 has been also found to control thrombospondin-1 (TSP-1) secretion and angiogenesis in renal cell carcinoma (RCC) (Veliceasa et al., 2007). TRPC4 loss has been lead to impaired Ca(2+) intake, misfolding, retrograde transport and diminished secretion of antiangiogenic TSP-1, thus enabling angiogenic switch during RCC progression. TRPC4 has been recently reported to be expressed in glioma cells (Wang et al., 2009), however at present no data on the role of this channel in the inhibition of glioma angiogenesis has been provided so far. Membrane-stretch activated TRPV calcium channels have been known to mediate the orientation of endothelial cells lining blood vessels thus influencing the angiogenesis. So, TRPV4 channels expressed in the plasma membrane of capillary endothelial cells is required for mechanical-induced changes in focal adhesion assembly, cell orientation and directional migration. Recent reports indicate that activation of the mechanosensitive TRPV4 in capillary endothelial cells, stimulates phosphatidylinositol 3-kinase-dependent activation and binding of additional β1 integrin receptors, which promotes cytoskeletal remodeling and cell reorientation. Inhibition of integrin activation using blocking Abs and knock-down of TRPV4 using siRNA, suppress capillary cell reorientation. Activation of TRPV4 channels by force transfer from integrins and CD98 may enable compartmentalization of calcium signaling within focal adhesions. This early-immediate calcium signaling response required the distal region of the β1 integrin cytoplasmic tail that contains a binding site for the integrin-associated transmembrane CD98 protein, and application of external force to CD98 within focal adhesions activated the same ultra-rapid calcium signaling response (Matthews et al., 2010). Thus, mechanical forces that physically deform extracellular matrix (ECM) guide capillary cell reorientation through an "integrin-to-integrin" signaling mechanism mediated by activation of mechanically gated TRPV4 channels on the cell surface (Thodeti et al., 2009). We have recently reported the expression of TRPV4 channels in glioma cell lines (Santoni et al., 2011), however the potential role of TRPV4 in the migration of endothelial cells during glioma angionenesis is at present unknown.

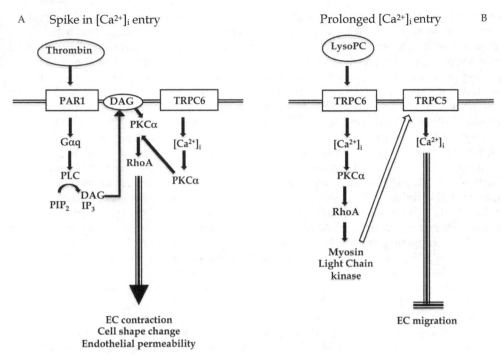

Fig. 3. Different modes of TRPC6 activation and cellular response, in glioma cells A) Spike in $[Ca^{2+}]_i$ entry induces endothelial cell (EC) contraction, cell shape and permeability; B) while prolonged $[Ca^{2+}]_i$ entry by LysoPC-induced TRPC6 activation inhibits EC migration.

4. TRPC and TRPM channels stimulate glioma cell migration and invasion

Glioblastoma multiforme is extremely invasive and consequently the clinical prognosis for patients is dismal. Invasion by glioma cells into regions of normal brain is driven by a multifactorial process involving cell interactions with ECM and with adjacent cells, as well as accompanying biochemical processes supportive of proteolytic degradation of ECM, and active cell movements (Bomben et al., 2010). These processes bear a striking resemblance to the robust inherent migration potential of glial cells during embryogenesis. Invasion and migration of glial tumors differ from other tumors where local spread is very limited and dissemination occurs hematogenously or via the lymphatic system. As they spread and form metastasis, glioma cells migrate through the narrow extracellular brain spaces often following the path of nerve fiber or blood vessels. Invading glioma cells commonly assume an elongated spindle-shaped morphology, suggesting that the cells have shrunk to fit into the narrow space into the brain (Sontheimer, 2008). Several studies have focused on the understanding of different molecular mechanisms expressed by invading tumor cells. Gliomas utilize a number of proteins and pathways to infiltrate the brain parenchyma including ion channels and calcium signaling pathways. Ion channels have recently involved in glioma invasion as a means to control cell volume or regulating Ca(2+) signaling pathways in invasive cells. Calcium signaling has been shown to play important roles in glioma cell invasion (Komuro & Kumada, 2005). Cell shrinkage by adaptation of cell size and volume to fit into narrow spaces is a prerequisite for cell movement and migration. Most immature cells that can migrate are well equipped to accumulate and release intracellular ions to shrink. How cell movement and invasion are coupled to the controlled activation of Ca(2+) channels is only partially understood (Mcferrin & Sontheimer, 2006). In glioma cells, invasion appears to involve a coordinated reduction in cell volume, which is mediated by the efflux of Cl⁻ and K⁺ through ion channels. The Cl⁻ efflux is accompanied by the movement of K⁺ ions. The principal pathway for K⁺ efflux from glioma cells appears to be via Ca(2+)-activated bradykinin (BK) channels, which have the unique ability to couple changes in intracellular Ca(2+) to changes in membrane K⁺ conductance and are expressed highly in glioma cells (Ransom & Sontheimer, 2001). In glioma cells, migration is accompanied by oscillatory changes in intracellular Ca(2+) in response to different stimuli (Grimaldi et al., 2003), which activate BK K⁺ channels, and the velocity of cell migration of glioma cells correlates with oscillatory changes in intracellular Ca(2+) concentration (Bordey et al., 2000). Among ion channels contributing to Ca(2+) signaling, cytoskeleton changes, movement and migration, the TRPM and TRPC channel families seem to play an important role. Thus, triggering of TRPM8 by the specific agonist, menthol (Wondergem & Bartley, 2009), as TRPC3 and TRPC6 (Kim et al., 2009) increases glioma cell [Ca(2+)]ᵢ that in turn activates BK channels. Thus. TRP-mediated activation of Ca(2+) influx appears to be the prerequisite for cell migration and this Ca(2+) signal is instructive with regards to cell volume changes that occur down-stream. Cell shape, adhesion and migration have been regulated by actomyosin contractility. TRPM7-like transcripts current has been identified in rat microglia (Jiang et al., 2003). TRPM7 plays a role in linking receptor-mediated signals to actomyosin remodelling and cell adhesion. Activation of TRPM7 by BK, leads to a Ca(2+) and kinase-dependent interaction with the actomyosin cytoskeleton. Overexpression of TRPM7, by increasing the intracellular Ca(2+) levels resulted in cell spreading, adhesion and formation of focal adhesions (Clark et al., 2006). The effects of TRPM7 on cell morphology is directly dependent on integrin activation or is associated to increase in cytosolic Ca(2+) concentrations that affect the actomyosin cytoskeleton. The integrin activation can lead to the remodeling of the actomyosin cytoskeleton that promotes cell spreading via outside-in signaling pathways. Alternatively, Ca(2+) is an important second messenger in actin remodeling including polymerization, severing of filaments and F-actin–membrane interactions. The TRPC channels play a role in store-operated calcium entry (SOCE), and in particular TRPC1 is involved in SOCE in glioma cells (Bomben & Sontheimer, 2010). TRPC1-dependent migration and chemotaxis have been reported in different cell types such as myoblasts (Louis et al., 2008), renal epithelial (Fabian et al., 2008) and nervous cells (Wang & Poo, 2005) (Fig.2). Recently, (Bomben & Sontheimer, 2010) showed that TRPC1 channel association with lipid rafts is essential for glioma chemotaxis in response to stimuli, such as EGF, but not chemokinesis. EGF stimulation affects both TRPC trafficking (Bezzerides et al., 2004) and activation (Beech, 2005; Liu et al., 2009), and TRPC1 channel localization to the leading edge of migrating glioma cells. TRPC1 channels co-localize with the lipid raft proteins, caveolin-1. Chemotaxis toward EGF was lost when TRPC channels were pharmacologically inhibited or by shRNA knock-down of TRPC1 channels, yet without affecting unstimulated cell motility. Lipid raft integrity was required for gliomas chemotaxis; thus disruption of lipid rafts not only impaired chemotaxis but also impaired TRPC currents and decreased store-operated calcium entry. TRPC6 is markedly up-regulated under hypoxia in a manner dependent on Notch activation. The Notch-regulated transcriptional targets that are responsible for the development of the aggressive and malignant phenotypes in GBM remain poorly characterized. Notch signaling mediates hypoxia-induced tumor migration and invasion under hypoxic environment (Sahlgren et al., 2008). TRPC6 has been found to markedly inhibited glioma cell migration and invasion in response to hypoxia by regulating actin cytoskeleton assembling and disassembling which control cell shape, allowing the cell to move along the surface. The last step of invasion requires cytoskeletal rearrangements and formation of lamillipodia and fillopodia for which the family of Rho GTPases plays an important role. Most Rho proteins, cycle between GTP-bound active and GDP-bound inactive state. From the family members, Rho stimulates formation of stress fibres and focal adhesion, Rac is required for the formation of lamellipodia and Cdc42 regulates cell polarity and fillopodia formation (Teodorczyk & Martin-Villalba, 2009). A role for TRPC6 in Rho activation and actin cytoskeleton rearrangements has been suggested (Albert & Large, 2003). The TRPC6-mediated Ca(2+) entry may contribute to invasion by promoting actin-myosin interactions and the formation and disassembly of cell-substratum adhesions that are important for glioma migration (Kim & Saffen, 2005). Moreover, a role for TRPC3 activation has been also proposed. Thus, Ca(2+) entry in type I astrocytes and rat C6 glioma cells induced by OAG was InsP3-independent and inhibited by a TRPC3 antisense (Grimaldi et al., 2003). In addition, TRPC3 is functionally involved in Ca(2+) entry and thrombin stimulated morphological changes (cell rounding) induced by PAR-1 activation in 1321N1 human astrocytoma cells (Nakao et al., 2008). Finally, GBM cells express TRPM8 mRNA and protein, and its involvement in menthol and hepatocyte growth factor/scatter factor (HGF/SF) increase of [Ca(2+)]i and glioma cell migration has been reported (Wondergem et al., 2008). Menthol a TRPM8 agonist, stimulated influx of Ca(2+), membrane current, and migration of human glioblastoma DBTRG cells. The effects on Ca(2+) and migration were enhanced by pre-treatment with HGF/SF. The effects on Ca(2+) also were greater in migrating cells compared with non-migrating cells. 2-Aminoethoxydiphenyl borate inhibited all menthol stimulations. In addition, menthol, by increasing [Ca(2+)]i, in human glioblastoma cells, resulted in activation of the large-conductance Ca(2+)-activated K+ membrane ion channels (BK channels). Kinetic analysis showed that menthol increased channel open probability and mean open frequency after 5 min, and this increase was abolished either by added paxilline, tetraethylammonium ion or by Ca(2+)-free external solution. In addition, inhibition of BK channels by paxillin reverses menthol-stimulated increase of [Ca(2+)]i and cell migration. Finally, menthol stimulated the rate of DBTRG cell migration into scratch wounds made in confluent cells, and this also was inhibited by paxilline or tetraethylammonium ion (Wondergem & Bartley, 2009). Invasion and metastasis are biologic hallmarks of malignant tumour. The invasion of ECM requires active degradation of ECM components. Tumour cells themselves secrete proteolytic enzymes (metalloproteinases, MMPs) or induce host cells to elaborate proteases (Pluda, 1997; Price et al., 1997; Liotta & Kohn, 1997). Glioma cells secrete MMPs to degradate the ECM surrounding invading cells (Levicar et al., 2003). In this regard, cannabidiol (CBD) has been found to impair the migration of U87 glioma cells in a cannabinoid receptor-independent manner (Vaccani et al., 2005), by increasing the tissue inhibitor of MMP1, (TIMP-1) (Ramer et al., 2010) and down-regulating the MMP-2 expression (Blazquez et al., 2008). Since CBD represents a specific ligand for TRPV2 (Qin et al., 2008), and being TRPV2 downregulated in the more invasive malignat gliomas (Nabissi et al., 2010), activation of this channel may represent an important target in anti-invasive chemotherapeutic strategy in GBM patients.

5. TRPV and TRPM channels trigger cell death in human glioma cells

Members of the TRPV and TRPM channels have been found to regulate apoptotic and necrotic cell death processes, respectively, as well as resistance to apoptotic stimuli in glioblastoma cells. In this regard, a role for TRPV1 in the apoptosis of glioma cells has been reported (Amantini et al., 2007). Thus, TRPV1 mRNA and protein expression was evidenced in normal astrocytes and glioma cells and tissues (Contassot et al., 2004; Amantini et al., 2007). TRPV1 expression inversely correlated with glioma grading, with a marked loss of TRPV1 expression in the majority of grade IV glioblastoma tissues. In addition, TRPV1 activation by the synthetic ligand, capsaicin (CPS) induced apoptosis of U373 glioma cells, and involved rise of Ca(2+) influx, p38MAPK activation, mitochondrial permeability transmembrane pore opening and transmembrane potential dissipation and caspase-3 activation (Amantini et al., 2007). Similarly, an other TRPV1 agonist, arachidonylethanolamide (AEA) induces apoptosis of human glioma cells in a TRPV1-dependent-manner (Contassot et al., 2004). Resistance of cancer cells to chemotherapeutic-induced cytotoxicity during tumor progression partially depends by a decrease sensitivity to CD95/Fas-induced apoptosis (Amantini et al., 2009). Induction of cell death by some cytotoxic drugs seems to depend to an intact Fas/FasL system. Tumour progression by exerting selective pressure alters Fas status and subsequently affects the sensitivity of cancer cells to chemotherapy (Sindhwani et al., 2001). Glioblastoma cells are resistant to Fas-induced cell death. We have recently reported that TRPV2 negatively controls glioblastoma survival as well as resistance to Fas/CD95-induced apoptosis in an ERK-dependent manner. Silencing of TRPV2 by RNA interference (siRNA) in U87 glioma cells down-regulated Fas/CD95 and procaspase-8 expression, and up-regulated Bcl-X$_L$ mRNA expression. Moreover, TRPV2 siRNA increased glioblastoma survival to Fas/CD95-induced apoptosis in an ERK-dependent manner (Nabissi et al., 2010). Inhibition of ERK activation by treatment of the siRNA-TRPV2 U87 glioma cells with the specific MEK-1 inhibitor PD98059, reduced Bcl-X$_L$ protein levels, promoted Fas/CD95 expression and restored Akt/PKB pathway activation leading to reduced cell survival and increased sensitivity to Fas/CD95-induced apoptosis (Nabissi et al., 2010). These events are consistent with previous evidence showing that PI3K pharmacological inhibitors inhibited calcium overload and cell death in TRPV2-transfected mouse cells (Penna et al., 2006). Consistently, TRPV2 transfection of the primary MZC glioblastoma cells also reduced glioma viability and increased spontaneous and Fas/CD95-induced apoptosis, by inducing Fas/CD95 expression (Nabissi et al., 2010). Among TRPM channels, a role for the Ca(2+) permeable TRPM2 channel in glioma cell death has been reported. Thus, insertion of TRPM2 in human A172 glioma cells enhanced cell death induced by H$_2$O$_2$ (Ishi et al., 2007).

6. TRP channels as cross-road of deregulated transcriptional activity in glioma stem like-cells

Evidence that malignant gliomas may arise from and contain a minority tumour cells with stem cell-like (GSCs) properties has been increased by the demonstration that GSCs maintain the potential for self-renewal and multi-lineage differentiation that recap the phenotype of the original glioma (Galli et al., 2004; Singh et al., 2003; Yuan et al., 2004), Since GSCs has been suggested to play an important role in glioma initiation, growth, and recurrence, it is extremely important to understand the signal pathways that contribute to their formation and maintenance, with the future aims to eliminate GSCs from the bulk tumor mass as a therapeutic strategy (Reya et al., 2001). Recent evidences adscript an emergent role of TRP channels in regulating neurogenesis (Tai et al., 2009) as well as neural differentiation (Shin et al., 2010), suggesting that deregulation of specific TRP target genes may be involved in gliomagenesis (Van Meir et al., 2010; Liu et al., 2010). In this regard, the expression of TRPV2 in normal neural stem/progenitor cells (NS/PC) from olfactory bulb and GSC lines derived from GBM patients, and a role of this TRP channel in the regulation of cellular proliferation and differentiation, have been observed (Nabissi et al., personal communication). Stem cells proliferation is maintained by a balance between proliferative and antiproliferative signals and any genetic or biochemical modifications that lead stem cells to become independent of growth signals, could induce an uncontrolled proliferation and possible tumorogenesis (Li & Neaves, 2006). GSCs divide core regulatory pathways with normal neural stem cells (NPSs), sharing developmental programs that lead NSCs to differentiate into astrocytes, oligodendrocytes and neurons (Galli et al., 2004; Singh et al., 2003), but induce in GSCs an aberrant differentiation (Cheng et al., 2010). GSCs are reported to express CD133 and nestin and to differentiate into cells expressing neuronal or glial cell markers upon growth factor depletion (Gunther et al., 2008). In addition to these NSC characteristics, glioma-derived neurospheres or CD133+ cells are tumorigenic and when transplanted into SCID mice formed secondary tumors with phenotypic and cytogenetic similarities to the patient tumor from which they were originally derived (Singh et al., 2003; Lee et al., 2006). Recent findings in GSCs demonstrated that the upregulation of classical pathways associated with neural development, as Notch, WNT, Hedgehog and TGFβ/BMT pathways (Clark et al., 2007; Silver & Steindler, 2009), induce in GSC-derived GBMs an invasive, angiogenetic, proliferative and chemoresistant phenotype (Sanai et al., 2005). So, modulation of these pathways may represent novel therapeutic approach for GBM. Notch is a family of hetero-dimeric transmembrane receptors composed of an extracellular domain responsible for ligand recognition, a transmembrane domain, and an intracellular domain involved in transcriptional regulation (Stockhausen et al., 2010). Notch proteins (and ligands)contain extracellular EGF-like repeats, which interact with the DSL domain of ligands. Activation of Notch upon ligand binding is accompanied by proteolytic processing that releases an intracellular domain of Notch (NICD) from the membrane tether. The NICD contains the RAM23 domain (RAM), which enhances interaction with the CSL protein, NLS (Nuclear Localization Signals), a CDC10/Ankyrin repeat domain ANK, which mediates interactions with CSL and other proteins, and a PEST domain rich in proline, glutamate, serine and threonine residues (Kopan, 2002). When Notch receptor is triggered by the ligands on the neighboring cells, the intracellular domain of the Notch receptor (NICD) is released from the membrane, after successive proteolytic cleavages by the γ-secretase complex. NICD then translocates into the nucleus and associates with the transcription factor RBP-J. This complex by recruiting other co-activators, stimulates the expression of downstream genes as Cyclin-D1, EGFR, and MAPK (Mitogen-Activated Protein Kinase) inducing cell proliferation, angiogenesis and chemoresistance, in GSCs (Stockhausen et al., 2010). Regarding the role of Notch signaling in GBM, gene microarray analysis have demonstrated that its expression in brain tumors correlated with good versus poor prognosis (Phillips et al., 2006). Moreover, in GBM tissue samples, high expression of Notch signal has been associated with high nestin levels, suggesting a correlation between GSCs and Notch expression (Purow et al., 2005; Lino et al.,2010; Boulay et al., 2007; Shih & Holland, 2006). Infact, Notch signaling plays a pivotal role in the maintenance of NSCs and leads to GSC-driven brain tumor development (Lino et al., 2010; Louvi & Artavanis-

Tsakonas, 2006). Recently, has been demonstrated that Notch activation is increased during hypoxia and hypoxia direct GBM to the development of an aggressive phenotype and resistance to radiation and chemotherapy (Flynn et al., 2008). Regarding the relationship between Notch signaling and TRP channels, a direct correlation has been demonstrated in human glioma cell lines where TRPC6 transcripts have been found to be increased under hypoxic condition and the involvement of Notch in hypoxia-induced TRPC6 expression in glioma has been demonstrated. Silencing of Notch1 gene inhibits TRPC6 expression suggesting that Notch1 is required for hypoxia-induced TRPC6 over-expression (Chigurupati et al., 2010). In response to hypoxia, the hypoxia inducing factors (HIF1-α and HIF-2α) are stabilized and as a consequence VEGF and TGFα are up-regulated (Birlik et al., 2006). Moreover, hypoxia-induced endothelial cell proliferation is associated with an increase of AP-1 expression, elevated store-operated calcium entry, and enhanced TRPC4 expression (Fantozzi et al., 2003), suggesting that additional TRP channels may regulate angiogenic signals (Fig.4). The interplay between GSCs and the endothelial compartement seems to be critical in gliomagenesis. Thus, GSCs closely interacting with the endothelial cells in vascular niche, promote angiogenesis through VEGF release (Bao et al., 2006a; Folkins et al., 2009). GSCs are reported to express CD133

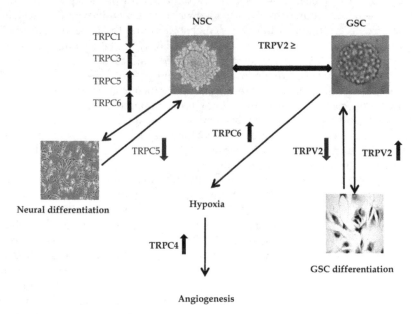

Fig. 4. The putative role of TRP channels in neural and glioma stem cell-like differentiation and angiogenesis. A schematic representation of different TRP members involved in the regulation of neuro- and glioma-genesis

and nestin (Yuan et al., 2004; Gunther et al., 2008) and have been demonstrated to have multipotent differentiative potential (Galli et al., 2004; Singh et al., 2003). Several authors have hypothesized that CD133+ tumor stem cells are the source of the recurrent tumors after treatment (Chua et al., 2008; Bleau et al., 2009) and the CD133+ cell population was enriched after radiation or chemotherapy and exhibited an increase in DNA repair capacity (Bao et al., 2006b). A series of pathways, including the Sonic hedgehog (Shh) and Notch, have been shown to be implicated in glioma's resistance to alkylating agents and/or the maintenance of brain tumor stem cells (Ulasov et al., 2011; Clement et al., 2007). Moreover, overexpression of *Dkk-1*, a gene encoding for a Wnt antagonist protein, has been shown to sensitize the U87 glioma cells to the cytotoxic effects of bis-chloronitrosourea (BCNU) and cisplatin (Shou et al., 2002). In this regard, an inverse correlation between TRPV2 and SHH and Notch pathways (Phillips et al., 2006; Nabissi et al., 2010) in regulating chemoresistance to the alkylating agent bis-chloronitrosourea (BCNU), can be supposed. TRPV2 expression progressively declined in high-grade glioma tissues as histological grade increased, while Notch and SHH signaling was activated in GBM. Knockdown of TRPV2 gene in gliomas increased the resistance to BCNU cytotoxicity which was associated with Ras/MEK/Erk and Akt overexpression in chemosensitive glioma cells, while TRPV2 overexpression augmented the chemosensitivity of resistant glioma cells to BCNU. In addition, down-regulation of TRPV2 reduced Fas expression and Fas-mediated apoptosis (Nabissi et al., 2010). Parallelely, upregulation of Notch 1, increased the resistance of glioma cell to apoptosis (Purow et al., 2005). Finally, forced Notch 1 overexpression in glioma cells increased the proliferation and the formation of nestin-positive, neurosphere-forming stem cells (Zhang et al., 2008). Overall, these data suggest that in gliomas, TRPV2 could be a downstream gene target of Notch signaling rescuing glioma cells to apoptosis and promoting cell proliferation.

7. Conclusions and prospectives

In this chapter, we have summarized current basic and translational changes and highlight the striking scientific advances regarding the expression and the function of the TRP channel family in glioma growth and progression, that promise to improve the clinical course of this lethal disease. These include a more comprisive view of the interplay between changes in TRP channel expression and functions (e.g., TRPC, TRPM and TRPV family) and alterations in transcriptional and growth factor pathways (e.g., Notch, PTEN, HIF-α, EGFR) driving the uncontrolled cellular proliferation, aberrant angiogenesis, intense migration and invasion, increased resistance to apoptosis. Clearly, the identification of cluster of TRP ion channels altered during glioma progression presents an opportunity for improving the understanding of this cancer. The progress and depth of understanding of the role of ion channels, including the TRP family in glioma, together with truly manipulable experimental models, now offer a real opportunities for the development of effective target therapy (Santoni & Farfariello, 2011). Despite significant gaps in our understanding, a wealth of information now exists about clinical and biological behaviour of these tumours, the genetic pathways involved in gliomagenesis and the nature and the role of their alterations. The challenge is now to integrate all of this knowledge in an interdisciplinary way to full understand this disease and how its heterogenicity contributes to the relatively poor therapeutic responses of GBM patients. In regard to stem cell issue, the fact that the glioma-like stem cells (GSCs) that play an important role in the development and recurrence of malignat glioma, not only express TRP channels, but also show functional alterations in their expression and transcriptional regulation, combined with the evidence that they displayed nearly identical Ca(2+) transients and pharmacological sensitivities to TRP channel antagonists (Nabissi et al., personal communication; Weick et al., 2009), may offer a new target for regulating GSC proliferation and developing novel therapeutic strategies. We are only at the begin of a new story; further studies on the expression and function of TRP channels in gliomas and GSCs must to be required to understand their contribute to malignant transformation and tumour progression, to delivery a specific target therapy in this devastating disease.

8. References

Albert, A.P. & Large, W.A. (2003). Synergism between inositol phosphates and diacylglycerol on native TRPC6-like channels in rabbit portal vein myocytes. *The Journal of Physiology*, Vol. 552, No. 3, pp. 789-795, ISSN 0022-3751

Amantini, C., Mosca, M., Nabissi, M., Lucciarini, R., Caprodossi, S., Arcella, A., Giangaspero, F. & Santoni, G. (2007). Capsaicin-induced apoptosis of glioma cells is mediated by TRPV1 vanilloid receptor and requires p38 MAPK activation. *Journal of Neurochemistry*, Vol. 102, No. 3, pp. 977-990, ISSN 0022-3042

Amantini, C., Ballarini, P., Caprodossi, S., Nabissi, M., Morelli, M.B., Lucciarini, R., Cardarelli, M.A., Mammana, G. & Santoni, G. (2009). Triggering of Transient Receptor Potential Vanilloid Type 1 (TRPV1) by Capsaicin induces Fas/CD95-mediated apoptosis of urothelial cancer cells in an ATM-dependent manner. *Carcinogenesis*, Vol. 30, No. 8, pp. 1320-1329, ISSN 0143-3334

Bao, S., Wu, Q., McLendon, R.E., Hao, Y., Shi, Q., Hjelmeland, A.B., Dewhirst, M.W., Bigner, D.D. & Rich, J.N. (2006b). Glioma stem cells promote radioresistance by preferential activation of the DNA damage response. *Nature*, Vol. 444, No. 7120, pp. 756-760, ISSN 0028-0836

Bao, S., Wu, Q., Sathornsumetee, S., Hao, Y., Li, Z., Hjelmeland, A.B., Shi, Q., McLendon, R.E., Bigner, D.D. & Rich, J.N. (2006a). Stem cell-like glioma cells promote tumor angiogenesis through vascular endothelial growth factor. *Cancer Research*, Vol. 66, No. 16, pp. 7843-7848, ISSN 0008-5472

Barajas, M., Andrade, A., Hernandez-Hernandez, O., Felix, R. & Arias-Montaño, J.A. (2008). Histamine-induced Ca2+ entry in human astrocytoma U373 MG cells: evidence for involvement of store-operated channels. *Journal of Neuroscience Research*, Vol. 86, No. 15, pp. 3456-3468, ISSN 0360-4012

Beech, D.J. (2005). TRPC1: store-operated channel and more. *Pflügers Archiv*, Vol. 451, No. 1, pp. 53-60, ISSN 0031-6768

Bement, W.M., Miller, A.L. & von Dassow, G. (2006). Rho GTPase activity zones and transient contractile arrays. *Bioessays*, Vol. 28, No. 10, pp.983-993, ISSN 0265-9247

Bezzerides, V.J., Ramsey, I.S., Kotecha, S., Greka, A. & Clapham, D.E. (2004). Rapid vesicular translocation and insertion of TRP channels. *Nature Cell Biology*, Vol. 6, No. 8, pp. 709-720, ISSN 1465-7392

Bidaux, G., Flourakis, M., Thebault, S., Zholos, A., Beck, B., Gkika, D., Roudbaraki, M., Bonnal, J.L., Mauroy, B., Shuba, Y., Skryma, R. & Prevarskaya, N. (2007). Prostate cell differentiation status determines transient receptor potential melastatin member 8 channel subcellular localization and function. *Journal of Clinical Investigation*, Vol. 117, No. 6, pp. 1647-1657, ISSN 0021-9738

Birlik, B., Canda, S. & Ozer, E. (2006). Tumour vascularity is of prognostic significance in adult, but not paediatric astrocytomas. *Neuropathology and Applied Neurobiology*, Vol. 32, No. 5, pp. 532-538, ISSN 0305-1846

Blázquez, C., Carracedo, A., Salazar, M., Lorente, M., Egia, A., González-Feria, L., Haro, A., Velasco, G. & Guzmán, M. (2008). Down-regulation of tissue inhibitor of metalloproteinases-1 in gliomas: a new marker of cannabinoid antitumoral activity? *Neuropharmacology*, Vol. 54, No. 1, pp. 235-243, ISSN 0952-2638

Bleau, A.M., Hambardzumyan, D., Ozawa, T., Fomchenko, E.I., Huse, J.T., Brennan, C.W. & Holland, E.C. (2009). PTEN/PI3K/Akt pathway regulates the side population phenotype and ABCG2 activity in glioma tumor stem-like cells. *Cell Stem Cell*, Vol. 4, No. 3, pp. 226-235, ISSN 1934-5909

Bomben, V.C. & Sontheimer, H. (2010). Disruption of Transient Receptor Potential Canonical Channel 1 causes incomplete cytokinesis and slows the growth of human malignant gliomas. *Glia*, Vol. 58, No. 10, pp. 1145-1156, ISSN 1098-1136

Bomben, V.C. & Sontheimer, H.W. (2008). Inhibition of transient receptor potential canonical channels impairs cytokinesis in human malignant gliomas. *Cell Proliferation*, Vol. 41, No. 1, pp. 98-121, ISSN 0960-7722

Bomben, V.C., Turner, K.L., Barclay, T.C. & Sontheimer, H. (2010). Transient Receptor Potential Canonical Channels are Essential for Chemotactic Migration of Human Malignant Gliomas. *Journal of Cellular Physiology* [Epub ahead of print], ISSN 1097-4652

Bordey, A., Sontheimer, H. & Trouslard, J. (2000). Muscarinic activation of BK channels induces membrane oscillations in glioma cells and leads to inhibition of cell migration. *Journal of Membrane Biology*, Vol. 176, No. 1, pp. 31-40, ISSN 0022-2631

Boulay, J.L., Miserez, A.R., Zweifel, C., Sivasankaran, B., Kana, V., Ghaffari, A., Luyken, C., Sabel, M., Zerrouqi, A., Wasner, M., Van Meir, E., Tolnay, M., Reifenberger, G. & Merlo, A. (2007). Loss of NOTCH2 positively predicts survival in subgroups of human glial brain tumors. *PLoS One*, Vol. 2, No. 6, pp. e576, ISSN 1932-6203

Brock, T.A., Dvorak, H.F. & Senger, D.R. (1991). Tumor-secreted vascular permeability factor increases cytosolic Ca^{2+} and von Willebrand factor release in human endothelial cells. *American Journal of Pathology*, Vol. 138, No. 1, pp. 213–221, ISSN 0002-9440

Bryant, J.A., Finn, R.S., Slamon, D.J., Cloughesy, T.F. & Charles, A.C. (2004). EGF activates intracellular and intercellular calcium signaling by distinct pathways in tumor cells. *Cancer Biology & Therapy*, Vol. 3, No. 12, pp. 1243-1249, ISSN 1538-4047

Buchholz,M. & Ellenrieder, V. (2007). An emerging role for Ca2+/calcineurin/NFAT siognaling in cancerogenesis. *Cell Cycle*, Vol. 6, No. 1, pp.16-19; ISSN 1551-4005

Butowiski, N.A., Sneed, P.K. & Chang, S.M. (2006). Diagnosis and treatment of recurrent high-grade astrocytoma. *Journal of Clinical Oncology*, Vol. 24, No. 8, pp. 1273-1280, ISSN 0732-183

Caprodossi, S., Lucciarini, R., Amantini, C., Nabissi, M., Canesin, G., Ballarini, P., Di Spilimbergo, A., Cardarelli, M.A., Servi, L., Mammana, G. & Santoni, G. (2008). Transient receptor potential vanilloid type 2 (TRPV2) expression in normal urothelium and in urothelial carcinoma of human bladder: correlation with the pathologic stage. *European Urology*, Vol. 54, No. 3, pp. 612–620, ISSN 0302-2838

Chaudhuri, P., Colles, S.M., Bhat, M., Van Wagoner, D.R., Birnbaumer, L. & Graham, L.M. (2008). Elucidation of a TRPC6-TRPC5 channel cascade that restricts endothelial cell movement. *Molecular Biology of the Cell*, Vol. 19, No. 8, pp. 3203-3211, ISSN 1059-1524

Cheng, H.W., James, A.F., Foster, R.R., Hancox, J.C. & Bates, D.O. (2006). VEGF activates receptor-operated cation channels in human microvascular endothelial cells.

Arteriosclerosis, Thrombosis, and Vascular Biology , Vol. 26, No. 8, pp. 1768–1776, ISSN 10795642

Cheng, L., Bao, S. & Rich, J.N. (2010). Potential therapeutic implications of cancer stem cells in glioblastoma. *Biochemical Pharmacology,* Vol. 80, No. 5, pp. 654-665, ISSN 0006-2952

Chigurupati, S., Venkataraman, R., Barrera, D., Naganathan, A., Madan, M., Paul, L., Pattisapu, J.V., Kyriazis, G.A., Sugaya, K., Bushnev, S., Lathia, J.D., Rich, J.N. & Chan, S.L. (2010). Receptor Channel TRPC6 Is a Key Mediator of Notch-Driven Glioblastoma Growth and Invasiveness. *Cancer Research,* Vol. 70, No. 1, pp. 418-427, ISSN 0008-5472

Chua, C., Zaiden, N., Chong, K.H., See, S.J., Wong, M.C., Ang, B.T. & Tang, C. (2008). Characterization of a side population of astrocytoma cells in response to temozolomide. *Journal of Neurosurgery,* Vol. 109, No. 5, pp. 856-866, ISSN 0022-3085

Clark, K., Langeslag, M., van Leeuwen, B., Ran, L., Ryazanov, A.G., Figdor, C.G., Moolenaar, W.H., Jalink, K. & van Leeuwen, F.N. (2006). TRPM7, a novel regulator of actomyosin contractility and cell adhesion. *The EMBO Journal,* Vol. 25, No. 2, pp. 290-301, ISSN 1469-221X

Clark, P.A., Treisman, D.M., Ebben, J. & Kuo, J.S. (2007). Developmental signaling pathways in brain tumor-derived stem-like cells. *Developmental Dynamics,* Vol. 236, No. 12, pp. 3297-3308, ISSN 1097-0177

Clement, V., Sanchez, P., de Tribolet, N., Radovanovic, I. & Ruiz i Altaba, A. (2007). HEDGEHOG-GLI1 signaling regulates human glioma growth, cancer stem cell self-renewal, and tumorigenicity. *Current Biology,* Vol. 17, No. 2, pp. 165-172, ISSN 0960-9822

Contassot, E., Wilmotte, R., Tenan, M., Belkouch, M.C., Schnüriger, V., de Tribolet, N., Burkhardt, K. & Dietrich, P.Y. (2004). Arachidonylethanolamide induces apoptosis of human glioma cells through vanilloid receptor-1. *Journal of Neuropathology & Experimental Neurology,* Vol. 63, No. 9, pp. 956–963, ISSN 0022-3069

Criscuolo, G.R., Lelkes, P.I., Rotrosen, D. & Oldfield, E.H. (1989). Cytosolic calcium changes in endothelial cells induced by a protein product of human gliomas containing vascular permeability factor activity. *Journal of Neurosurgery,* Vol. 71, No. 6, pp. 884-891, ISSN 0022-3050

Criscuolo, G.R., Merrill, M.J. & Oldfield, E.H. (1988). Further characterization of malignant glioma-derived vascular permeability factor. *Journal of Neurosurgery,* Vol. 69, No. 2, pp. 254-262, ISSN 0022-3050

Ding, X., He, Z., Zhou, K., Cheng, J., Yao, H., Lu, D., Cai, R., Jin, Y., Dong, B., Xu, Y. & Wang, Y. (2010). Essential role of TRPC6 channels in G2/M phase transition and development of human glioma. *Journal of the National Cancer Institute,* Vol. 102, No. 14, pp. 1052-1068, ISSN 0027-8874

Duncan, L.M., Deeds, J., Hunter, J., Shao, J., Holmgren, L.M., Woolf, E.A., Tepper, R.I. & Shyjan, A.W. (1998). Down-regulation of the novel gene melastatin correlates with potential for melanoma metastasis. *Cancer Research,* Vol. 58, No. 7, pp. 1515–1520, ISSN 0008-5472

Eggert, U.S., Mitchinson, T.J. & Field, C.M. (2006). Animal cytokinesis: from parts list to mechanism. *Annual Review of Biochemistry,* Vol. 75, pp. 543-566, ISSN 0066-4154

Fabian, A., Fortmann, T., Dieterich, P., Riethmuller, C., Schon, P., Mally, S., Nilius, B. & Schwab, A. (2008). TRPC1 channels regulate directionality of migrating cells. *Pflügers Archives,* Vol. 457, No. 2, pp. 475-484, ISSN 0031-6768

Faehling, M., Koch, E.D., Raithel, J., Trischler G. & Waltenberger, J. (2001). Vascular endothelial growth factor-A activates Ca^{2+}-activated K$^+$ channels in human endothelial cells in culture. *The International Journal of Biochemistry & Cell Biology*, Vol. 33, No. 4, pp. 337–346, ISSN 1357-2725

Faehling, M., Kroll, J., Fohr, K.J., Fellbrich, G., Mayr, U., Trischler, G. & Waltenberger, J. (2002). Essential role of calcium in vascular endothelial growth factor A-induced signaling: mechanism of the antiangiogenic effect of carboxyamidotriazole. *The FASEB Journal*, Vol. 16, No. 13, pp. 1805–1807, ISSN 0892-6638

Fantozzi, I., Zhang, S., Platoshyn, O., Remillard, C.V., Cowling, R.T. & Yuan, J.X. (2003). Hypoxia increases AP-1 binding activity by enhancing capacitative Ca2+ entry in human pulmonary artery endothelial cells. *American Journal of Physiology Lung Cellular and Molecular Physiology*, Vol. 285, No. 6, pp. L1233-1245, ISSN 1522-1504

Flynn, J.R., Wang, L., Gillespie, D.L., Stoddard, G.J., Reid, J.K., Owens, J., Ellsworth, G.B., Salzman, K.L., Kinney, A.Y. & Jensen, R.L. (2008). Hypoxia-regulated protein expression, patient characteristics, and preoperative imaging as predictors of survival in adults with glioblastoma multiforme. *Cancer*, Vol. 113, No. 5, pp. 1032-1042, ISSN 1097-0142

Folkins, C., Shaked, Y., Man, S., Tang, T., Lee, C.R., Zhu, Z., Hoffman, R.M. & Kerbel, R.S. (2009). Glioma tumor stem-like cells promote tumor angiogenesis and vasculogenesis via vascular endothelial growth factor and stromal-derived factor 1. *Cancer Research*, Vol. 69, No. 18, pp. 7243-7251, ISSN 0008-5472

Freichel, M., Suh, S.H., Pfeifer, A., Schweig, U., Trost, C., Weissgerber, P., Biel, M., Philipp, S., Freise, D., Droogmans, G., Hofmann, F., Flockerzi, V. & Nilius, B. (2001). Lack of an endothelial store-operated Ca2+ current impairs agonist-dependent vasorelaxation in TRP4−/− mice. *Nature Cell Biology*, Vol. 3, No. 2, pp. 121–127, ISSN 1465-7392

Furnari, F.B., Fenton, T., Bachoo, R.M., Mukasa, A., Stommel, J.M., Stegh, A., Hahn, W.C., Ligon, K.L., Louis, D.N., Brennan, C., Chin, L., DePinho, R.A. & Cavenee, W.K. (2007). Malignant astrocytic glioma: genetics, biology, and paths to treatment. *Genes & Devevelopment*, Vol. 21, No. 21, pp. 2683-2710, ISSN 0890-9369

Galli, R., Binda, E., Orfanelli, U., Cipelletti, B., Gritti, A., De Vitis, S., Fiocco, R., Foroni, C., Dimeco, F. & Vescovi, A. (2004). Isolation and characterization of tumorigenic, stem-like neural precursors from human glioblastoma. *Cancer Research*, Vol. 64, No. 19, pp. 7011-21, ISSN 0008-5472

Ge, R., Tai, Y., Sun, Y., Zhou, K., Yang, S., Cheng, T., Zou, Q., Shen, F. & Wang, Y. (2009). Critical role of TRPC6 channels in VEGF-mediated angiogenesis. *Cancer Letters*, Vol. 283:, No. 1, pp. 43–51, ISSN 0304-3835

Gkika, D. & Prevarskaya, N. (2009). Molecular mechanisms of TRP regulation in tumor growth and metastasis. *Biochimica et Biophysica Acta*, Vol. 1793, No. 6, pp. 953–958, ISSN 0304-4165

Glotzer, M. (2005). The molecular requirements for cytokinesis. *Science*, Vol. 307, No. 5716, pp.1735-1739, ISSN 0036-8075

Grimaldi, M., Maratos, M. & Verma, A. (2003). Transient receptor potential channel activation causes a novel form of [Ca 2+]I oscillations and is not involved in capacitative Ca 2+ entry in glial cells. *Journal of Neuroscience*, Vol. 23, No. 11, pp. 4737-4745, ISSN 0270-6474

Gunther, H.S., Schmidt, N.O., Phillips, H.S., Kemming, D., Kharbanda, S., Soriano, R., Modrusan, Z., Meissner, H., Westphal, M. & Lamszus, K. (2008). Glioblastoma-

derived stem cell-enriched cultures form distinct subgroups according to molecular
and phenotypic criteria. *Oncogene*, Vol. 27, No. 20, pp. 2897-2909, ISSN 0950-9232

Gustafsson, M.V., Zheng, X., Pereira, T., Gradin, K., Jin, S., Lundkvist, J., Ruas, J.L.,
Poellinger, L., Lendahl, U. & Bondesson, M. (2005). Hypoxia requires notch
signaling to maintain the undifferentiated cell state. *Developmental Cell*, Vol. 9, No.
5, pp. 617–628, ISSN 1534-5807

Hamdollah Zadeh, M.A., Glass, C.A., Magnussen, A., Hancox, J.C. & Bates, D.O. (2008).
VEGF-mediated elevated intracellular calcium and angiogenesis in human
microvascular endothelial cells in vitro are inhibited by dominant negative TRPC6.
Microcirculation, Vol. 15, No. 7, pp. 605–614, ISSN 1549-8719

Höckel, M. & Vaupel, P. (2001). Biological consequences of tumor hypoxia. *Seminars in
Oncology*, Vol.28, No.2 Suppl8, pp. 36–41, ISSN 0093-7754

Hofmann, T., Schaefer, M., Shultz, G. & Gudermann, T. (2002). Subunit composition of
mammalian transient receptor potential channels in living cells. *Proceedings of the
National Academy of Sciences of the United States of America*, Vol. 99, No. 11, pp. 7461–
7466, ISSN 0027-8424

Huncharek, M. & Muscat, J. (1998). Treatmentbof recurrent high grade astrocytoma; results
of a systematic review of 1,415 patients. *Anticancer Research*, Vol. 18, No. 2B,
pp.1303-1311, ISSN 0250-7005

Ishii, M., Oyama, A., Hagiwara, T., Miyazaki, A., Mori, Y., Kiuchi, Y. & Shimizu, S. (2007).
Facilitation of H2O2-induced A172 human glioblastoma cell death by insertion of
oxidative stress-sensitive TRPM2 channels. *Anticancer Research*, Vol. 27, No. 6B, pp.
3987-3992, ISSN 0250-7005

Jho, D., Mehta, D., Ahmmed, G., Gao, X.P., Tiruppathi, C., Broman, M. & Malik, A.B. (2005).
Angiopoietin-1 opposes VEGF-induced increase in endothelial permeability by
inhibiting TRPC1-dependent Ca$_2$ influx. *Circulation Research*, Vol. 96, No. 12, pp.
1282–1290, ISSN 0009-7330

Jiang, X., Newel, E.W. & Schlichter, L.C. (2003). Regulation of a TRPM7-like current in rat
brain microglia. *Journal of Biological Chemistry*, Vol. 278, No. 44, pp. 42867-42876,
ISSN 0021-9258

Kanamori, M., Kawaguchi, T., Nigro, J.M., Feuerstein, B.G., Berger, M.S., Miele, L. & Pieper,
R.O. (2007). Contribution of Notch signaling activation to human glioblastoma
multiforme. *Journal of Neurosurgery*, Vol. 106, No. 3, pp. 417–427, ISSN 0022-3085

Kawasaki, J., Hirano, K., Hirano, M., Nishimura, J., Nakatsuka, A., Fujishima, M. & Kanaide,
H. (2000). Dissociation between the Ca$^{(2+)}$ signal and tube formation induced by
vascular endothelial growth factor in bovine aortic endothelial cells. *European
Journal of Pharmacology*, Vol. 398, No. 1, pp. 19–29, ISSN 0014- 2999

Kim, J.Y. & Saffen, D. (2005). Activation of M1 muscarinic acetylcholine receptors stimulates
the formation of a multiprotein complex centered on TRPC6 channels. *Journal of
Biological Chemistry*, Vol. 280, No. 36, (September 2005), pp. 32035-47, ISSN 0021-
9258

Kim, E.Y., Alvarez-Baron, C.P. & Dryer, S.E. (2009). Canonical transient receptor potential
channel (TRPC)3 and TRPC6 associate with large-conductance Ca2+-activated K+
(BKCa) channels: role in BKCa trafficking to the surface of cultured podocytes.
Molecular Pharmacology, Vol. 75, No. 3, pp. 466-477, ISSN 0026-895X

Kini, V., Chavez, A. & Mehta, D. (2010). A new role for PTEN in regulating transient
receptor potential canonical channel 6-mediated Ca2+ entry, endothelial

permeability, and angiogenesis. *Journal of Biological Chemistry*, Vol. 285, No. 43, pp. 33082-33091, ISSN 0021-9258

Kiselyov, K., Soyombo, A. & Muallem, S. (2007). TRPpathies. *The Journal of Physiology*, Vol. 578, No. 3, pp. 641–653, ISSN 0022-3751

Komuro, H. & Kumada, T. (2005). Ca2+ transients control CNS neuronal migration. *Cell Calcium*, Vol. 37, No. 5, pp. 387-393, ISSN 0143-4160

Kopan, R. (2002). Notch: a membrane-bound transcription factor. *Journal of Cell Science*, Vol. 115, No. 6, pp. 1095-1097, ISSN 0021-9533

Kunzelmann, K. (2005). Ion channels and cancer. *Journal of Membrane Biology*, Vol. 205, No. 3, pp. 159-173, ISSN 0022-2631

Kuwahara, K., Wang, Y., McAnally, J., Richardson, J.A., Bassel-Duby, R., Hill, J.A. & Olson, E.N. (2006). TRPC6 fulfills a calcineurin signaling circuit during pathologic cardiac remodeling. *Journal of Clinical Investigation*, Vol. 116, No. 12, pp. 3114-3126, ISSN 0021-9738

Kuwahara, M. & Kuwahara, M. (2006). Store-mediated calcium entry in pleural mesothelial cells. *European Journal of Pharmacology*, Vol. 542, No. 1-3, pp. 16-21, ISSN 0014- 2999

Lee, J., Kotliarova, S., Kotliarov, Y., Li, A., Su, Q., Donin, N.M., Pastorino, S., Purow, B.W., Christopher, N., Zhang, W., Park, J.K. & Fine, H.A. (2006). Tumor stem cells derived from glioblastomas cultured in bFGF and EGF more closely mirror the phenotype and genotype of primary tumors than do serum-cultured cell lines. *Cancer Cell*, Vol. 9, No. 5, pp. 391-403, ISSN 1535-6108

Levicar, N., Nuttall, R.K. & Lah, T.T. (2003). Proteases in brain tumour progression. *Acta Neurochirurgica*, Vol. 145, No. 9, pp. 825-838, ISSN 0001-6268

Li, L. & Neaves, W.B. (2006). Normal stem cells and cancer stem cells: the niche matters. *Cancer Research*, Vol. 66, No. 9, pp. 4553-4557, ISSN 0008-5472

Lino, M.M., Merlo, A. & Boulay, J.L. (2010). Notch signaling in glioblastoma: a developmental drug target? *BMC Medicine*, Vol. 8, pp. 72, ISSN 1741-7015

Liotta, L.A. & Kohn, E.C. (1997). Invasion and metastasis. In: *Cancer Medicine 4th ed.*, Holland, J.F., Bast, R.C.J., Morton, D.L., Frei, III E., Kufe, D.W. & Weichselbaum, R.R. (Ed.), pp. 165-180, Williams & Wilkins, ISBN 0-683-04095-2, Baltimore

Lipskaia, L. & Lompré, A.M. (2004). Alteration in temporal kinetics of Ca2+ signaling and control of growth and proliferation. *Biology of the Cell*, Vol. 96, No. 1, pp. 55-68, ISSN 0248-4900

Liu, D., Yang, D., He, H., Chen, X., Cao, T., Feng, X., Ma, L., Luo, Z., Wang, L., Yan, Z., Zhu, Z. & Tepel, M. (2009). Increased transient receptor potential canonical type 3 channels in vasculature from hypertensive rats. *Hypertension*, Vol. 53, No. 1, pp. 70-76, ISSN 0263-6352

Liu, Y., Shete, S., Hosking, F., Robertson, L., Houlston, R. & Bondy, M. (2010). Genetic advances in glioma: susceptibility genes and networks. *Current Opinion in Genetics & Development*, Vol. 20, No. 3, pp. 239-44, ISSN 0959-437X

Louis, M., Zanou, N., Van Schoor, M. & Gailly, P. (2008). TRPC1 regulates skeletal myoblast migration and differentiation. *Journal of Cell Science*, Vol. 121, pp. 23-29, ISSN 0021-9533

Louvi, A. & Artavanis-Tsakonas, S. (2006). Notch signalling in vertebrate neural development. *Nature Reviews Neuroscience*, Vol. 7, No. 2, pp. 93-102, ISSN 1471-0048

Lutsenko, S.V., Kiselev, S.M. & Severin, S.E. (2003). Molecular mechanisms of tumor angiogenesis. *Biochemistry (Moscow)*, Vol. 68, No. 3, pp. 286-300, ISSN: 0006-2979

Malarkey, E.B., Ni, Y. & Parpura, V. (2008). Ca2+ entry through TRPC1 channels contributes to intracellular Ca2+ dynamics and consequent glutamate release from rat astrocytes. *Glia*, Vol. 56, No. 8, pp- 821-835, ISSN 1098-1136

Matthews, B.D., Thodeti, C.K., Tytell, J.D., Mammoto, A., Overby, D.R. & Ingber, D.E. (2010). Ultra-rapid activation of TRPV4 ion channels by mechanical forces applied to cell surface beta1 integrins. *Integrative Biology*, Vol. 2, No. 9, pp. 435-42, ISSN 0973-8363

Mcferrin, M.B. & Sontheimer, H. (2006). A role for ion channels in glioma cell invasion. *Neuron Glia Biology*, Vol. 2, No. 1, pp. 39-49, ISSN 1740-925X

Mehta, D., Ahmmed, G.U., Paria, B., Holinstat, M., Voyno-Yasenetskaya, T., Tiruppathi, C., Minshall, R.D. & Malik, A.B. (2003). RhoA interaction with inositol 1,4,5-trisphosphate receptor and transient receptor potential channel-1 regulates Ca2+ entry. Role in signaling increased endothelial permeability. *Journal of Biological Chemistry*, Vol. 278, No. 35, pp. 33492–33500, ISSN 0021-9258

Montell, C. (2003). Thermosensation: hot findings make TRPNs very cool. *Current Biology*, Vol. 13, No. 12, pp. R476–R478, ISSN 0960-9822

Mosieniak, G., Pyrzynska, B. & Kaminska, B. (1998). Nuclear factor of activated T cells (NFAT) as a new component of the signal transduction pathway in glioma cells. *Journal of Neurochemistry*, Vol. 71, No. 1, pp. 134-141, ISSN 0022-3042

Nabissi, M., Morelli, M.B., Amantini, C., Farfariello, V., Ricci-Vitiani, L., Caprodossi, S., Arcella, A., Santoni, M., Giangaspero, F., De Maria, R. & Santoni, G. (2010). TRPV2 channel negatively controls glioma cell proliferation and resistance to Fas-induced apoptosis in ERK-dependent manner. *Carcinogenesis*, Vol. 31, No. 5, pp. 794-803, ISSN 0143-3334

Nakao, K., Shirakawa, H., Sugishita, A., Matsutani, I., Niidome, T., Nakagawa, T. & Kaneko, S. (2008). Ca2+ mobilization mediated by transient receptor potential canonical 3 is associated with thrombin-induced morphological changes in 1321N1 human astrocytoma cells. *Journal of Neuroscience Research*, Vol. 86, No. 12, pp. 2722-2732, ISSN 0360-4012

Nilius, B., Droogmans, G. & Wondergem, R. (2003). Transient receptor potential channels in endothelium: solving the calcium entry puzzle? *Endothelium*, Vol. 10, No. 1, pp. 5-15, ISSN 1029-2373

Nilius, B., Owsianik, G., Voets, T. & Peters, J.A. (2007). Transient receptor potential cation channels in disease. *Physiological Reviews*, Vol. 87, No. 1, pp. 165–217, ISSN 0031-9333

Odell, A.F., Scott, J.L. & Van Helden D.F. (2005). Epidermal growth factor induces tyrosine phosphorylation, membrane insertion, and activation of transient receptor potential channel 4. *Journal of Biological Chemistry*, Vol. 280, No. 45, pp. 37974-37987, ISSN 0021-9258

Onohara, N., Nishida, M., Inoue, R., Kobayashi, H., Sumimoto, H., Sato, Y., Mori, Y., Nagao, T. & Kurose, H. (2006). TRPC3 and TRPC6 are essential for angiotensin II-induced cardiac hypertrophy. *EMBO Journal*, Vol. 25, No. 22, pp. 5305-5316, ISSN 1469-221X

Palma, L., Celli, P., Maleci, A., Di Lorenzo, N. & Cantore, G. (1989). Malignant monstrocellular brain tumours. A study of 42 surgically treated cases. *Acta Neurochirurgica*, Vol. 97, No. 1-2, pp. 17-25, ISSN 0001- 6268

Penna, A., Juvin, V., Chemin, J., Compan, V., Monet, M. & Rassendren, F.A. (2006). PI3-kinase promotes TRPV2 activity independently of channel translocation to the plasma membrane. *Cell Calcium*, Vol. 39, No. 6, pp. 495-507, ISSN 0143-4160

Phillips, H.S., Kharbanda, S., Chen, R., Forrest, W.F., Soriano, R.H., Wu, T.D., Misra, A., Nigro, J.M., Colman, H., Soroceanu, L., Williams, P.M., Modrusan, Z., Feuerstein, B.G. & Aldape, K. (2006). Molecular subclasses of high-grade glioma predict prognosis, delineate a pattern of disease progression, and resemble stages in neurogenesis. *Cancer Cell*, Vol. 9, No. 3, pp. 157-173, ISSN 1535-6108

Pluda, J.M. (1997). Tumor-associated angiogenesis: mechanisms, clinical implications, and therapeutic strategies. *Seminars in Oncology*, Vol. 24, No. 2, pp. 203-218, ISSN 0093-7754

Pocock, T.M., Williams, B., Curry, F.E. & Bates, D.O. (2000). VEGF and ATP act by different mechanisms to increase microvascular permeability and endothelial [Ca(2+)](i). *American Journal of Physiology Heart and Circulatory Physiology*, Vol. 279, No. 4, pp. H1625-1634, ISSN 0363-6135

Pocock, T.M. & Bates, D.O. (2001). In vivo mechanisms of vascular endothelial growth factor-mediated increased hydraulic conductivity of Rana capillaries. *The Journal of Physiology*, Vol. 534, No. 2, pp. 479–488, ISSN 0022-3751

Pocock, T.M., Foster, R.R. & Bates, D.O. (2004). Evidence of a role for TRPC channels in VEGF-mediated increased vascular permeability in vivo. *American Journal of Physiology Heart and Circulatory Physiology*, Vol. 286, No. 3, pp. H1015–H1026, ISSN 0363-6135

Prevarskaya, N., Zhang, L. & Barritt, G. (2007). TRP channels in cancer. *Biochimica and Biophysica*, Vol. 1772, No. 8, pp. 937–946, ISSN 0006-3002

Price, J.T., Bonovich, M.T. & Kohn, E.C. (1997). The biochemistry of cancer dissemination. *Critical Reviews in Biochemistry and Molecular Biology*, Vol. 32, No. 3, pp. 175–253, ISSN 1040-9238

Purow, B.W., Haque, R.M., Noel, M.W., Su, Q., Burdick, M.J., Lee, J., Sundaresan, T., Pastorino, S., Park, J.K., Mikolaenko, I., Maric, D., Eberhart, C.G. & Fine, H.A. (2005). Expression of Notch-1 and its ligands, Delta-like-1 and Jagged-1, is critical for glioma cell survival and proliferation. *Cancer Research*, Vol. 65, No. 6, pp. 2353-2363, ISSN 0008-5472

Qin, N., Neeper, M.P., Liu, Y., Hutchinson, T.L., Lubin, M.L. & Flores, C.M. (2008). TRPV2 is activated by cannabidiol and mediates CGRP release in cultured rat dorsal root ganglion neurons. *Journal of Neuroscience*, Vol. 28, No. 24, pp. 6231-6238, ISSN 0270-6474

Ramer, R., Merkord, J., Rohde, H. & Hinz, B. (2010). Cannabidiol inhibits cancer cell invasion via upregulation of tissue inhibitor of matrix metalloproteinases-1. *Biochemical Pharmacology*, Vol. 79, No. 7, pp. 955-966, ISSN 0006-2952

Ransom, C.B. & Sontheimer, H. (2001). BK channels in human glioma cells. *Journal of Neurophysiology*, Vol. 85, No. 2, pp. 790-803, ISSN 0022-3077

Reya, T., Morrison, S.J., Clarke, M.F. & Weissman, I.L. (2001). Stem cells, cancer, and cancer stem cells. *Nature*, Vol. 414, No. 6859, pp. 105-111, ISSN 0028-0836

Sahlgren, C., Gustafsson, M.V., Jin, S., Poellinger, L. & Lendahl, U. (2008). Notch signaling mediates hypoxia-induced tumor cell migration and invasion. *Proceedings of the National Academy of Sciences of the United States of America*, Vol. 105, No. 17, pp. 6392–6397, ISSN 0027-8424

Sanai, N., Alvarez-Buylla, A. & Berger, M.S. (2005). Neural stem cells and the origin of gliomas. *The New England Journal of Medicine*, Vol. 353, No. 8, pp. 811-822, ISSN 0028-4793

Santoni, G., Farfariello, V. & Amantini, C. (2011). TRPV Channels in Tumor Growth and Progression. *Advances in Experimental Medicine and Biology*, Vol. 704, pp. 947-967, ISSN 0065-2598

Santoni, G. & Farfariello, V. (2011). TRP Channels and Cancer: New Targets for Diagnosis and Chemotherapy. *Endocrine, Metabolic & Immune Disorders- Drug Targets*, Vol. 11, No. 1, pp. 54-57, ISSN 1871-5303

Schönherr, R. (2005). Clinical relevance of ion channels for diagnosis and therapy of cancer. *Journal of Membrane Biology*, Vol. 205, No. 3, pp. 175-184, ISSN 0022-2631

Schwartzbaum, J.A., Fischer, J.L., Aldape, K.D. & Wrensch,M. (2006). Epiodemiology and molecular pathology of glioma. *Nature Clinical Practice Neurology*, Vol. 2, No. 9, pp. 494-503, ISSN 1745-8358

Semenza, G.L. (2003). Targeting HIF-1 for cancer therapy. *Nature Reviews Cancer*, Vol. 3, No. 10, pp. 721–732, ISSN 1474-175X

Shih, A.H. & Holland, E.C. (2006). Notch signaling enhances nestin expression in gliomas. *Neoplasia*, Vol. 8, No. 12, pp. 1072-1082, ISSN 1522-8002

Shin, H.Y., Hong, Y.H., Jang, S.S., Chae, H.G., Paek, S.L., Moon, H.E., Kim, D.G., Kim, J., Paek, S.H. & Kim, S.J. (2010). A role of canonical transient receptor potential 5 channel in neuronal differentiation from A2B5 neural progenitor cells. *PLoS One*, Vol. 5, No. 5, pp. e10359, ISSN 1932-6203

Shirakawa, H., Nakagawa, T. & Kaneko, S. (2010). Pathophysiological roles of transient receptor potential channels in glial cells. *Yakugaku Zasshi*, Vol. 130, No. 3, pp. 281-287, ISSN 0031-6903

Shou, J., Ali-Osman, F., Multani, A.S., Pathak, S., Fedi, P. & Srivenugopal, K.S. (2002). Human Dkk-1, a gene encoding a Wnt antagonist, responds to DNA damage and its overexpression sensitizes brain tumor cells to apoptosis following alkylation damage of DNA. *Oncogene*, Vol. 21, No. 6, pp. 878-889, ISSN 0950-9232

Silver, D.J. & Steindler, D.A. (2009). Common astrocytic programs during brain development, injury and cancer. *Trends in Neurosciences*, Vol. 32, No. 6, pp. 303-311, ISSN 0166-2236

Sindhwaani, P., Hampton, J.A., Baig, M.M., Keck, R. & Selman, S.H. (2001). Curcumin prevents intravesical tumor implantation of the MBT-2 tumor cell line in C3H mice. *Journal of Urology*, Vol. 166, No. 4, pp. 1498-501, ISSN 0022-5347

Singh, I., Knezevic, N., Ahmmed, G.U., Kini, V., Malik, A.B. & Mehta, D. (2007). $G\alpha_q$-TRPC6-mediated Ca^{2+} Entry Induces RhoA Activation and Resultant Endothelial Cell Shape Change in Response to Thrombin. *The Journal of Biological Chemistry*, Vol. 282, No. 11, pp. 7833-7843, ISSN 0021-9258

Singh, S.K., Clarke, I.D., Terasaki, M., Bonn, V.E., Hawkins, C., Squire, J. & Dirks, P.B. (2003). Identification of a cancer stem cell in human brain tumors. *Cancer Research*, Vol. 63, No. 18, pp. 5821-5828, ISSN 0008-5472

Song, L.L., Peng, Y., Yun, J., Rizzo, P., Chaturvedi, V., Weijzen, S., Kast, W.M., Stone, P.J., Santos, L., Loredo, A., Lendahl, U., Sonenshein, G., Osborne, B., Qin, J.Z., Pannuti, A., Nickoloff, B.J. & Miele, L. (2008). Notch-1 associates with IKKα and regulates IKK activity in cervical cancer cells. *Oncogene*, Vol. 27, No. 44, pp. 5833–5844, ISSN 0950-9232

Sontheimer, H. (2008). An Unexpected Role for Ion Channels in Brain Tumor Metastasis. *Experimental Biology and Medicine (Maywood)*, Vol. 233, pp. 779-791, ISSN 1573-8221

Sontheimer, H. (2010). An unexpected role for ion channels in brain tumor metastasis. *Experimental Biology and Medicine*, Vol. 233, No. 7, pp. 779-791, ISSN 1535-3702

Stark, G.R. & Taylor, W.R. (2006). Control of the G2/M transition. *Molecular Biotechnology*, Vol. 32, No. 3, pp. 227-248, ISSN 1073-6085

Stockhausen, M.T., Kristoffersen, K. & Poulsen, H.S. (2010). The functional role of Notch signaling in human gliomas. *Neuro-Oncology*, Vol. 12, No. 2, pp. 199-211, ISSN 0167 -594X

Tai, Y., Feng, S., Du, W. & Wang, Y. (2009). Functional roles of TRPC channels in the developing brain. *Pflügers Archiv*, Vol. 458, No. 2, pp. 283-289, ISSN 0031-6768

Teodorczyk, M. & Martin-Villalba, A. (2009). Sensing Invasion: Cell Surface Receptors Driving Spreading of Glioblastoma. *Journal of Cellular Physiology*, Vol. 222, No. 1, pp. 1-10, ISSN 1097-4652

Thebault, S., Flourakis, M., Vanoverberghe, K., Vandermoere, F., Roudbaraki, M., Lehen'kyi, V., Slomianny, C., Beck, B., Mariot, P., Bonnal, J.L., Mauroy, B., Shuba, Y., Capiod, T., Skryma, R. & Prevarskaya, N. (2006). Differential role of transient receptor potential channels in Ca2+ entry and proliferation of prostate cancer epithelial cells. *Cancer Research*, Vol. 66, No. 4, pp. 2038–2047, ISSN 0008-5472

Thodeti, C.K., Matthews, B., Ravi, A., Mammoto, A., Ghosh, K., Bracha, A.L. & Ingber, D.E. (2009). TRPV4 channels mediate cyclic strain-induced endothelial cell reorientation through integrin-to-integrin signaling. *Circulation Research*, Vol. 104, No. 9, pp. 1123-30, ISSN 0009-7330

Tiruppathi, C., Freichel, M., Vogel, S.M., Paria, B.C., Mehta, D., Flockerzi, V. & Malik, A.B. (2002). Impairment of store-operated Ca2+ entry in TRPC4−/− mice interferes with increases in lung microvascular permeability. *Circulation Research*, Vol. 91, No. 1, pp. 70–76, ISSN 0009-7300

Tsavaler, L., Shapero, M.H., Morkowski, S. & Laus, R. (2001). Trp-p8, a novel prostate-specific gene, is up-regulated in prostate cancer and other malignancies and shares high homology with transient receptor potential calcium channel proteins. *Cancer Research*, Vol. 61, No. 9, pp. 3760–3769, ISSN 0008-5472

Ulasov, I.V., Nandi, S., Dey, M., Sonabend, A.M. & Lesniak, M.S. (2011). Inhibition of Sonic hedgehog and Notch pathways enhances sensitivity of CD133(+) glioma stem cells to temozolomide therapy. *Molecular Medicine*, Vol. 17, No. 1-2, pp. 103-112, ISSN 1076-1551

Vaccani, A., Massi, P., Colombo, A., Rubino, T. & Parolaro, D. (2005). Cannabidiol inhibits human glioma cell migration through a cannabinoid receptor-independent mechanism. *British Journal of Pharmacology*, Vol. 144, No. 8, pp. 1032-1036, ISSN 1476- 5381

Van Meir, E.G., Hadjipanayis, C.G., Norden, A.D., Shu, H.K., Wen, P.Y. & Olson, J.J. (2010). Exciting new advances in neuro-oncology: the avenue to a cure for malignant glioma. *CA Cancer Journal for Clinicians*, Vol. 60, No. 3, pp. 166-193, ISSN 0007-9235

Veliceasa, D., Ivanovic, M., Hoepfner, F.T., Thumbikat, P. Volpert, O.V. & Smith, N.D. (2007). Transient potential receptor channel 4 controls thrombospondin-1 secretion and angiogenesis in renal cell carcinoma. *FEBS Journal*, Vol. 274, No. 24, pp. 6365-6377, ISSN 1742-464X

Wang, G.X. & Poo, M.M. (2005). Requirement of TRPC channels in netrin-1-induced chemotropic turning of nerve growth cones. *Nature*, Vol. 434, No. 7035, pp. 898-904, ISSN 0028-0836

Wang, B., Li, W., Meng, X. & Zou, F. (2009). Hypoxia up-regulates vascular endothelial growth factor in U-87 MG cells: involvement of TRPC1. Neuroscience Letters ISSN 0304-3940

Weick, J.P., Austin Johnson, M. & Zhang, S.C. (2009). Developmental regulation of human embryonic stem cell-derived neurons by calcium entry via transient receptor potential channels. *Stem Cells*, Vol. 27, No. 12, pp. 2906-2916, ISSN 1549-4918

Wisnoskey, B.J., Sinkins, W.G. & Schilling, W.P. (2003). Activation of vanilloid receptor type 1 in the endoplasmic reticulum fails to activate store-operated Ca2+ entry. *Biochemical Journal*, Vol. 372, No. 2, pp. 517-528, ISSN 0264-6021

Wissenbach, U., Niemeyer, B.A., Fixemer, T., Schneidewind, A., Trost, C., Cavalie, A., Reus, K., Meese, E., Bonkhoff, H. & Flockerzi, V. (2001). Expression of CaT-like, a novel calcium-selective channel, correlates with the malignancy of prostate cancer. *Journal of Biological Chemistry*, Vol. 276, No. 22, pp. 19461-19468, ISSN 0021-9258

Wondergem, R. & Bartley, J.W. (2009). Menthol increases human glioblastoma intracellular Ca2+, BK channel activity and cell migration. *Journal of Biomedical Science*, Vol. 16, No. 1, pp. 90, ISSN 1021- 7770

Wondergem, R., Ecay, T.W., Mahieu, F., Owsianik, G. & Nilius, B. (2008). HGF/SF and menthol increase human glioblastoma cell calcium and migration. *Biochemical and Biophysical Research Communications*, Vol. 372, No. 1, pp. 210-215, ISSN 0006-291X

Wu, H.M., Yuan, Y., Zawieja, D.C., Tinsley, J. & Granger, H.J. (1999). Role of phospholipase C, protein kinase C, and calcium in VEGF-induced venular hyperpermeability. *American Journal of Physiology*, Vol. 276, No. 2, pp. H535-H542, ISSN 0363-6135

Xin, H., Tanaka, H., Yamaguchi, M., Takemori, S., Nakamura, A. & Kohama, K. (2005). Vanilloid receptor expressed in the sarcoplasmic reticulum of rat skeletal muscle. *Biochemical and Biophysical Research Communications*, Vol 332, No. 3, pp. 756-762, ISSN 0006-291X

Xu, X.Z., Moebius, F., Gill, D.L. & Montell, C. (2001). Regulation of melastatin, a TRP-related protein, through interaction with a cytoplasmic isoform. *Proceedings of the National Academy of Sciences of the United States of America*, Vol. 98, No. 19, pp. 10692-10697, ISSN 0027-8424

Yang, H., Mergler, S., Sun, X., Wang, Z., Lu, L., Bonanno, J.A., Pleyer, U. & Reinach, P.S. (2005). TRPC4 knockdown suppresses epidermal growth factor-induced store-operated channel activation and growth in human corneal epithelial cells. *Journal of Biological Chemistry* Vol. 280, No. 37, pp. 32230-32237, ISSN 0021-9258

Yu, P.C., Gu, S.Y., Bu, J.W. & Du, J.L. (2010). TRPC1 is essential for in vivo angiogenesis in zebrafish. *Circulation Research*, Vol. 106, No. 7, pp. 1221-1232, ISSN 0009-7330

Zhang, X.P., Zheng, G., Zou, L., Liu, H.L., Hou, L.H., Zhou, P., Yin, D.D., Zheng, Q.J., Liang, L., Zhang, S.Z., Feng, L., Yao, L.B., Yang, A.G., Han, H. & Chen, J.Y. (2008). Notch activation promotes cell proliferation and the formation of neural stem cell-like colonies in human glioma cells. *Molecular and Cellular Biochemistry*, Vol. 307, No. 1-2, pp. 101-108, ISSN 0300-8177

8

Role of the Centrosomal MARK4 Protein in Gliomagenesis

Ivana Magnani, Chiara Novielli and Lidia Larizza
Università degli Studi di Milano
Italy

1. Introduction

Human gliomas are the most frequent tumours of the central nervous system (Kleihues & Cavenee, 2000). They are of neuroectodermal origin and present as different histological types and malignancy grades (Louis et al., 2007).

According to the WHO (world health organization) system, astrocytoma, oligodendroglioma and mixed oligoastrocytoma are classified as differentiated gliomas, while anaplastic glioma and glioblastoma show increasing grades of malignancy (Box 1).

HUMAN GLIOMAS ARE A HETEROUGENEOUS GROUP OF GLIAL NEOPLASMS:

astrocytoma ⎫
oligodendroglioma ⎬ differentiated gliomas
mixed oligoastrocytoma ⎭
anaplastic glioma   different grades of malignancy
glioblastoma   grade IV

Box 1.

Gliomas are composed of different cell types displaying, even within low-grade tumours, a wide spectrum of heterogeneity regarding morphology, genotype, invasive potentiality, and treatment sensitivity (Noble & Dietrich, 2004). The development and progression of glioma malignancies is driven by accumulation of genomic alterations, including both mutations and chromosomal instability (CIN).

2. Chromosomal instability (CIN) in glioma

CIN refers to the rate of lost or gained chromosomes and/or structural chromosome anomalies and ploidy changes during cell divisions (Geigl et al., 2008; Lengauer et al., 1998). Structural chromosome anomalies (translocations, deletions, insertions, inversion and additions) may be balanced or unbalanced and involve one or more chromosomes (Bayani et al., 2007). Chromosomal instability in glioma is mainly characterized by aneuploidy (Bigner et al., 1988; Hecht et al., 1995; Jenkins et al., 1989; Lindstrom et al., 1991; Magnani et al., 1994; Park et al., 1995; Thiel et al., 1992) affecting in particular glioblastoma, the most malignant glioma. Gliomas frequently display near-diploid (2n+/-) and/or near-tri-tetraploid (3n+/-)/(4n+/-) karyotypes, implicating aberrant mitotic divisions, in addition to chromosomal rearrangements. Highly polyploid subpopulations and the presence of apoptotic nuclei are also reported (Figures 1a-d).

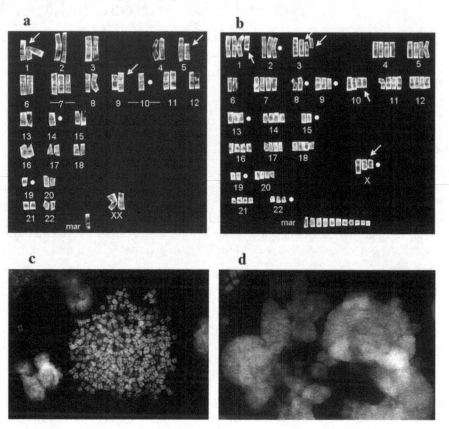

Fig. 1. (a) The G-banded, near diploid karyotype of MI-4 GBM (glioblastoma multiforme) cell line (Magnani et al., 1994), showing trisomy of chromosome 7, monosomy of chromosome 10 and a complex rearrangement involving chromosomes 1, 9 and 19. (b) The G-banded, near tetraploid karyotype of MI-4 cell line, displaying several chromosome losses and structural rearrangements including marker chromosomes. (c) Representative polyploid metaphase from MI-60 GBM cell line, characterized by a high frequency of hyperdiploid cells. (d) Apoptotic and large nuclei of MI-60 cell line.

Low-grade astrocytomas and oligodendrogliomas (WHO grades I-II) show a number of chromosome aberrations quite low. When present, they involve the gain of chromosome 7, the loss of chromosomes 10, 22 and one sex chromosome (see Figures 1a, b), while structural changes affect in particular 1p (Figure 2a) and 9p (Figure 2b) chromosome arms.
These chromosome abnormalities are qualitatively similar to those found in anaplastic astrocytoma (WHO grade III) and glioblastoma (WHO grade IV), but their frequency is

increased in the latter and multiple chromosomal rearrangements are also present. The finding of common abnormalities associated to both low- and high-grade glioma has suggested a progressive chromosomal evolution during tumour growth (Bigner et al., 1988; Jenkins et al., 1989; Magnani et al., 1994; Thiel et al., 1992) even though it has been demonstrated that a subset of glioblastomas arises clonally *de novo*, further emphasizing the genetic heterogeneity of glioma (Kleihues & Ohgaki, 2000; von Deimling et al., 1993). Given that numerical CIN features many cancer cells, it has been hypothesized that it may have a primary role in tumorigenesis (Duesberg et al., 2006; Weaver et al., 2007). Recently it has been shown that the main pathway to aneuploidy in cancer cells is triggered by extra centrosomes that, increasing improper merotelic attachments of kinetochores to spindle microtubules, cause chromosome mis-segregation (Meraldi et al., 2002) (Figure 3) (see Box 3 for centrosomes and Box 4 for mitotic spindle).

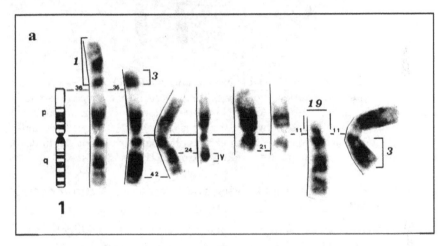

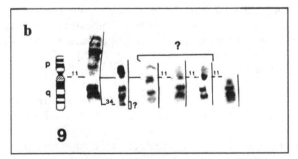

Fig. 2. (a) Chromosome 1 rearrangements of both p and q arms observed in different glioma cell lines by G-banding. (b) Rearrangements of chromosome 9p, sharing the loss of p21 band, observed in different glioblastoma cell lines by G-banding.

At early mitosis, the merotelic orientation escapes the spindle mitotic checkpoint thus representing the major mechanism of chromosome mis-segregation in non-cancer cells. Usually these errors are corrected before cells enter anaphase, to preserve genome stability (Cimini et al., 2004).

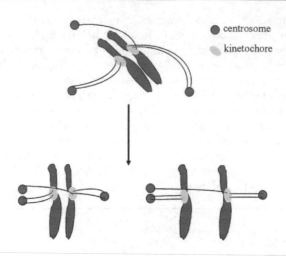

Fig. 3. Proposed events of lagging chromosomes in cancer cells with extra centrosomes through merotelic kinetochore orientation. (top) In the presence of extra centrosomes (three instead of two, as example), merotelic kinetochore orientation may occur: one kinetochore is bound by spindle microtubules from two centrosomes (right) instead of just one (left). (bottom) As cells move to mitosis and cluster extra centrosomes in a bipolar spindle, many attachment errors persist into anaphase, leading to lagging chromosomes.

3. Tetraploidy, centrosome amplification and spontaneous chromosomal instability in glioma

A relationship between extra centrosomes and the formation of multipolar spindles in cancer cells has been proposed by different authors (Basto et al., 2008; Cimini et al., 2004; Saunders, 2005; Sluder & Nordberg, 2004). Multipolarity in cancer cells is considered an essential transient stage prior to clustering extra centrosomes in a bipolar fashion (Brinkley, 2001). Multiple centrosomes have been detected in many types of cancer cells including glioma (Figure 4) and strongly linked to aneuploidy in a variety of studies (D'Assoro et al., 2002; Ganem et al., 2009; Ghadimi et al., 2000; Katsetos et al., 2006; Lingle et al., 2002; Magnani et al., 2009; Pihan et al., 1998).

A positive linear correlation between the percentage of cells with supernumerary centrosomes and the extent of aneuploidy within a panel of glioblastoma cell lines is shown in Figure 5.

In tumour development, aneuploidy is frequently preceded by tetraploidy, often with prolonged tetraploid precancerous status, a feature that makes it of central importance to cancer research (Margolis et al., 2003). It has been proposed that failure of cytokinesis is a key step in the formation of tetraploid karyotypes and in tumour initiation (Fujiwara et al., 2005). A tetraploid cell inherits twice the normal complement of centrosomes, a condition assessed to generate chromosomes mis-segregation in subsequent cell divisions (Ganem et al., 2007). However, tetraploid cells are observed in some normal tissues including liver and heart, indicating that cytokinesis is physiologically regulated. The possible fate of a tetraploid progeny is shown in Figure 6.

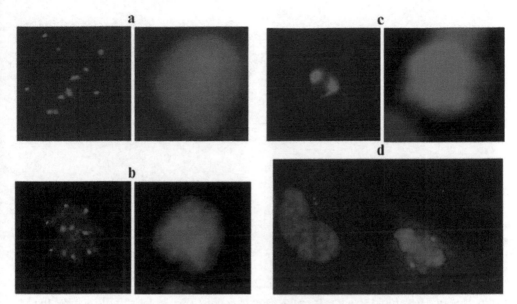

Fig. 4. Immunofluorescence with anti-γtubulin antibody (red) of representative glioblastoma cell lines, showing (a) multiple centrosomes; (b) multipolar spindles; (c) a mitotic bipolar spindle in which centrosomes are larger than the normal one (likely extra centrosomes clustered into two spindle poles), a condition that favours mitotic stability and neoplastic growth; (d) normal centrosomes and a mitotic bipolar spindle configuration. The nuclei are counterstained with DAPI (4′,6-di amidino-2-phenyl indole) (blue).

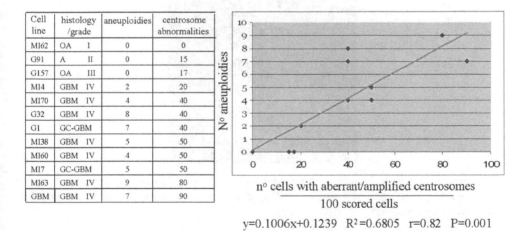

Cell line	histology /grade		aneuploidies	centrosome abnormalities
MI62	OA	I	0	0
G91	A	II	0	15
G157	OA	III	0	17
MI4	GBM	IV	2	20
MI70	GBM	IV	4	40
G32	GBM	IV	8	40
G1	GC-GBM		7	40
MI38	GBM	IV	5	50
MI60	GBM	IV	4	50
MI7	GC-GBM		5	50
MI63	GBM	IV	9	80
GBM	GBM	IV	7	90

$$\frac{n° \text{ cells with aberrant/amplified centrosomes}}{100 \text{ scored cells}}$$

$y=0.1006x+0.1239 \quad R^2=0.6805 \quad r=0.82 \quad P=0.001$

Fig. 5. Regression analysis between aneuploidies and centrosome aberrations in glioma cell lines, showing a statistically significant positive correlation. OA: oligoastrocytomas; A: astrocytomas; GBM: glioblastoma multiforme; GC-GBM: giant cell-GBM.

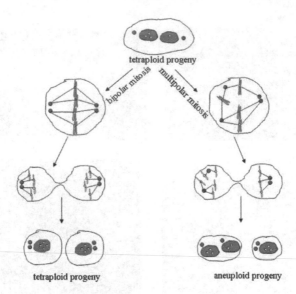

Fig. 6. Fate of a tetraploid cell: if extra centrosomes coalesce, a bipolar spindle assures the progeny maintains a tetraploid set, while lack of this *escamotage* gives rise to aneuploid progeny through a multipolar mitosis.

Binucleated tetraploid cells with multiple centrosomes are frequently observed in glioma cell lines, as illustrated by a representative image in Figure 7.

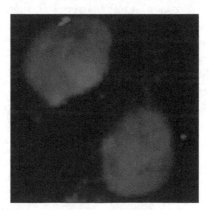

Fig. 7. Immunofluorescence with anti-γtubulin antibody (red) of a binucleated, tetraploid-derived glioblastoma cell line, showing coalesced centrosomes in one (left) of the two nuclei. Nuclei are counterstained with DAPI (blue).

To measure the occurrence of DNA damage in once-divided binucleated (BN) cells, the cytokinesis-block micronucleus cytome (CBMN Cyt) assay, an established biomarker to detect spontaneous genomic instability (Fenech, 2007), can be used. Application of CBMN Cyt to a series of glioma cell lines evidenced a high rate of micronuclei (MNi), a biomarker of chromosome breakage and/or whole chromosome loss, and chromosome aberrations such as nucleoplasmic bridges (NPBs), a biomarker of DNA misrepair and/or telomere end-fusions determining the furrow regression, and nuclear buds (NBUDSs), a biomarker of elimination of amplified DNA and/or DNA repair complexes (Figure 8a, b).

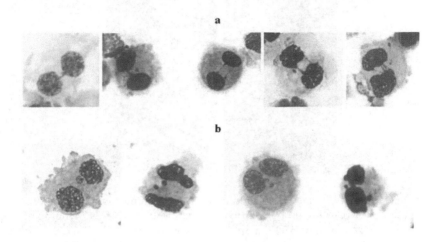

Fig. 8. Photomicrographs of glioma cell lines showing (a) typical binucleated cells with nucleoplasmic bridges and (b) binucleated cells with micronuclei and nuclear buds.

Thus, binucleated tetraploid cells may be transmitted to the progeny and enhance subsequent rounds of aberrant mitosis.

4. Cytogenomics of gliomas

Chromosomal instability can be detected by different techniques, including conventional karyotyping, fluorescence *in situ* hybridization (FISH), spectral karyotyping (SKY) and array-based comparative genomic hybridization (aCGH) analyses.

The classic assay to monitor and quantify chromosome aberrations is karyotyping (see Figure 2).

The *in situ* hybridization technique with fluorescently labelled probes targeting specific chromosomes is commonly applied on fixed glioma cells, allowing the analysis of chromosomes of interest cell by cell. Examples of FISH analysis in glioma cell lines are shown in Figure 9.

Aneuploidies are rapidly detectable by interphase FISH as well as by quantification of micronuclei formed by chromosomes that lagged behind during a previous mitosis (Figure 10).

The technique of array-CGH is considered the most powerful tool for identifying copy number changes of genetic material, since it combines high resolution and large scale genomic analysis, characteristics that are not combined by conventional approaches. Since it allows a quantification of amplifications and deletions, pointing through human genome databases directly to the affected genes, aCGH technology is more and more used in the study of tumours for the identification of potentially causative cancer genes.

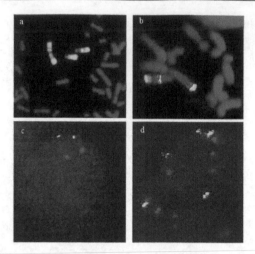

Fig. 9. Partial karyotype of MI-4 GBM cell line displaying chromosome 1 alterations by (a) whole chromosome 1 painting probe and (b) dual colour FISH of YACs 745h6, spanning the 1p36.3 breakpoint (green), and 957f12, mapping to 1p36.1 (red), showing a transposition of 1p36.1 material to der (1)(p22). DNA is counterstained with DAPI (blue). Interphase dual colour FISH of RP11-111p21, mapping to 3p21 control clone (red), and RP11-172g5, mapping to 3q26.3 (green), (c) in a normal diploid cell and (d) in MI-60 GBM cell line showing amplification of the region targeted by RP22-172g5 (green).

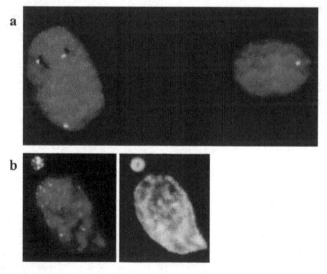

Fig. 10. (a) Interphase FISH with centromeric probes of chromosomes 7 and 10 showing trisomy of chromosome 7 and monosomy of chromosome 10 in MI-4 GBM cell line. (b) Interphase FISH with whole chromosome 19 painting probe showing a micronucleus labelled by chromosome 19 material. DNA is counterstained with DAPI (blue).

aCGH studies have been applied to gliomas and have successfully complemented previously published metaphase-CGH, SKY and LOH (loss of heterozigosity) analyses (Bredel et al, 2005; Cowell et al., 2004a, 2004b; Kitange et al., 2005; Nigro et al., 2005). Integration of the results has demonstrated an excellent correlation between the findings obtained through this genomic approach and those obtained by alternative techniques, stressing the usefulness and overall accuracy of aCGH as compared to classic previously widely employed analyses (Cowell et al., 2004a, 2004b). Comparative analysis of elaborated aCGH data led to identify copy number changes shared by various glioma grades as well as aberrations apparently related to progression to glioblastoma (GBM) (Roversi et al., 2006).

5. Non-random chromosomal aberrations in gliomas: The 19q13 abnormalities

Over the last decade, molecular approaches including mutation screening, LOH and aCGH analyses have led to identify the most frequently recurring genomic imbalances associated with each WHO glioma subtype (Kitange et al., 2005; Koschny et al., 2002; Shapiro, 2002) and hence the driver genes acting in pathways involved in glioma development, either in the initiation stages (Tp53 and Ras by PDGF-NF1) or in malignant progression (Rb-CDKN2-CDK4) (Collins, 2004; Zhu & Parada, 2002). Comprehensive genomic characterization by integrative analysis of DNA copy number, gene expression and DNA methylation aberrations in >200 glioblastomas has then refined the definition of human glioblastoma genes and core pathways (The Cancer Genome Atlas [TGCA] Research Network, 2008). Deletion of chromosome 19q is nevertheless of particular interest, as it is shared by all three glioma subtypes, occurring in approximately 75% of oligodendrogliomas, 45% of mixed oligoastrocytomas and 40% of astrocytomas (von Deimling et al., 1992, 1994), where it is associated with the transition from low-grade to anaplastic tumours (Ohgaki et al., 1995; Ritland et al., 1995; Smith et al., 1999) (Box 2).

The presence on chromosome 19 of TSGs relevant to glioma development has been inferred from LOH and cytogenetic studies

Molecular results (LOH studies)

Total loss of chromosome 19 is an unusual event in glial tumors, whereas partial genetic deletions at 19q13 are more frequently observed.

LOH on chromosome 19q13 is associated with astrocytomas, oligodendrogliomas and mixed gliomas

Cytogenetic results

Clustering of breakpoints at 19q13 is shared by all three histological types

No appreciable loss of genetic material from chromosome 19, even though microdeletions at the site of breakage cannot be ruled out

Box 2. TSGs: tumour suppressor genes.

At the cytogenetic level, chromosome 19q abnormalities are more frequently detectable in GBM than in low grade glioma, with 19q13 as the most affected region, as shown in Table1.

Case no.	Diagnosis	Partial Karyotypes
D-245	GBM	49,XY,... +19
D-250	GBM	47,XY,... +19
D-256	GBM	44,XY,... t(9;19)(p13;q13)⋆
D-290	GBM	45,X,−X,... t(1;19)(q21;q13) ⋆
D-299	GBM	46,XY,... der(19)t(17,19)(q11;q13)⋆
D-304	AMG	43,XY,... −19
D-316	GBM	46,XX,... der(19)t(10;19)(q11;q11)
D-340	GBM	66∼77,XXYY,... −19,−19,der(11)t(11q19p)×2, der(11)t(11p19q),der(11)t(11;19)(cen;q13)⋆
D-320	GBM	47,XX,... der(19)t(5;10;19)(q15−21;q11−26;q13)⋆
nr	GBM	47,XX,... der(19)t(19; ?)(q13;?)⋆
nr	GBM	79∼83,Y,... −19,−19,der(19)t(19;?)(q13.3;?)×2 ⋆
37	PA	46,... der(19)t(19;?)(q13.1,?),der(19)t(19;?)(p13.3;?)⋆
43	O	83∼88,XXYY,... −19,der(19)t(19;?)(q13.3;?)⋆
nr	GBM	39∼45,der(X)t(X;?),... der(19)t(19;?)(p13;?)
39	GBM	43,X,−X,... tdic(19;22)(p13.3;q13)⋆
33	GBM	43,XX,... +19
36	GBM	44,XY,... der(19)t(9;19)(q13;q13)⋆
37	GBM	47∼48,XY,... +19
40	AA	65∼75,XY,... +19,+19
34	GBM	44,XX,... der(19)t(12;19)(q13;q13) ⋆
nr	GBM	82∼90,... del(19)(q13.1)⋆
5 MI	AA	80∼86,XXXX,... +19
85 SJ	AA	48,XY,... +19
56 AW	GBM	47,XY,... +19
MI-4	GBM	47,XX,... der(1)t(1;19)(p10,q10)
MI-32	GBM	47,XX,... del(19)(q13.2)⋆
MI-14	GBM	86∼89,X,−X,... −19,−19
nr	O	45,XY,... der(1)t(1;19)(p11,q11)
T-60	GBM	45∼46,XX,... −19,der(19)t(19;?)
3/T110	AO	44∼46,XY,... −19
26/G227	GBM	44∼45,X,−Y,... der(19)t(14;19)(q11.2;p13.1)
31/T35	GBM	41∼45,XY,... der(19)t(14;19)(q13;q13.1)⋆
36/T66	GBM	48∼52,XY,... der(19)t(1;19)(q21;q13)⋆
nr	PXA	46,XY,... t(1;11;19)(q24;q23;q13)⋆
2	GBM	44,XX,... t(1;19)(q23;q13)⋆
nr	GBM	... t(10;19)(q24;q13)⋆

Table 1. Cytogenetic alterations of chromosome 19 in gliomas; 19q13 alterations are marked by red stars. GBM: glioblastoma multiforme; AMG: anaplastic mixed glioma; PA: pilocytic astrocytoma; O: oligodendroglioma; AA: anaplastic astrocytoma; AO: anaplastic oligodendroglioma; PXA: pleomorphic xanthoastrocytoma; nr: not reported.

Furthermore, similarly to oligodendroglioma, combined LOH of 1p and 19q was found to define a small subset of GBM patients with a significantly better survival, even if their tumours were not morphologically distinguishable from the bulk of GBMs (Schmidt et al., 2002). This finding has been translated into significant advance in the prognosis and treatment of oligodendrogliomas (van den Bent, 2004). A candidate tumour suppressor region has been assigned by LOH to 19q13.3 (Hartmann et al., 2002), but no positional or functional candidate gene in this band has yet been appointed.

Only recently an integrated analysis of human glioblastoma multiforme with the application of next generation sequencing technology disclosed a new marker associated with an increase in overall survival, represented by recurrent mutations in the active site of isocitrate dehydrogenase 1 (*IDH1*) in a large fraction of young patients with secondary GBM (Parsons et al., 2008).

6. Identification of *MARK4* gene through refined FISH mapping of 19q13 breakpoints

FISH studies of structural 19q chromosomal rearrangements in glioma (Magnani et al., 1999) and a detailed analysis of the breakpoints underlying the 19q13 alterations in the MI-4 glioblastoma cell line, led to identify a 19q13.2 intrachromosomal duplication of the MAP/microtubule affinity-regulating kinase 4 (*MARK4*) gene (Beghini et al., 2003) (Figure 11). Genomic profiling by means of array-CGH interrogation of 25 primary glioma cell lines including the MI-4 GBM cell line (Roversi et al., 2006) revealed that the BAC clone encompassing *MARK4* at 19q13.2 (Figure 12) is included in a "gain" region in a few of the tested cell lines and confirmed *MARK4* duplication in the MI-4 glioblastoma cell line (Figure 13).

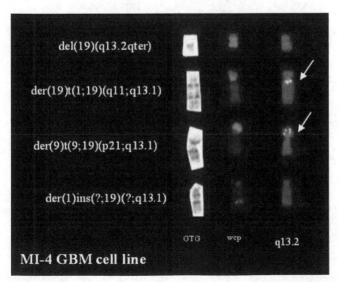

Fig. 11. 19q13.2 intrachromosomal duplication of *MARK4* in the MI-4 GBM cell line detected by G-banding and FISH analysis using a whole chromosome painting 19 probe and a *MARK4*-specific cosmid clone.

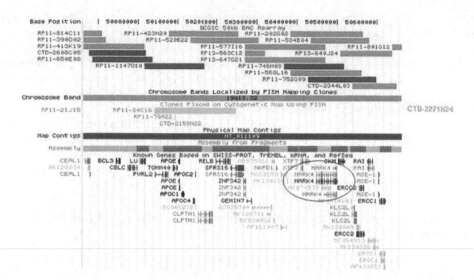

Fig. 12. *MARK4* genomic region (http://genome.ucsc.edu/). Clones of chromosome 19q full coverage (blue) overlapping *MARK4* gene are circled in red: the gene is entirely encompassed by BAC clones RP11-746H08, RP11-568L16, RP11-202G02, RP11-752G09 RP11-584B04, RP13-647G21 and partially encompassed by RP11-577I16.

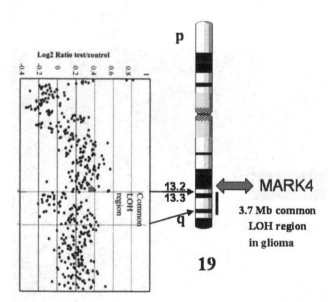

Fig. 13. (left) Chromosome 19q array-CGH of MI-4 GBM cell line, showing duplicated *MARK4* gene (red star) and the common LOH region in glioma. (right) Schematic representation of *MARK4* position on chromosome 19, at the boundary of 19q13.3 LOH region.

The combined FISH and array-CGH results provided the rationale for investigating a possible role of the serine-threonine kinase MARK4 in glioma. It's worth of note that this gene, belonging to the so called "kinome", maps at the centromeric boundary of the 19q13.3 LOH region in glioma.

7. The family of MARK kinases

MARK4 (MAP/microtubule affinity-regulating kinase 4) is a member of the MARKs family, constituted in mammals by four serine-threonine kinases (MARK1-4) which are able to phosphorylate the microtubule-associated proteins (MAPs, including Tau, MAP2, MAP4 and doublecortin) (Drewes et al., 1997). Microtubules (MTs) are cytoskeleton cylindrical structures formed by α and β tubulin dimers; dimers can quickly assemble or disassemble, causing the microtubules to grow or shorten and making them very dynamic. MAPs association stabilizes the MTs; when MARK kinases link a phosphate group to MAPs (phosphorylation), MAPs cannot associate to MTs any longer, thus microtubules become more instable and disassemble (Figure 14).

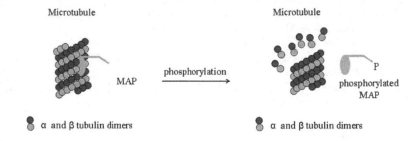

Fig. 14. Schematic representation of microtubules. Assembled α and β tubulin dimers form the microtubules, stabilized by MAP association. When MAPs are phosphorylated, they are no more able to bind microtubules, which disassemble.

7.1 MARKs protein structure

All MARK proteins have a very conserved structure, consisting of six sequence segments (Marx et al., 2010) (Figure 15):

- the N-terminal header, whose role is unknown;
- the catalytic or kinase domain, containing both the activation/inactivation loop (MARK kinases are in turn activated/inactivated by phosphorylation/dephosphorylation) and the catalytic loop, by which MARKs transfer a phosphate group to substrate proteins;
- a linker, that is a highly and negatively charged motif resembling the common docking (CD) site in MAP kinases; it may bind interactors;
- the UBA domain, a small globular domain with sequence homology to ubiquitin-associated proteins; it may exert an autoregulatory function through interaction with the catalytic domain;
- a spacer, the most variable region among MARK members; it is probably important for regulating MARK activity since it holds phosphorylation sites;
- the C-terminal tail, consisting of the kinase-associated (KA1) domain, whose function is still uncertain. It is characterized by a hydrophobic portion surrounded by positively

charged residues, which may interact with negatively charged regions of cytoskeletal proteins, MARK catalytic domain or MARK CD domain (Tochio et al., 2006) with an inhibitory effect. It has been proposed it could be involved in protein localization to the membrane, being identified as a domain that binds membrane anionic phospholipids, in particular phosphatidylserine (Moravcevic et al., 2010).

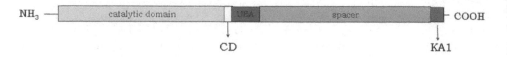

Fig. 15. Schematic representation of MARK protein structure. Boxes are not drawn to scale.

7.2 MARKs regulation
Being composed of several domains, MARK proteins are regulated by multiple mechanisms. All MARKs are activated by liver kinase B (LKB1) and MARK kinase (MARKK) by phosphorylation on the threonine residue in the activation loop (Timm et al., 2008); in addition, phosphorylation by CaMKI (calcium/calmodulin-dependent protein kinase I) activates MARK2 (Matenia & Mandelkow, 2009). On the contrary, phosphorylation by the glycogen synthase kinase 3β (GSK3β) on the serine residue in the activation loop, by aPKC (atypical protein kinase C) in the spacer region or by Pim1 kinase, down-regulates MARK activity (Matenia & Mandelkow, 2009; Timm et al., 2008). Finally, interaction between MARK catalytic domain and other proteins/MARK domains (such as 14-3-3 proteins, PAK5, MARK UBA and KA1 domains) inhibits MARK activity (Marx et al., 2010).

7.3 MARKs functions
Since MARK kinases regulate the affinity between MAPs and MTs, they are implicated in several cellular processes involving the microtubules, such as cytoskeleton dynamics, neuron motility (Schaar et al., 2004), and microtubule-dependent transport of proteins, vesicles and organelles (Mandelkow et al., 2004). Microtubules also play an important role in centrosome formation (Box 3) and in the correct distribution of the chromosomes in the two daughter cells during cell division (mitosis and cytokinesis; Box 4).

Tau is a microtubule-associated protein particularly expressed in the central nervous system. The aggregation of hyperphosphorylated *Tau* has been demonstrated to form insoluble neurofibrillary tangles (Chin et al., 2000; Gamblin et al., 2003) which are characteristic of Alzheimer's disease. MARKs role in this pathology has been evaluated in many studies, demonstrating, as an example, MARK co-localization with neurofibrillary tangles (Chin et al., 2000).

MARK2 is involved in establishing cell polarity, cooperating in the organization of the epithelial structure of liver, kidney and stomach (Cohen et al., 2004; Matenia & Mandelkow, 2009), and regulating axon formation in neuronal cells (Chen et al., 2006). Experiments in mice demonstrated that MARK2 is also implicated in many physiological functions, such as fertility, homeostasis of the immune system, memory, growth and metabolism (Bessone et al., 1999; Hurov et al., 2001; Hurov & Piwnica-Worms, 2007; Segu et al., 2008). MARK3 plays an important role in cell signaling and cell cycle control: phosphorylation of some proteins by MARK3 induces their binding to 14-3-3 proteins thus regulating many cellular pathways (Bachmann et al., 2004; Müller et al., 2001).

8. MARK4

MARK4 is the less characterized member among MARK proteins. It has been discovered by Kato and colleagues in 2001 among a few genes whose expression resulted significantly increased in hepatocarcinoma cells with elevated β-catenin levels in their nucleus (Kato et al., 2001).

MARK4 gene is located on chromosome 19q13.2, consists of 18 exons and encodes at least two isoforms, namely MARK4S and MARK4L, originated by alternative splicing (Kato et al., 2001) (Figure 16). mRNA splicing is a complex process consisting in the removal of introns, which are non-coding sequences, and in the joining of exons, the coding sequences, to generate the "edited" mRNA ready to be translated into a protein.

* MARK4S ("short") protein is the native isoform, consisting of all the 18 exons, and is 688 aminoacid-long with predicted molecular weight of 75.3 kilo Daltons (kDa);
* MARK4L protein derives from skipping of exon 16, which causes a shift of the reading frame[1] with a downstream stop codon, originating a longer protein (752 aminoacids; predicted molecular weight: 82.5 kDa).

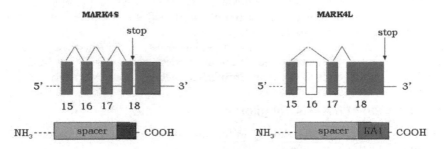

Fig. 16. Alternative splicing of exon 16 gives origin to MARK4 isoforms. When exon 16 is included in the mRNA, the stop codon is inside exon 18 and the encoded protein, MARK4S, lacks the KA1 domain at the C-terminal tail (left); when exon 16 is skipped, a shift of the reading frame occurs, changing the stop codon and generating a longer MARK4L protein, which has the classical KA1 domain (right).

Both MARK4L and S share the same protein structure of MARKs, with 90% sequence homology in the kinase domain. The two isoforms differ in the C-terminal tail, since MARK4L includes the kinase-associated 1 domain as the other MARK proteins, whereas MARK4S contains a domain with no homology to any known structure (Kato et al., 2001; Moroni et al., 2006) (Figure 16). Actually, MARK4 has less sequence homology in the C-terminus compared to the other MARKs; nevertheless MARK4L tail seems to fold in a similar shape, suggesting that the role of the C-terminal region may apply also to MARK4L (Marx et al., 2010).

---

[1] The mRNA sequence is "read" by an enzyme which matches a determinate "codon", made by three nucleotides, with its respective aminoacid. There are two particular codons, namely the start and the stop codon, which mark the beginning and the end of the protein.

8.1 MARK4 regulation

Phosphorylation by LKB1, in the activation loop, activates MARK4, while polyubiquitination of MARK4 inhibits the kinase activation (Al-Hakim et al., 2008). Furthermore, as MARK4 interacts with aPKC (Brajenovic et al., 2008), it could be phosphorylated and inactivated by this kinase as reported for MARK2 and MARK3.

8.2 MARK4 interactors and hypothetical functions

By tandem affinity purification and immunoprecipitation experiments, near twenty proteins have been identified as putative MARK4 interactors (Brajenovic et al., 2008). Among them, PKCλ and Cdc42 are implicated in cell polarity control and TGFβIAF (transforming growth factor β-inducing anti-apoptotic factor) is thought to be a hortologue of Miranda, a protein involved in the asymmetric division of neuroblasts in *Drosophila*. MARK4 interacts with the 14-3-3η isoform (Angrand et al., 2006; Brajenovic et al., 2008) of 14-3-3 proteins, which control multiple cellular processes by binding phosphorylated proteins and could directly regulate MARK4 or act as bridges among different pathways. Other MARK4 interactors are ARHGEF2, a cytoskeleton binding protein, and Phosphatase 2A, which is associated to microtubules and regulates *Tau* (Brajenovic et al., 2008). MARK4 protein has been also found to co-localize and co-precipitate in complex with α, β, and γ tubulin, myosin and actin (Brajenovic et al., 2008; Trinczek et al., 2004).

As the other MARK members, MARK4 phosphorylates MAPs, increasing microtubule dynamics; therefore, as also suggested by the interactions above reported, MARK4 may be involved in many processes involving microtubules, such as cytoskeleton dynamics.

9. Up-regulation of MARK4L in glioma

MARK4 gene is expressed ubiquitously in human tissues, with particularly elevated levels in brain and testis (Kato et al., 2001).

Few *MARK4* expression studies are reported in literature; they were performed with non-quantitative methods, such as northern blot (Kato et al., 2001; Schneider et al., 2004; Trinczek et al., 2004) and semi-quantitative competitive PCR (polymerase chain reaction) (Moroni et al., 2006), on different organisms (human, rat and mouse tissues) not always allowing to discern between the two MARK4 isoforms. MARK4 transcriptional variants are differentially regulated in human tissues, especially in the central nervous system: MARK4S is the predominant isoform in mouse and human brain, while MARK4L has been found highly expressed in neural progenitors and in gliomas (Beghini et al., 2003; Moroni et al., 2006).

By a semi-quantitative approach MARK4L has been found up-regulated in glioma tissue samples (fragments of glial tumours excised from patients) and glioma cell lines, of different malignancy grades, including the MI-4 GBM cell line carrying the *MARK4* duplicated gene as detected by FISH and aCGH analysis. MARK4L has been also found highly expressed in neural progenitors and down-regulated during their glial differentiation into astrocytes, suggesting that it might be necessary for proliferation, being thus highly enriched in proliferating or undifferentiated cells (Beghini et al., 2003) (Figure 17).

Protein kinase activation, often caused by gene amplification and/or mutation, is frequently associated to cancer initiation and progression, as most kinases are involved in cell proliferation. Although array-CGH analyses on glioma cell lines showed that the BAC clone encompassing *MARK4* at 19q13.2 is included in a "gain" region in a few of the tested cell lines, it did not evidence *MARK4* copy number variations, except for the MI-4 GBM cell line (Roversi et al., 2006). Only a few *MARK4* alterations are reported in the literature, namely two missense mutations (aminoacidic substitution) in exon 12 (R377Q and R418C in the spacer region), two silent mutations (no aminoacidic substitution) in exons 5 (Y137Y) and 9 (I286I) (kinase domain), while one intronic mutation (exon 8 +5 C>T; kinase domain) has been found in a few tumour samples (Greenman et al., 2007). In addition, only a splice-site mutation (exon 13 +1 G>A; spacer region) has been identified in one among 91 glioblastoma samples (TGCA Research Network, 2008). However, CpG methylation and/or promoter amplification have not yet been investigated. Based on this evidence, neither amplification nor mutations of *MARK4* gene seem to be the cause of its reported sustained expression in glioma samples.

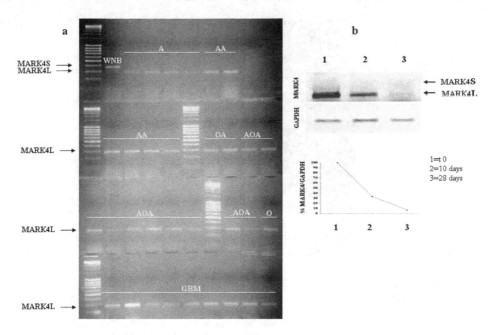

Fig. 17. (a) Semi-quantitative Reverse Transcription-PCR of MARK4S and MARK4L isoforms in whole normal brain (WNB) and in 32 glioma cell lines, subdivided according to WHO grade (A: astrocytoma; AA: anaplastic astrocytoma; OA: oligoastroctytoma; AOA: anaplastic oligoastrocytoma; O: oligodendroglioma; GBM: glioblastoma multiforme). (b) Downregulation of MARK4L expression during glial differentiation of human neural progenitors: semi-quantitative RT-PCR (top) and graph representation (bottom) of MARK4L expression in neural progenitors at times 0, 10 and 28 days of induced differentiation.

10. MARK4 sub-cellular localization in glioma cell lines

Recently, immunofluorescence analyses with a specific anti-MARK4L antibody highlighted multiple sub-cellular localizations for the endogenous MARK4L protein in glioma cell lines (Magnani et al., 2009).

10.1 Centrosome localization

It has been assessed that, under microtubule-stabilizing conditions, MARK4L localizes in the perinuclear region of glioma cell lines. By co-localization experiments with both anti-MARK4L and anti-γtubulin (the main centrosomal protein) antibodies, this perinuclear localization has been demonstrated to correspond to the centrosome (Magnani et al., 2009), as shown in Figure 18 (Box 3). This result confirms previous data referring to exogenous MARK4 protein conjugated to GFP (green fluorescent protein), which has been shown to co-localize with microtubules and centrosomes of CHO (Chinese hamster ovary) and neuroblastoma cell lines (Trinczek et al., 2004), in contrast to MARK1, MARK2 and MARK3 that exhibit uniform cytoplasmic localization. Furthermore, it has been demonstrated that the association with the centrosome is independent from microtubules, since it is not abolished when microtubules are depolimerized by nocodazole treatment (Magnani et al., 2009).

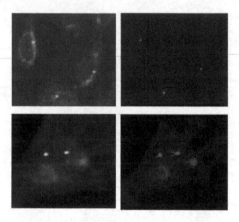

Fig. 18. Anti-MARK4L (green; left) and anti-γtubulin (red; right) antibodies showing co-localization signals in interphase (top) and mitotic (bottom) centrosomes of glioma cell lines.

The centrosome

The centrosome is a little organelle, not bound by membrane, positioned centrally in the cell near the nucleus. It is the primary MicroTubule Organizing Center (MTOC), as it can nucleate and organize microtubules. It consists of two distinct domains:
• the centriolar domain, including the centrioles, which are cylindrical organelles important for centrosome organization and replication. Each centriole consists of 9 triple microtubules;
• the pericentriolar domain, consisting of many fibers and proteins that surround the centriole. In this domain microtubules are nucleated, by associating α and β-tubulin dimers from a γ-tubulin ring (Doxsey, 2001).
The centrosome plays a key role in organizing the interphase cytoskeleton (regulating cell polarity, adhesion and motility) and the mitotic spindle (Kramer et al., 2002). It also contributes to cell cycle progression and cytokinesis (Martinez-Garay et al., 2006) and is involved in cell cycle transitions, in the cellular response to stress and signal transduction (Doxsey et al., 2005). The centrosomes duplicate only once in the cell cycle, during G1/S transition and in S phase, and form a strictly bipolar spindle during mitosis.

Box 3.

The endogenous MARK4L localizes both at normal interphase centrosomes (Figure 18) as well as at the aberrant centrosomes frequently observed in glioma cell lines (see Figure 4), suggesting a possible link between the alternatively spliced kinase and the mitotic instability frequently observed in human glioma. Two abnormal centrosome configurations are reported: a random one (multiple centrosomes randomly distributed) and a clustered one (multiple centrosomes collected in a single large aggregate) (Magnani et al., 2009), as depicted in Figure 19.

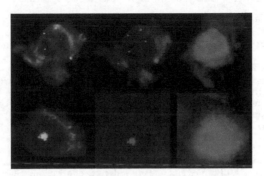

Fig. 19. Anti-MARK4L (green; left) and anti-γtubulin (red; middle) antibodies showing co-localization signals in abnormal centrosomes of glioma cell lines. Both the abnormal centrosome configurations are reported: the random one (top) and the clustered one (bottom). The nuclei are counterstained with DAPI (blue, right).

10.2 Midbody localization

The centrosome association is maintained during the entire course of mitosis, as MARK4L co-localizes with γtubulin in all the cell cycle phases. The anti-MARK4L antibody is also detected in the midbody, a microtubule structure forming at the contact point between the two daughter cells at the end of the cell division. These data demonstrate that the kinase is endogenously associated with the centrosomes during the whole cell cycle and concentrates thereafter into the midbody during cytokinesis (Magnani et al., 2009) (Figure 20) (Box 4).

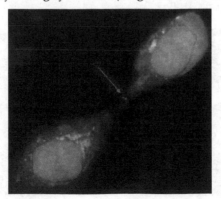

Fig. 20. Co-localization of MARK4L (green) and γtubulin (red) proteins at the midbody (arrow) during the cytokinesis of a glioma cell. The nuclei are counterstained with DAPI (blue).

Cell cycle, cytokinesis and midbody

The cell cycle corresponds to the life of a cell, beginning from its formation from a mother cell to its division into two daughter cells or to its death.

It consists of two main phases, interphase (subdivided in G1, S and G2 phases) and M phase (mitosis+cytokinesis). During interphase the cell grows and doubles its structures and DNA content; during the M phase the cell splits into two daughter cells.

In mitosis the two centrosomes move to opposite poles in the cell (asters) and organize the mitotic spindle, formed by bundles of microtubules getting off the centrosomes. The spindle binds chromosomes and segregate them toward one aster or the other, splitting the genetic material between the two poles.

During cytokinesis, the mitotic spindle locates the cleavage furrow, which will divide the cell, in a point which is equidistant from the two asters. In this furrow, a contractile ring of actin and myosin grows up and shrinks, causing the "stricture" of the cell, until the two opposing surfaces of the membrane come in contact and merge, closing and delimiting the two daughter cells (Bringmann, 2005).

Initially the two daughter cells are connected by a narrow intercellular bridge, whose core is the midbody, consisting of microtubules and a dense matrix (Mullins & McIntosh, 1982). The diameter of the intercellular bridge then decreases until it vanishes, making the two daughter cells effectively separated. The midbody is finally discarded and undergoes degradation (Mullins & Biesele, 1977). The midbody is thought to have an important role in maintaining a bipolar spindle and in correctly separating the cytoplasm between the two daughter cells.

Box 4.

10.3 Nucleolar localization

Under standard immunofluorescence conditions, anti-MARK4L antibody is also detected in the nucleoli (Box 5).

Silver-colloid method, which allows visualizing the nucleolar organizing regions (NORs), and co-localization experiments with anti-nucleolin (a nucleolar protein) antibody allowed to assess that the nuclear structures bound by MARK4L antibody are indeed the nucleoli (Magnani et al., 2009) (Figure 21) (Box 5).

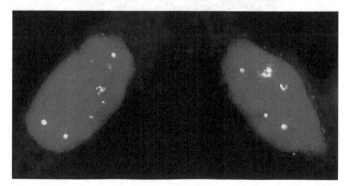

Fig. 21. Co-localization of MARK4L (green) and nucleolin (red) proteins in the nucleoli of glioma cells. The nuclei are counterstained with DAPI (blue).

The nucleolus

The nucleolus is a sub-nuclear organelle not surrounded by membranes and whose main function is ribosome biogenesis (ribosomes are involved in protein synthesis). It originates at the end of mitosis from the Nucleolus Organizing Regions (NORs), which are clusters of genes (rDNA), codifying for ribosomal RNA (rRNA), located on the acrocentric chromosomes.

The nucleolus consists of three main components, each with a different role in the formation of ribosomes, here defined starting from the inside of the nucleolus to outside:

• the fibrillar center, which is a NOR (rDNA);

• the dense fibrillar component, consisting of pre-rRNA;

• the granular component, whose granular appearance is conferred by the presence of ribosomal subunits.

The transcription of the rDNA leads to the formation of pre-rRNAs, which then undergo rearrangements and are assembled with ribosomal proteins to form the pre-ribosomes. The pre-ribosomal particles then move into the cytoplasm, passing through the nuclear pores (Carmo-Fonseca et al., 2000; Schwarzacher & Wachtler, 1983).

Besides this traditional ribosome biogenesis activity, the nucleolus is characterized by multiple functions, including the response to cellular stress, the regulation of cell cycle (Visintin & Amon, 2000) and cell growth (Zhang et al., 2010) and of post-translational modifications (phosphorylation and sumoylation) of proteins.

Box 5.

The overall immunofluorescence data on endogenous MARK4L protein confirm the previous evidence on its centrosome association and highlight two novel localization sites of MARK4L: the nucleolus and the midbody (Magnani et al., 2009).

Immunoblotting with anti-MARK4L antibody on centrosomes, midbody and nucleoli isolated by biochemical fractionation from glioblastoma cell lines confirmed the presence of MARK4L protein in each fraction, validated by antibodies specific for each cell structure: anti-γtubulin antibody for centrosomes, anti-βtubulin for the midbody (βtubulin, together with αtubulin, accounts for 30% of midbody proteins) and anti-nucleolin for the nucleolus (Magnani et al., 2009).

The localization pattern of MARK4L delineated by the above studies suggests that the kinase may take part in cell cycle progression and influence the microtubules, particularly those affecting the centrosome and midbody.

MARK4L association with the nucleolus in glial tumours is very interesting, since MARK4L could have a functional impact on this organelle, being requested for its building and maintenance like other protein kinases, as well as it could be spatially regulated by alternate translocation in and out the nucleolus. Many proteins are indeed sequestered in the nucleolus and then released according to a temporally regulated activity, since they must exert their function in certain phases of the cell cycle (Visintin & Amon, 2000). Last, the nucleolar localization of a protein may also influence its stability, protecting the protein from proteasomal degradation, since proteasomes are present in the nucleoplasm but not in nucleoli (Wojcik & DeMartino, 2003).

11. Conclusion

A few remarks can be drawn from the above synthesis on cytogenomics of human gliomas and the *MARK4* cell cycle gene as a likely "player" in gliomagenesis.

Gliomas are one of the most intractable tumours due to their "complex identity": as it has been beautifully underlined, the generation - since the earliest glioma stages - of multiple cell populations with different genotypic and phenotypic features makes unlikely to succeed therapeutic strategies targeting only clones with "dominant" or "average" characteristics of the cell population (Noble & Dietrich, 2004). The intrinsic genomic heterogeneity of human glioma has first been disclosed cytogenetically, as documented by a huge number of studies which across two decades have used the cytogenetic tools suitable to monitor the intratumour cell heterogeneity and to discern "recurrent" and potentially causative chromosomal rearrangements. A few of these rearrangements entered the diagnostic and prognostic flow chart of gliomas, others allowed to identify crucial genes which mutations or imbalance are the signature of a specific glioma type or glioma malignancy stage. In line with a research pathway that has been reiterated for several genes of relevance in cancer, focus on *MARK4* has been pinpointed by cytogenetics and deepened by multiple tools ranging from gene-targeted molecular to genomic and cytogenomic analyses. Despite its nature of serine-threonine kinase gene, *MARK4* has not be found mutated or affected by copy number alterations in glioma, while its encoded proteins represented by two different isoforms, MARK4S and MARK4L, could be featured as a potential target of dysregulation in tumours due to its dual nature. The latter isoform, produced by alternative splicing, has been found up-regulated in glioma and shown to display sub-cellular localizations, namely the centrosome, the midbody and the nucleolus, which strictly associate it with the process of cell division. Interestingly, alternative mRNA splicing has been considered a mechanism not only increasing proteomic complexity but also involved in cancer, through mechanisms of oncogenes/tumour suppressors activation/inactivation or through the generation of CIN (López-Saavedra & Herrera, 2010). CIN is a general property of aneuploid cancer cells and is generated by defects in different processes, among which the regulation of the number of centrosomes, the dynamics of microtubules attachment to the kinetochores and the overall control of cell cycle. Defects in centrosomal number and structure have been well documented in gliomas (D'Assoro et al., 2002; Katsetos et al., 2006; Magnani et al., 2009) raising the issue whether the increased MARK4L isoform, a gene involved in microtubule dynamics, may concur to errors in chromosomal segregation driving gliomagenesis.

Recent application of multidimensional technological approaches has comprehensively highlighted the scenario of glioma genes and core pathways. However, despite the impressive advances, the links between genes alteration and cellular behavior are yet hampered by the multiplicity of the genetic lesions and the interconnections among the different affected pathways. Hopefully ongoing and next years research will compose the puzzle promising to translate into the clinical set the unraveled glioma pathomechanisms.

12. Acknowledgement

We thank the *Associazione italiana per la ricerca sul cancro* (AIRC) for supporting this work (grant n 4217 to LL for 2008).

13. Methods

13.1 Cell cultures and preparation of human metaphase chromosomes

Glioma cell lines were derived from primary tumour post-surgery specimens and subsequently maintained by serial passages in RPMI 1640 medium containing 5% Fetal Calf Serum at 37°C in a 5% CO_2 atmosphere. Most of the cell lines were used within the first 30 passages.

Metaphase spreads were obtained on both fresh tumours and cultured cell lines, harvested when "peak" mitotic activity was observed; usually, a 16-hour treatment with Colcemid at a final concentration of 0.01-0.02 mg/ml is employed (Magnani et al., 1994).

13.2 Fluorescence in situ hybridization (FISH) analysis

Fluorescence hybridization with genomic DNA has proven to be a powerful tool for identification of chromosome rearrangements in cancer cells. Potential applications include detection of chromosome-specific aneuploidy in metaphase and interphase cells, quantification of the frequency of chromosome translocations and/or aneuploidy as a measure of genetic damage, and detection of diagnostically and prognostically relevant chromosomal lesions. Detection of translocations between human metaphase chromosomes is possible by using cocktails of chromosome-specific sequences that hybridize more or less uniformly along the chromosome. Depending on the aberration, its detection may be by visual fluorescence microscopy (see Figures 9, 10). In brief: slides carrying interphase or metaphase spreads are washed in 2x SSC (1 x SSC is 0.15 M NaCl/0.015 M sodium citrate), dehydrated in an ethanol series and denatured [70% (vol/vol) formamide/2x SSC (final concentration), pH 7, at 70°C for 2 min]. The hybridization mix consists of (final concentrations) 50% formamide, 2x SSC, 20% dextran sulfate, carrier DNA (sonicated herring sperm DNA), and biotin-labeled human genomic DNA. The mixture is applied to the slides under a glass coverslip. After overnight incubation at 37°C, the slides are washed at 45°C (50% formamide/2x SSC, pH 7), and immersed in BN buffer (0.1 M sodium bicarbonate, 0.05% Nonidet P-40, pH 8). The slides are never allowed to dry after this step. The coverslips are then removed and fluorescein-avidin DCS is applied. The coverslips are put back in their original places and the slides incubated 20 min at 37°C. They are then washed in BN buffer at 45°C. The intensity of biotin fluorescence is amplified by adding a layer of biotinylated goat anti-avidin antibody followed, after washing as above, by another layer of fluorescein-avidin DCS. After washing in BN buffer a fluorescence anti-fade solution is added. The DNA counterstain [4,6-diamidino-2-phenylindole (DAPI) or propidium iodide] is included in the anti-fade solution (Magnani et al., 1999; Pinkel et al., 1986).

13.3 Immunofluorescence

Immunofluorescence analyses enable to visualize, by fluorescence microscopy, the sub-cellular localization of a specific protein in cultured cells. The target protein is recognized by an antibody, which in turn is conjugated to a fluorochrome emitting fluorescent light. Briefly, cells are grown on glass chamber slides, then permeabilized (with solvents that extract lipids from the membranes allowing antibodies to reach a sub-cellular structure) and fixed (in order to protect the cell structure from eventual damages and to "freeze" cells in their current state). Afterwards, cells are incubated with bovine serum albumin (BSA) to block non-specific binding of antibodies. Glass slides are then incubated with a primary antibody specific to the target protein, then with a secondary antibody conjugated to the fluorochrome and finally observed under the microscope (Magnani et al., 2009).

13.4 Biochemical fractionation and immunoblotting

By biochemical fractionation we mean the whole techniques that allow to separate and isolate intact cellular components. It usually consists in carefully breaking the cell membrane with homogenizers and isotonic/hypotonic solutions, so that intact organelles can come out, and in separating cellular components by centrifugation, on the basis of differences in their mass and specific weight. Centrosome, midbody and nucleoli isolation protocols are described in Magnani et al., 2009 and based on methods respectively by Moudjou & Bornens, 1994; Chu & Sisken, 1977; Muramatsu et al., 1963. In particular, for midbody isolation cells are synchronized in mitosis by nocodazole treatment and then released from mitotic arrest in nocodazole-free medium, so that after 30 minutes near 90% of cells had formed the midbody.

After membrane breaking, all the passages are done at 4°C and with protease inhibitors, in order to prevent protein degradation, possibly exerted by released proteases. Proteins extracted from centrosome, midbody and nucleolus fractions are then analyzed by immunoblotting. Proteins are first separated, according to their molecular weight, by SDS-PAGE (Sodium Dodecyl Sulphate – PolyAcrilamide Gel Electrophoresis): this technique allows proteins to migrate, driven by electric current, in a porous gel, with speed depending exclusively on their size. Afterwards, separated proteins are transferred onto a membrane, incubated with a blocking solution (BSA or milk) to prevent non-specific binding of antibodies and then incubated with appropriate antibodies (immunoblotting). The primary antibody is specific to the target protein and is recognized by the secondary antibody conjugated to HRP (horse radish peroxidase). Antibodies are detected by covering the membrane with a peroxide/enhancer solution, which is oxidized by HRP and emits light signals.

14. References

Al-Hakim, A.K.; Zagorska, A.; Chapman, L.; Deak, M.; Peggie, M. & Alessi, D.R. (2008). Control of AMPK-related kinases by USP9X and atypical Lys^{29}/Lys^{33}-linked polyubiquitin chains. *The Biochemical Journal*, Vol.411, pp. 249-260, ISSN 0264-6021

Angrand, P.O.; Segura, I.; Völkel, P.; Ghidelli, S.; Terry, R.; Brajenovic, M.; Vintersten, K.; Klein, R.; Superti-Furga, G.; Drewes, G.; Kuster, B.; Bouwmeester, T. & Acker-Palmer, A. (2006). Transgenic mouse proteomics identifies new 14-3-3-associated proteins involved in cytoskeletal rearrangements and cell signaling. *Molecular and Cellular Proteomics*, Vol.5, No.12, pp. 2211-2227, ISSN 1535-9484

Bachmann, M.; Hennemann, H.; Xing, P.X.; Hoffmann, I. & Möröy, T. (2004). The oncogenic serine/threonine kinase Pim-1 phosphorylates and inhibits the activity of Cdc25C-associated kinase 1 (C-TAK1): a novel role for Pim-1 at the G2/M cell cycle checkpoint. *Journal of Biological Chemistry*, Vol. 279, pp. 48319-48328, ISSN 0021-9258

Basto, R.; Brunk, K.; Vinadogrova, T.; Peel, N.; Franz, A.; Khodjakov, A. & Raff, J.W. (2008). Centrosome amplification can initiate tumorigenesis in flies. *Cell*, Vol. 133, pp. 1032-1042, ISSN 0092-8674

Bayani, J.; Selvarajah, S.; Maire, G.; Vukovic, B.; Al-Romaih, K.; Zielenska, M. & Squire, J.A. (2007). Genomic mechanisms and measurement of structural and numerical instability in cancer cells. *Seminars in Cancer Biology* , Vol.17, pp. 5-18, ISSN 1044-579X

Beghini, A.; Magnani, I.; Roversi, G.; Piepoli, T.; Di Terlizzi, S.; Moroni, R.F.; Pollo, B.; Fuhrman Conti, A.M.; Cowell, J.K.; Finocchiaro, G. & Larizza, L. (2003). The neural progenitor-restricted isoform of the MARK4 gene in 19q13.2 is upregulated in human gliomas and overexpressed in a subset of glioblastoma cell lines. *Oncogene,* Vol. 22, pp. 2581-2591, ISSN 0950-9232

Bessone, S.; Vidal, F.; Le Bouc, Y.; Epelbaum, J.; Bluet-Pajot, M.T. & Darmon, M. (1999) EMK protein kinase-null mice: dwarfism and hypofertility associated with alterations in the somatotrope and prolactin pathways. *Developmental Biology*, Vol. 214, pp. 87-101, ISSN 0012-1606

Bigner, S.H.; Mark, J.; Burger, P.C.; Mahaley, M.S.Jr.; Bullard, D.E.; Muhlbaier, L.H. & Bigner, D.D. (1988). Specific chromosomal abnormalities in malignant human gliomas. *Cancer Research* , Vol.88, pp. 405-411, ISSN 0008-5472

Brajenovic, M.; Joberty, G.; Küster, B.; Bouwmeester, T. & Drewes, G. (2004). Comprehensive proteomic analysis of human Par protein complexes reveals an interconnected protein network. *The Journal of Biological Chemistry*, Vol. 279, No.13, pp. 12804-12811, ISSN 1083-351X

Bredel, M.; Bredel, C.; Juric, D.; Harsh, G.R.; Vogel, H.; Recht, L.D. & Sikic, B.I. (2005). High-resolution genome-wide mapping of genetic alterations in human glial brain tumors. *Cancer Research*, Vol. 10, pp. 4088-4096, ISSN 0008-5472

Bringmann, H. (2005). Cytokinesis and the spindle midzone. *Cell cycle*, Vol. 4, No.12, pp. 1709-1712, ISSN 1551-4005

Brinkley, B.R. (2001). Managing the centrosome numbers game: from chaos to stability in cancer cell division. *Trends in Cell Biology* , Vol.11 , pp. 18–21, ISSN 0962-8924

Carmo-Fonseca, M.; Mendes-Soares, L. & Campos, I. (2000). To be or not to be in the nucleolus. *Nature Cell Biology* , Vol. 2, No.6, pp. E107-112, ISSN 1097 -6256

Chen, Y.M.; Wang, Q.J.; Hu, H.S.; Yu, P.C.; Zhu, J., Drewes, G.; Piwnica-Worms, H. & Luo, Z.G. (2006). Microtubule affinity-regulating kinase 2 functions downstream of the PAR-3/PAR-6/atypical PKC complex in regulating hippocampal neuronal polarity. *Proceedings of the National Academy of Science of the United States of America*, Vol. 103, pp. 8534-8539, ISSN 0027-8424

Chin, J; Knowles, R.B.; Schneider, A.; Drewes, G.; Mandelkow, E.M. & Hyman, B.T. (2000). Microtubule-Affinity Regulating Kinase (MARK) is tightly associated with neurofibrillary tangles in Alzheimer brain: a fluorescence energy transfer study. *Journal of Neuropathology and Experimental Neurology*, Vol. 59, No.11, pp. 966-971, ISSN 0022-3069

Chu, L.K. & Sisken, J.E. (1977). The isolation and preliminary electrophoretic analysis of the mitotic spindle from cultured mammalian cells. *Experimental Cell Research*, Vol. 107, pp. 71-77, ISSN 0014-4827

Cimini, D.; Cameron, L.A. & Salmon, E.D. (2004). Anaphase spindle mechanics prevent mis-segregation of merotelically oriented chromosomes. *Current Biology*, Vol. 23, pp. 2149-2155, ISSN 0960-9822

Cohen, D.; Brennwald, P.J.; Rodriguez-Boulan, E. & Müsch, A. (2004). Mammalian PAR-1 determines epithelial lumen polarity by organizing the microtubule cytoskeleton. *Journal of Cell Biology*, Vol. 164, pp. 717-727, ISSN 1540-8140

Collins, V.P. (2004). Brain tumours: classification and genes. *Journal of Neurology, Neurosurgery & Psychiatry*, Vol. 75, (Suppl 2), pp. 2-11, ISSN 0022-3050

Cowell, J. K.; Barnett, G.H. & Nowak, N.J. (2004a). Characterization of the 1p/19q chromosomal loss in oligodendrogliomas using comparative genomic hybridization arrays (CGHa). *Journal of Neuropathology & Experimental Neurology*, Vol. 63, pp. 151-158, ISSN 0022-3069

Cowell, J.K.; Matsui, S.; Wang, Y.D.; LaDuca, J.; Conroy, J.; McQuaid D. & Nowak N.J. (2004b). Application of bacterial artificial chromosome array-based comparative genomic hybridization and spectral karyotyping to the analysis of glioblastoma multiforme. *Cancer Genetics and Cytogenetics*, Vol. 151, pp.36- 51, ISSN 0165-4608

D'Assoro, A.B.; Lingle, W.L. & Salisbury, J.L. (2002). Centrosome amplification and the development of cancer. *Oncogene*, Vol. 21, pp. 6146-6153. Review, ISSN 0950-9232

Doxsey, S. (2001). Re-evaluating centrosome function. *Nature*, Vol.2, No.9, pp. 688-698, ISSN 0028-0836

Doxsey, S.; McCollum, D. & Theurkauf, W. (2005). Centrosomes in cellular regulation. *Annual Review of Cell and Developmental Biology*, Vol. 21, pp.411-434, ISSN 1081-0706

Drewes, G.; Ebneth, A.; Preuss, U.; Mandelkow, E.M. & Mandelkow, E. (1997). MARK, a novel family of protein kinases that phosphorylate microtubule-associated proteins and trigger microtubule disruption. *Cell*, Vol. 89, pp.297-308, ISSN 0092-8674

Duesberg, P.; Li, R.; Fabarius, A. & Hehlmann, R. (2006). Aneuploidy and cancer: from correlation to causation. *Contributions to Microbiology*, Vol.13, pp. 16-44, ISSN 1420-9519

Fenech, M. (2007). Cytokinesis-block micronucleus cytome assay. *Nature Protocols*, Vol.2, pp. 1084-1104, ISSN 1754-2189

Fujiwara, T.; Bandi, M.; Nitta, M.; Ivanova, E.V.; Bronson, R.T. & Pellman, D. (2005). Cytokinesis failure generating tetraploids promotes tumorigenesis in p53-null cells. *Nature*, Vol. 437, 1043-1047, ISSN 0028-0836

Gamblin, T.C.; Chen, F.; Zambrano, A.; Abraha, A.; Lagalwar, S.; Guillozet, A.L.; Lu, M.; Fu, Y.; Garcia-Sierra, F.; LaPointe, N.; Miller, R.; Berry, R.W.; Binder, L.I. & Cryns, V.L. (2003) Caspase cleavage of tau: linking amyloid and neurofibrillary tangles in Alzheimer's disease. *Proceedings of the National Academy of Sciences of the United States of America*, Vol. 100, No. 17, pp. 10032-10037, ISSN 0027-8424

Ganem, N.J.; Storchova, Z. & Pellman, D. (2007). Tetraploidy, aneuploidy and cancer. *Current Opinion in Genetics & Development*, Vol. 17, pp. 157-162, Review, ISSN 0959-437X

Ganem, N.J.; Godinho, S.A. & Pellman, D. (2009). A mechanism linking extra centrosomes to chromosomal instability. *Nature*, Vol. 460, pp.278-282 , ISSN 0028-0836

Geigl, J.B.; Obenauf, A.C.; Schwarzbraun, T. & Speicher, M.R. (2008). Defining 'chromosomal instability'. *Trends in Genetics*, Vol. 24, pp. 64-69, ISSN 0168-9525

Ghadimi, B.M.; Sackett, D.L.; Difilippantonio, M.J.; Schröck, E.; Neumann, T.; Jauho, A.; Auer, G. & Ried, T. (2000). Centrosome amplification and instability occurs exclusively in aneuploid, but not in diploid colorectal cancer cell lines, and correlates with numerical chromosomal aberrations. *Genes Chromosomes and Cancer*, Vol. 27, pp.183-190, ISSN 1045-2257

Greenman, C.; Stephens, P.; Smith, R.; Dalgliesh, G.L.; Hunter, C.; Bignell, G.; Davies, H.; Teague, J.; Butler, A.; Stevens, C.; Edkins, S.; O'Meara, S.; Vastrik, I.; Schmidt, E.E.; Avis, T.; Barthorpe, S.; Bhamra, G.; Buck, G.; Choudhury, B.; Clements, J.; Cole, J.; Dicks, E.; Forbes, S.; Gray, K.; Halliday, K.; Harrison, R.; Hills, K.; Hinton, J.; Jenkinson, A.; Jones, D.; Menzies, A.; Mironenko, T.; Perry, J.; Raine, K.; Richardson, D.; Shepherd, R.; Small, A.; Tofts, C.; Varian, J.; Webb,T.; West, S.; Widaa, S.; Yates, A.; Cahill, D.P.; Louis, D.N.; Goldstraw, P.; Nicholson, A.G.; Brasseur, F.; Looijenga, L.; Weber, B.L.; Chiew, Y.E.; De Fazio, A.; Greaves, M.F.; Green, A.R.; Campbell, P.; Birney, E.; Easton, D.F.; Chenevix-Trench, G.; Tan, M.H.; Khoo, S.K.; Teh, B.T.; Yuen, S.T.; Leung, S.Y.; Wooster, R.; Futreal, P.A. & Stratton, M.R. (2007). Patterns of somatic mutation in human cancer genomes. *Nature*, Vol. 446, pp.153-158, ISSN 0028-0836

Hartmann, C.; Johnk, L.; Kitange, G.; Wu, Y.; Ashworth, L.K.; Jenkins, R.B. & Louis, D.N. (2002). Transcript Map of the 3.7-Mb D19S112–D19S246. *Cancer Research*, Vol.62, pp. 4100-4108, ISSN 0008-5472

Hecht, B.K.; Turc-Carel, C.; Chatel, M.; Grellier, P.; Gioanni, J.; Attias, R.; Gaudray, P. & Hecht, F. (1995). Cytogenetics of malignant gliomas: I. The autosomes with reference to rearrangements. *Cancer Genetics and Cytogenetics*, Vol. 84, pp. 1-8, ISSN 0165- 4608

Hurov, J.B.; Stappenbeck, T.S.; Zmasek, C.M.; White, L.S.; Ranganath, S.H.; Russell, J.H.; Chan, A.C.; Murphy, K.M. & Piwnica-Worms, H. (2001). Immune system dysfunction and autoimmune disease in mice lacking Emk (Par-1) protein kinase. *Molecular Cell Biology*, Vol. 21, pp.3206-3219, ISSN 1098-5549

Hurov, J. & Piwnica-Worms, H. (2007). The Par-1/MARK family of protein kinases: from polarity to metabolism. *Cell cycle*, Vol.6, pp. 1966-1969, ISSN 1538-4101

Jenkins, R.B.; Kimmel, D.W.; Moertel, C.A.; Schultz, C.G.; Scheithauer, B.W.; Kelly, P.J. & Dewald, G.W. (1989). A cytogenetic study of 53 human gliomas. *Cancer Genetics and Cytogenetics*, Vol. 39, pp. 253-279, ISSN 0165- 4608

Kato, T.; Satoh, S.; Okabe, H.; Kitahara, O.; Ono, K.; Kihara, C.; Tanaka, T.; Tsunoda, T.; Yamaoka, Y.; Nakamura, Y. & Furukawa, Y. (2001). Isolation of a novel human gene, MARKL1, homologous to MARK3 and its involvement in hepatocellular carcinogenesis. *Neoplasia*, Vol. 3, No.1, pp. 4-9, ISSN 1522-8002

Katsetos, C.D.; Reddy, G.; Dráberová, E.; Smejkalová, B.; Del Valle, L.; Ashraf, Q.; Tadevosyan, A.; Yelin, K.; Maraziotis, T.; Mishra, O.P.; Mörk, S.; Legido, A.; Nissanov, J.; Baas, P.W.; de Chadarévian, J.P. & Dráber, P. (2006). Altered cellular distribution and subcellular sorting of gamma-tubulin in diffuse astrocytic gliomas and human glioblastoma cell lines. *Journal of Neuropathology and Experimental Neurology*, Vol. 65, pp. 465–477, ISSN 0022-3069

Kitange, G.; Misra, A.; Law, M.; Passe, S.; Kollmeyer, T.M.; Maurer, M.; Ballman, K.; Feuerstein, B.G. & Jenkins, R.B. (2005). Chromosomal imbalances detected by array comparative genomic hybridization in human oligodendrogliomas and mixed oligoastrocytomas. *Genes Chromosomes and Cancer*, Vol. 42, pp. 68-77, ISSN 1045-2257

Kleihues, P. & Cavenee, W.K. (2000). *Pathology and Genetics of Tumours of the Nervous System*, IARC Press, ISBN 92 83 22409 4, Lyon, France

Kleihues, P.& Ohgaki, H. (2000). Phenotype vs genotype in the evolution of astrocytic brain tumors. *Toxicologic Pathology*, Vol. 28, No.1, pp. 164-170, ISSN 0192-6233

Koschny, R.; Koschny, T.; Froster, U.G.; Krupp, W. & Zuber, M.A. (2002). Comparative genomic hybridization in glioma: a meta-analysis of 509 cases. *Cancer Genetics and Cytogenetics*, Vol. 135, pp. 147-159, ISSN 0165- 4608

Kramer, A.; Neben, K. & Ho, AD. (2002). Centrosome replication, genomic instability and cancer. *Leukemia,* Vol. 16, pp. 767-775 , ISSN 0887-6924

Lengauer, C.; Kinzler, K.W. & Vogelstein B. (1998). Genetic instabilities in human cancers. *Nature*, Vol. 396, pp. 643-649, ISSN 0028-0836

Lindstrom, E.; Salford, L.G. Heim S, Mandahl N, Stromblad S, Brun A, Mitelman F. (1991): Trisomy 7 and sex chromosome loss need not be representative of tumor parenchyma cells in malignant glioma. *Genes, Chromosomes and Cancer*, Vol. 3, pp. 474-479, ISSN 1045-2257

Lingle, W.L.; Barrett, S.L.; Negron, V.C.; D'Assoro, A.B.; Boeneman, K.; Liu, W.; Whitehead, C.M.; Reynolds, C. & Salisbury, J.L. (2002). Centrosome amplification drives chromosomal instability in breast tumor development. *Proceedings of the National Academy of Science of the United States of America*, Vol. 99, pp.1978-1983, ISSN 0027-8424

López-Saavedra, A. & Herrera, L.A. (2010). The role of alternative mRNA splicing in chromosome instability. *Mutation research*, Vol. 705, pp.246-51, ISSN 0027-5107

Louis, D.N.; Ohgaki, H.; Wiestler, O.D.; Cavenee, W.K.; Burger, P.C.; Jouvet, A.; Scheithauer, B.W. & Kleihues, P. (2007). The 2007 WHO Classification of Tumours of the Central Nervous System. *Acta Neuropathologica*, Vol. 114, No.2, pp. 97-109, ISSN 0001-6322

Magnani, I.; Guerneri, S.; Pollo, B.; Cirenei, N.; Colombo, B.M.; Broggi, G.; Galli, C.; Bugiani, O.; DiDonato, S.; Finocchiaro, G. & Fuhrman Conti, A.M. (1994). Increasing complexity of the karyotype in 50 human gliomas. *Cancer Genetics and Cytogenetics*, Vol. 75, pp. 77-89, ISSN 0165-4608

Magnani, I.; Chiariello, E.; Furhrman Conti, A.M. & Finocchiaro, G. (1999). A recurrent 19q11-12 breakpoint suggested by cytogenetic and fluorescence in situ hybridization analysis of three glioblastoma cell lines. *Cancer Genetics and Cytogenetics*, Vol. 110, pp.82-86, ISSN 0165-4608

Magnani, I.; Novielli, C.; Bellini, M.; Roversi, G.; Bello, L. & Larizza, L. (2009). Multiple localization of endogenous MARK4L protein in human glioma. *Cellular Oncology*, Vol.31, pp. 357-370, ISSN 1570-5870

Mandelkow, E.M.; Thies, E.; Trinczek, B.; Biernat, J. & Mandelkow, E. (2004). MARK/PAR1 kinase is a regulator of microtubule-dependent transport in axons. *The Journal of Cell Biology*, Vol. 167, No.1, pp. 99-110, ISSN 0021-9525

Margolis, R.L.; Lohez, O.D. & Andreassen, P.R. (2003). G1 tetraploidy checkpoint and the suppression of tumorigenesis. *Journal of Cellular Biochemistry*, Vol. 88, pp. 673-683, Review, ISSN 1097-4644

Martinez-Garay, I.; Rustom, A.; Gerdes, H.H. & Kutsche, K. (2006). The novel centrosomal associated protein CEP55 is present in the spindle midzone and the midbody. *Genomics*, Vol. 87, pp. 243-253, ISSN 0888-7543

Marx, A.; Nugoor, C.; Panneerselvam, S. & Mandelkow, E. (2010). Structure and function of polarity-inducing kinase family MARK/Par-1 within the branch of AMPK/Snf1-related kinases. *The FASEB Journal*, Vol. 24, pp. 1637-1648, ISSN 0892-6638

Matenia, D. & Mandelkow, E.M. (2009). The tau of MARK: a polarized view of the cytoskeleton. *Trends in biochemical sciences*, Vol. 34, No.7, pp. 332-342, ISSN 0968-0004

Meraldi, P.; Honda, R. & Nigg, E.A. (2002). Aurora-A overexpression reveals tetraploidization as a major route to centrosome amplification in p53-/- cells. *The EMBO Journal*, Vol. 21, pp. 483-492, ISSN 0261-4189

Moravcevic, K.; Mendrola, J.M.; Schmitz, K.R.; Wang, Y.H.; Slochower, D.; Janmey, P.A. & Lemmon, M.A. (2010). Kinase associated-1 domains drive MARK/PAR1 kinases to membrane targets by binding acidic phospholipids. *Cell*, Vol. 143, pp.966-977, ISSN 0092-8674

Moroni, R.F.; De Biasi, S.; Colapietro, P.; Larizza, L. & Beghini, A. (2006). Distinct expression pattern of microtubule-associated protein/microtubule affinity-regulating kinase 4 in differentiated neurons. *Neuroscience*, Vol. 143, pp. 83-94, ISSN 0306-4522

Moudjou, M. & Bornens, M. (1994). Method of centrosome isolation from cultured animal cells. In: *Cell biology: a laboratory handbook*, Celis J.E., pp.595-604, Academic Press, (Ed.), ISBN 0-12-164715-3, San Diego, CA

Müller, J.; Ory, S.; Copeland, T.; Piwnica-Worms, H. & Morrison, D.K. (2001). C-TAK1 regulates Ras signalling by phophorylating the MAPK scaffolds, KSR1. *Molecular Cell*, Vol. 8, pp. 983-993, ISSN 1097-2765

Mullins, J.M. & Biesele, J.J. (1977). Terminal phase of cytokinesis in D-98S cells. *The Journal of Cell Biology*, Vol. 73, pp. 672-684, ISSN 0021-9525

Mullins, J.M. & McIntosh, J.R. (1982). Isolation and initial characterization of the mammalian midbody. *The Journal of Cell Biology*, Vol. 94, pp.654-661, ISSN 0021-9525

Muramatsu, M.; Smetana, K. & Busch, H. (1963). Quantitative aspects of isolation of nucleoli of the Walker carcinosarcoma and liver of the rat. *Cancer Research*, Vol. 23, pp. 510-518, ISSN 0008-5472

Nigro, J.M.; Misra, A.; Zhang, L.; Smirnov, I.; Colman, H.; Griffin, C.; Ozburn, N.; Chen, M.; Pan, E.; Koul, D.; Yung, W.K.; Feuerstein, B.G. & Aldape, K.D. (2005). Integrated array-comparative genomic hybridization and expression array profiles identify clinically relevant molecular subtypes of glioblastoma. *Cancer Research*, Vol. 65, 1678-1686, ISSN 0008-5472

Noble, M. & Dietrich, J. (2004). The complex identity of brain tumors: emerging concerns regarding origin, diversity and plasticity. *TRENDS in Neurosciences*, Vol. 27, No.3, 148-154, ISSN 0166-2236

Ohgaki, H.; Schauble, B.; zur Hausen, A.; von Ammon, K. & Kleihues, P. (1995). Genetic alterations associated with the evolution and progression of astrocytic brain tumours. *Virchows Archive*, Vol. 427, pp. 113-118, ISSN 0945-6317

Park, H.S.; Maeda, T.; Mohapatra, G.; Waldman, F.M.; Davis, R.L. & Feuerstein, B.G. (1995). Heterogeneity, poliploidy, aneusomy and 9p deletion in human glioblastoma multiforme. *Cancer Genetics and Cytogenetics*, Vol. 83, pp. 127-135, ISSN 0165-4608

Parsons, D.W.; Jones, S.; Zhang, X.; Lin, J.C.; Leary; R.J.; Angenendt, P.; Mankoo, P.; Carter, H.; Siu, I.M.; Gallia, G.L.; Olivi, A.; McLendon, R.; Rasheed, B.A.; Keir, S.; Nikolskaya, T.; Nikolsky, Y.; Busam, D.A.; Tekleab, H.; Diaz, L.A. Jr.; Hartigan, J.; Smith, D.R.; Strausberg, R.L.; Marie, S.K.; Shinjo, S.M.; Yan, H.; Riggins, G.J.; Bigner, D.D.; Karchin, R.; Papadopoulos, N.; Parmigiani, G.; Vogelstein, B.; Velculescu, V.E. & Kinzler, K.W. (2008). An integrated genomic analysis of human glioblastoma multiforme. *Science*, Vol. 321, pp.1807-1812, ISSN 0036-8075

Pihan, G.A.; Purohit, A.; Wallace, J.; Knecht, H.; Woda, B.; Quesenberry, P. & Doxsey, S.J. (1998). Centrosome defects and genetic instability in malignant tumors. *Cancer Research*, Vol. 58, pp. 3974-3985, ISSN 0008-5472

Pinkel, D.; Straume, T. & Gray, J.W. (1986). Cytogenetic analysis using quantitative, high-sensitivity, fluorescence hybridization. *Proceedings of the National Academy of Science of the United States of America*, Vol. 83, pp. 2934-2938, ISSN 0027-8424

Ritland, S.R.; Ganju, V. & Jenkins, R.B. (1995). Region-specific loss of heterozygosity on chromosome 19 is related to the morphologic type of human glioma. *Genes, Chromosomes and Cancer*, Vol. 12, pp. 277-282, ISSN 1045-2257

Roversi, G.; Pfundt, R.; Moroni, R.F.; Magnani, I.; van Reijmersdal, S.; Pollo, B.; Straatman, H.; Larizza, L. & Schoenmakers, E.F. (2006). Identification of novel genomic markers related to progression to glioblastoma through genomic profiling of 25 primary glioma cell lines. *Oncogene*, Vol. 9, pp. 1571-1583, ISSN 0950-9232

Saunders, W. (2005). Centrosomal amplification and spindle multipolarity in cancer cells. *Seminars in Cancer Biology*, Vol. 15, pp. 25-32, Review, ISSN 1044-579X

Schaar, B.T.; Kinoshita, K. & McConnell, S.K. (2004). Doublecortin microtubule affinity is regulated by a balance of kinase and phosphatase activity at the leading edge of migrating neurons. *Neuron*, Vol. 41, pp. 203-213, ISSN 0896-6273

Schmidt, M.C.; Antweiler, S.; Urban, N.; Mueller, W.; Kuklik, A.; Meyer-Puttlitz, B; Wiestler, O.D.; Louis, D.N.; Fimmers, R. & von Deimling, A. (2002). Impact of genotype and morphology on the prognosis of glioblastoma. *Journal of Neuropathology & Experimental Neurology*, Vol.61, pp. 321-328, ISSN 0014-4886

Schneider, A.; Laage, R.; von Ahsen, O.; Fischer, A.; Rossner, M.; Scheek, S.; Grünewald, S.; Kuner, R.; Weber, D.; Krüger, C.; Klaussner, B.; Götz, B.; Hiemisch, H.; Newrzella, D.; Martin-Villalba, A.; Bach, A. & Schwaninger, M. (2004). Identification of regulated genes during permanent focal cerebral ischemia: characterization of the protein kinase 9b5/MARKL1/MARK4. *Journal of Neurochemistry*, Vol. 88, pp. 1114-1126, ISSN 1474-1644

Schwarzacher, H.G. & Wachtler, F. (1983). Nucleolus organizer regions and nucleoli. *Human genetics*, Vol. 63, pp. 89-99, ISSN 0340-6717

Segu, L.; Pascaud, A.; Costet, P.; Darmon, M. & Buhot, M.C. (2008). Impairment of spatial learning and memory in ELKL Motif Kinase 1 (EMK1/MARK2) knockout mice. *Neurobiology of aging*, Vol. 29, pp. 231-24, ISSN 0197-4580

Shapiro, J.R. (2002). Genetic alterations associated with adult diffuse astrocytic tumors. *American Journal of Medical Genetics*, Vol.115, pp. 194-201, ISSN 1552-4833

Sluder, G. & Nordberg, J.J. (2004). The good, the bad and the ugly: the practical consequences of centrosome amplification. *Current Opinion in Cell Biology*, Vol. 16, pp.49-54, Review, ISSN 09550674

Smith, J.S.; Alderete, B.; Minn, Y.; Borell, T.J.; Perry, A.; Mohapatra, G.; Hosek, S.M.; Kimmel, D.; O'Fallon, J.; Yates, A.; Feuerstein, B.G.; Burger, P.C.; Scheithauer, B.W. & Jenkins, R.B. (1999). Localization of common deletion regions on 1p and 19q in human gliomas and their association with histological subtype. *Oncogene*, Vol. 18, pp. 4144-4155, ISSN 0950-9232

The Cancer Genome Atlas (TGCA) Research Network. (2008). Comprehensive genomic characterization defines human glioblastoma genes and core pathways. *Nature*, Vol. 455, No.7216, pp. 1061-1068, ISSN 0028-0836

Thiel, G.; Losanowa, T.; Kintzel, D.; Nisch, G.; Martin, H.; Vorpahl, K. & Witkowski, P. (1992). Karyotypes in 90 human gliomas. *Cancer Genetics and Cytogenetics*, Vol. 58, pp. 109-120, ISSN 0165- 4608

Timm, T.; Marx, A.; Panneerselvam, S.; Mandelkow, E. & Mandelkow, E.M. (2008). Structure and regulation of MARK, a kinase involved in abnormal phosphorylation of Tau protein. *BMC Neuroscience*, Vol. 9, Suppl 2, S9, ISSN 1471-2202

Tochio, N.; Koshiba, S.; Kobayashi, N.; Inoue, M.; Yabuki, T.; Aoki, M.; Seki, E.; Matsuda, T.; Tomo, Y.; Motoda, Y.; Kobayashi, A.; Tanaka, A.; Hayashizaki, Y.; Terada, T.; Shirouzu, M.; Kigawa, T. & Yokoyama, S. (2006). Solution structure of the kinase-associated domain 1 of mouse microtubule-associated protein/microtubule affinity-regulating kinase 3. *Protein science*, Vol. 15, 2534-2543, ISSN 1469-896X

Trinczek, B.; Brajenovic, M.; Ebneth, A. & Drewes, G. (2004). MARK4 is a novel Microtubule-associated Proteins/Microtubule Affinity-regulating Kinase that binds to the cellular microtubule network and to centrosomes. *The Journal of Biological Chemistry*, Vol. 279, No. 7, pp. 5915-5923, ISSN 0021-9258

van den Bent, M.J.(2004). Advances in the biology and treatment of oligodendrogliomas. *Current Opinion in Neurology*, Vol. 17, pp.675-680, Review, ISSN 13507540

Visintin, R. & Amon, A. (2000). The nucleolus: the magician's hat for cell cycle tricks. *Current Opinion in Cell Biology*, Vol. 12, No. 3, pp. 372-37, ISSN 09550674

von Deimling, A.; Louis, D.N.; von Ammon, K.; Petersen, I.; Wiestler, O.D. & Seizinger, B.R. (1992). Evidence for a tumor suppressor gene on chromosome 19q associated with human astrocytomas, oligodendrogliomas, and mixed gliomas. *Cancer Research*, Vol. 52, pp.4277-4279, ISSN 0008-5472

von Deimling, A.; von Ammon, K.; Schoenfeld, D.; Wiestler, O.D.; Seizinger, B.R.& Louis, D.N. (1993). Subsets of glioblastoma multiforme defined by molecular genetic analyis. *Brain Pathology*, Vol. 3, pp.19-26, ISSN 1750-3639

von Deimling, A.; Nagel, J.; Bender, B; Lenartz, D.; Schramm, J.; Louis, D.N. & Wiestler, O.D.(1994). Deletion mapping of chromosome 19 in human gliomas. *International Journal of Cancer*, Vol. 57, pp.676-680, ISSN 1097-0215

Weaver, B.A.; Silk, A.D.; Montagna, C.; Verdier-Pinard, P.& Cleveland, D.W. (2007). Aneuploidy acts both oncogenically and as a tumor suppressor. *Cancer Cell* , Vol.11, No.1, pp. 25-36 , ISSN 1535-6108

Wojcik, C. & DeMartino, G.N. (2003). Intracellular localization of proteasomes. *The International Journal of Biochemistry & Cell Biology*, Vol. 35, No.5, pp. 579-5, ISSN 1357-2725 89

Zhang, H.; Ma, X.; Shi, T.; Song, Q.; Zhao, H. & Ma, D. (2010). NSA2, a novel nucleolus protein regulates cell proliferation and cell cycle. *Biochemical and Biophysical Research Communications*, Vol. 391, No.1, p. 65, ISSN 0006-291X

Zhu, Y. & Parada, L.F. (2002). The molecular and genetic basis of neurological tumours. *Nature Reviews Cancer* , Vol. 2, pp. 616-626 , ISSN 1474-175X

9

The Role of Stem Cells in the Glioma Growth

Sergio Garcia, Vinicius Kannen and Luciano Neder
Faculty of Medicine of Ribeirao Preto
University of Sao Paulo
Brazil

1. Introduction

Malignant glioma is the most common type of primary brain tumor and represents one of the most lethal cancers. In contrast to the long-standing and well-defined histopathology, the underlying molecular and genetic bases for gliomas are less known. (Collins, 2004; Dai & Holland, 2001).

As some other human cancers, particularly central nervous tumors are highly heterogeneous. Primarily because of its diffuse nature, relatively little is known about the processes by which they develop (Hulleman & Helin, 2005). Thus, the traditional evolution concept of tumors arising from a single mutated cell has limitations in explaining the heterogeneity observed in a single tumor nest.

Recent decades have seen only limited progress in treatment trials and basic research on human glioma, the most common central nervous malignancy (Huang et al., 2008). Unfortunately, for such gliomas, tumor recurrence after treatment is the rule due to the infiltrative nature of these tumors and the presence of cellular populations with ability to escape therapies and drive tumor recurrence and progression. At least in some cases, these resistant cells exhibit stem cell properties (Frosina, 2011). For these reasons the comprehension of the current knowledge of cancer stem cells (CSC) in relation to gliomas origin, growth and treatment is crucial. As the stem cells (for glioma, neuronal stem cells) are more susceptible to mutation, they become altered easily for their genetic composition and therefore act as the source of cancer/glioma cells. They are not actually a separate cell type and in most cases they are misinterpreted as cancer stem cells (in brain, they are glioma stem cells).

2. Glioma and the concept of cancer stem cells

For a long time it has been known that there are subpopulations of cells within solid tumors that contain different biological behaviors. Among these subpopulations, accumulating evidence supports the existence of the so-called cancer stem cells (CSCs), because these tumor cells possess stem cell properties, possibly being responsible for the initiation, growth and recurrence of tumors. Apparent similarities with non-transformed stem cells, including high self-renewal capacity and the ability to generate differentiated progeny of several cellular lineages, have led to the proposal that stem cell-like cancer cells may either originate from adult undifferentiated stem and progenitor cells or that these properties are being expressed as an effect of the genetic alterations which drive tumorigenicity (Reya et al., 2001; Gilbertson, 2006; Das et al., 2008). Basically, the CSCs, which have also been described as tumor initiating cells or tumor propagating cells, are tumor cells that self-renew and propagate tumors phenotypically similar to the parental tumor (Li et al., 2009). Furthermore, recent studies have suggested that CSC cause tumor recurrence based on their resistance to radiotherapy and chemotherapy (Inoue et al, 2010).

Although considerable controversy still surrounds the existence, behaviors and even the nomenclature of CSCs, there is no doubt that populations of cells with stem-like properties do exist inside several solid and non-solid tumors, including brain cancers. So, despite the fact that CSCs in solid tumors have not yet been precisely identified, the "CSC hypothesis" opens a new paradigm in understanding the biology of cancers. For this reason, the search for the tumor stem cells that may originate and perpetuate the tumor growth has been receiving great attention in the literature (Sanchez-Martin, 2008), but the available knowledge on this issue with regards to the gliomas is scant. Particularly, the exact identity and cell(s) of origin of the so-called glioma stem cell remains elusive (Park & Rich, 2009). Vescovi (2006) offered a functional definition of brain tumor stem cells, namely: brain tumor cells should qualify as stem cells if they show cancer-initiating ability upon orthotopic implantation, extensive self-renewal ability demonstrated either ex vivo or in vivo, karyotypic or genetic alterations, aberrant differentiation properties, capacity to generate non-tumorigenic end cells, and multilineage differentiation capacity. Furthermore, parallels between normal neurogenesis and brain tumorigenesis have been proposed (Singh et al., 2004). It has been more recently confirmed that cancer stem cells from glioblastomas share some characteristics with normal neural stem cells including the expression of neural stem cell markers, the capacity for self-renewal and long term proliferation, the formation of neurospheres, and the ability to differentiate into multiple nervous system lineages (astrocytic, oligodendrocytic and/or neuronal differentiation) (Li et al., 2009).

Among the so far evaluated stem cell markers, the transmembrane protein CD133 has been widely used to isolate putative CSC populations in several cancer types. In fact, CD133 is currently one of the best markers to characterize CSCs (Singh et al., 2004). In both human glioblastomas (GBMs) and medulloblastomas, the expression of the neural stem cell marker CD133 (also known as prominin 1) has been associated with both tumor initiation capacity and radioresistance (Pérez Castillo et al., 2008). Extensive computational comparisons with a compendium of published gene expression profiles revealed that the CD133 gene signature transcriptionally resembles human embryonic stem cells and in vitro cultured GBMs stem cells (GSC), and this signature successfully distinguishes GBMs from lower-grade gliomas. Moreover, the CD133 gene signature identifies an aggressive subtype of GBMs seen in younger patients with a shorter survival (Yan et al., 2011), confirming previous observations that Glioma stem cells are more aggressive in recurrent tumors (Huang et al., 2008). Nevertheless, it must be pointed out that the use of CD133 as a unique glioma stem cell marker is probably not sufficient to tag the whole self-renewing tumor cell reservoir (Clément et al., 2009).

Holmberg et al (2011) have recently characterized human gliomas in various malignancy grades according to the expression of stem cell regulatory proteins. These authors have shown that cells in high grade glioma co-express an array of markers defining neural stem cells (NSCs) and that these proteins can fulfill similar functions in tumor cells as in NSCs. In contrast to NSCs, the glioma cells co-express neural proteins together with pluripotent stem cell markers, including the transcription factors as Oct4, Sox2, Nanog and Klf4. In line with these findings, in high grade gliomas, mesodermal- and endodermal-specific transcription factors were detected together with neural proteins, a combination of lineage markers not normally present in the central nervous system. These findings demonstrate a general deregulated expression of neural and pluripotent stem cell traits in malignant human gliomas.

3. Stem cells and the origin of gliomas

Primarily because of the diffuse nature of gliomas, relatively little is known about the processes by which they develop (Hulleman & Helin, 2005). The concept of stem cells originating gliomas is gaining increased recognition in neuro-oncology (Richj & Eyler, 2008). Until recently, the paradigm of a tumor-initiating stem cell was confined to hematopoietic malignancies where the hierarchical lineages of stem progenitor cells are well established. Nevertheless, the demonstration of persistent stem cells and cycling progenitors in the adult brain is coupled with the expansion of the cancer stem cell concept to solid tumors, leading to the exploration of "stemness" within gliomas. Emerging data are highly suggestive of the subsistence of transformed multipotential cells within a glioma, with a subfraction of cells exhibiting increased efficiency at tumor initiation stage. However, data in support of the true glioma stem cells are inconclusive to date, particularly in respect to the functional characterization of these cells. (Panagiotakos & Tabar, 2007).

Thus, it may be considered that currently it is conceivable thought that malignant gliomas may arise from neural stem cells and appear to contain tumor stem cells. It is thought that normal stem cells live in protected pockets of the body called *niches*, where they divide infrequently to avoid accumulating damaging mutations. Upon injury or in response to normal stimuli, stem cells are mobilized to divide (Gilbertson, 2006). Hence, parallel to the role that normal stem cells play in organogenesis, stem cells are thought to be crucial for tumorigenesis.

The normal adult neural stem cells (NSCs) arise from radial glia (RG) within the central nervous system (Weiner, 2008). The RG progeny includes all the main lineages of the CNS: neurons, astrocytes, oligodendrocytes, ependymocytes and adult neural stem cells (Malatesta et al. 2003). By comparing the gene expression profiles of ependymomas with those of cells in the normal developing nervous system, it was possible to identify the RG as candidate stem cells of this brain tumor (Gilbertson, 2006). Furthermore, RG cells produce neurons in addition to glia during central nervous system development in all vertebrates and are also involved in reparative process (Weiner, 2008).

Until recently, it was thought that ependymomas originated from neuroepithelial cells, glioblastomas from abnormal astrocytes, and medulloblastomas from primitive cells in the external granular layer, but there is now evidence that all tumors can originate from a special type of stem cell called "radial glial cell" (RGC). It is interesting to note that in the human brain, most of stem cells are located in the subventricular zones (SVZ). Both supra- and infratentorially and when stimulated with carcinogens, cells in the SVZ become tumorigenic faster than those located elsewhere. In the SVZ, stem cells exist in the form of RGCs, which remain quiescent until they receive transformational signals. It is not clear whether RGCs, after receiving transformation signals, return to their initial stem cell configuration and then become tumorigenic or they transform to tumor progenitor cells directly. In the cerebellum, depending upon the signals received, RGCs and stem cells may give origin to either ependymoma or medulloblastoma.

Tumours with the highest incidence in humans— medulloblastomas and glioblastomas — both originate from abnormal brain stem cells. . Not surprising, both of these tumors are CD133-positive, containing great neuronal differentiation, which makes them prone to be diffuse and resistant to treatment (Castilo, 2010).

4. Gliomas and the field cancerization concept

It is universally accepted that tumors growth as a clonal evolution from a single cell (Nowell, 1976). The "field cancerization theory" was introduced more than fifty years ago by Slaugher et al (1953), when studying the presence of histologically abnormal tissue surrounding carcinomas. In a classic report on oral cancer, Slaughter called "field cancerization" – a process of repeated exposure of a region's entire tissue area to carcinogenic insult (e.g., tobacco and alcohol), which increases the tissue's risk for developing multiple independent premalignant and malignant foci. The field cancerization hypothesis states that multiple cells form independent tumors on one given tissue, since carcinogenic exposure affects multiple cells in the field (Slaughter *et al.*, 1953), and predicts that second primary or synchronous tumours arise from independent genetic events (Garcia et al., 1999). The field cancerization theory may be explained by the concept that a given stem cell that acquires genetic alterations may form a "patch", a clonal unit of altered daughter cells. The proliferation of these patch cells forms expanding fields which gradually displace the normal tissue and, by clonal divergence, ultimately leads to the development of one or more tumors within a contiguous field of preneoplastic cells (Garcia et al., 1999). An important clinical implication is that fields often remain after surgery of the primary tumor and may lead to new cancers, designated presently by clinicians as "a second primary tumor" or "local recurrence," depending on the exact site and time interval (Braakhuis et al., 2003; Ryan, 2007). We had previously discussed how mutated clones from mutated stem cells may spread on tissues and that the field cancerization theory implies that the mutated genotype and molecular changes occur before the appearance of histopathological evidence of malignant cells (Garcia et al., 1999). Therefore, this "anomaly" might be due to changes that occur in a "premalignant" neoplastic condition that was histologically identified as "normal". In the clinical aspect, the field cancerization may have an etiologic role in a substantial number of recurrences. For example, a surgical resection margin that includes a genetically altered field can explain the occurrence of scar recurrence. This explanation suggests that molecular profiling of surgical margins will help reduce scar recurrences. Since multiple independent patches of cancer fields may be present in the same organ exposed to the same insults, clean molecular margins may not necessarily prevent recurrences in the residual organ (Dakubo et al., 2007). Similarly to gliomas, tumor recurrence is a major clinical concern for patients with urothelial carcinoma of the urinary bladder. Traditional morphological analysis is of limited utility for identifying cases in which recurrence will occur. However, recent studies have suggested that urothelial carcinogenesis occurs as a 'field effect' that can involve any number of sites in the bladder mucosa. Accumulating evidence supports the notion that resident urothelial stem cells in the affected field are transformed into cancer stem cells by acquiring genetic alterations that lead to tumor formation through clonal expansion (Cheng et al., 2009).

The available information in regards to the existence of a field phenomenon in gliomas is scant. In malignant gliomas, the high recurrence rates, the characteristically heterogeneous features and frequent diffuse spread within the brain have raised the question of whether malignant gliomas arise monoclonally from a single precursor cell or polyclonally from multiple transformed cells forming confluent clones (Inoue et al., 2008). To address this issue, Kattar et al (1997) have evaluated the clonality of low-grade and malignant gliomas by using polymerase chain reaction (PCR)-based assay for nonrandom X chromosome inactivation using surgical and autopsy material. The same pattern of nonrandom X chromosome inactivation was present in all areas of fifteen of 19 tumors, which were considered as monoclonal, suggesting that low-grade and malignant gliomas are, at least, usually monoclonal tumors, and extensively infiltrating tumors must result from migration of tumor cells.

Gliomatosis cerebri may shed some light in this issue. It is a rare condition in which the brain is infiltrated by an exceptionally diffusely growing of malignant glial cell population involving at least 2 lobes, though often more extensive, sometimes even affecting infratentorial regions. Kross et al (2002) have evaluated the existence of field cancerization in this affection, since gliomatosis cerebri may initiate as an oligoclonal process or result from collision of different gliomas. It was hypothesized that the presence of an identical set of genetic aberrations throughout the lesion would point to monoclonality of the process. In contrast, the finding of non-identical genetic changes in widely separated regions within the neoplasm would support the concept of collision of different mutated clones. For such, the authors used one autopsy case of gliomatosis cerebri, from which tissue samples were randomly taken from 24 locations throughout the brain and used for genetic investigation. With this aim, genome-wide screening for chromosomal aberrations was accomplished by comparative genomic hybridization (CGH). The authors found a wide distribution of particular sets of genetic aberrations, supporting the concept of monoclonal tumor proliferation (Kross et al., 2002). Nevertheless, it has been observed and well documented in one clinical case that on the long term, after initial treatment for gliomatosis cerebri, one glioblastoma multiforme has developed, and in a location separate from the initial lesion, suggesting that different clonal origin may had occurred (Inoue et al., 2008). More recently, Chen et al (2010) showed that the capacities for self-renewal and tumour initiation in GBM need not be restricted to a uniform population of stemlike cells.

5. The contribution of studies in animal models: Unifying the cancer stem cells and field cancerization concepts

Many genetic alterations have been identified in human gliomas, however, establishing unequivocal correlation between these genetic alterations and gliomagenesis requires accurate animal models for these cancers (Dai & Holland, 2001). Indeed, it is useful and necessary to have animal models for CNS tumors studies allowing to be carried out in different stages of tumor growth, especially in early stages, rare to be detected and observed in clinical practice (Bulnes-Sesma, 2006).

Experimental models of gliomagenesis most commonly used alkylating agents such as N-ethyl N-nitrosourea (ENU), which has been considered as a suitable model to study malignant changes. These changes were reported to appear firstly as early neoplastic proliferation (ENP) center, which continues in following stages subsequently progressing to "microtumors" until a tumor in itself. (Koestner et al., 1971; Naito et al., 1984).

By using the experimental model of gliomagenesis induced by the N-ethyl N-nitrosourea, we were able to detect putative tumor stem cells in early oncogenesis, yielding to analyze a field cancerization process and observe a close morphological relationship between metallothionein (MT) positive cells and blood vessels. With this aim, we have developed an experimental model to track putative mutated stem cells, using the ENU experimental model and metallothioneins (MT) immunostaining. MTs are metal binding proteins that take part in the homeostasis of the ions of the metals which are necessary for the proper metabolism of the organism (zinc, copper), disintoxication of metals and protect the tissues from the effects of free radicals, radiation and from mutagens (Thirumoorthy et al., 2007). MT expression is present in a significant portion of especially malignant brain tumors. In astrocytic tumors an acquired enhanced ability to produce MT has been observed as the malignant potential of a tumor increases (Hiura et al., 1998), and MT might be involved in poor response to antineoplastic drugs (Maier et al., 1997). In the murine colonic mucosa, the crypt restricted immunopositivity for MT has been shown to be reliable marker of stem cell mutation that may be induced early after mutagen treatment and that can be assayed in paraffin-fixed tissue sections (Cook et al., 2000). We have observed that 30 days after the treatment of rats with ENU, the main location of the MT positive cells have striking similarity to that of the RG cells and that the frequency of these cells (a) is strongly correlated with the increased appearing of ENP centers and new blood vessels, (b) is augmented at higher levels in long-term observation, i.e., 180 days after the carcinogen administration, (c) is related to a high staining intensity in both nucleus and cytoplasm, and (d) is very similar to the pattern of immunostaining that was observed in the nervous tissue surrounding gliomas, which were originated at an average of 321 days after the ENU administration (Fernandes-da-Silva et al., 2009). The mechanisms and reasons why MT is expressed in the preneoplastic and neoplastic lesions remain to be fully elucidated. It has been hypothesized that mutation-induced MT overexpression may interfere with the function of zinc finger DNA binding transcription factors (Zeng et al., 1991), which have been implicated in transcriptional control of various genes, including TP53, involved in cell proliferation and apoptosis. These MT-mediated effects on gene transcription are thought to confer a selective growth or survival advantage (or both) on the mutated cells (Bruewer, 2002).

6. Glioma, stem cells niche and angiogenesis

Recently in a review article, Gilbertson & Rich JN (2007) address a number of key questions which remain to be answered: do all cancer stem cells require the support of aberrant niches? Are cancer stem cell niches the primary drivers of tumor development, or are they recruited by pre-formed cancer stem cells? How do cancer stem cells and their niches subvert the tight regulatory conditions that characterize normal stem cell niches?

The stem cells of glioblastoma seem to be dependent on signals from aberrant vascular niches that mimic the normal neural stem cell niche (Gilbertson & Rich, 2007). Stem cells of various tissues are tightly regulated by the immediate microenvironment or stem cell niche (Moore & Lemischka, 2006), which is provided by capillaries in specific locations (Riquelme et al., 2008). This organization places the stem cells in close proximity to endothelial and other vascular cells, facilitating cross-talking among these cell types and affecting stem cell fate choices (Gilbertson, 2006). It is well-known that stem cells and their microenvironments may influence each other (Scadden, 2006). In fact, Cues within the niche, from cell–cell interactions to diffusible factors, are spatially and temporally coordinated to regulate proliferation and neurogenesis, ultimately (Riquelme et al., 2008).

In ENU treated rats, we have observed the existence of a close morphological relationship between MT positive cells and blood vessels. What is the relationship between them? It is known that MT is involved in the regulation of the functions of endothelial cells as well as in their protection against cytotoxic agents (Kaji et al., 1993). MT knock-out (MT-KO) mice presented dramatically decreased IL-6-induced angiogenesis caused by cortical freeze injury, suggesting that the MT have major regulatory functions in the angiogenesis process (Penkowa et al., 2000). In fact, human CD133+ Glioma CSCs are capable of producing vascular endothelial growth factor (VEGF) and thus may play an important role in glioma angiogenesis (Yao et al.,2008).

7. The concept of stemness, modulation of csc and glioma treatment

Understanding the characteristics and function of CSCs has shed light on their roles in glioma progression, including the implications for prognosis and treatment resistance. The original use of the term stemness was derived from a number of articles aimed to look for genes that could be expressed in general stem cell populations. The *stemness hypothesis* states that all stem cells use common mechanisms to regulate self-renewal and multi-lineage potential. This hypothesis has been debated and so far no conclusive evidence for a set of genes expressed in all stem cells. Certainly, identifying genes regulating stem cell properties will greatly improve our understanding of the molecular mechanisms regulating stem cell functions, our ability to manipulate stem cell fate, and the roles of stem cells in cancer (Koeva et al., 2011). Interestingly, overexpression of the transcription factor NANOG in gliomas and its close relationship with the undifferentiated state of glioma cells in vivo and in vitro indicated that NANOG may contribute to the existence of brains CSCs and may be related to tumorigenesis of the cerebrum by maintaining the undifferentiated state of glioma cells (Niu et al., 2011).

The new concept stemness is closely related to the observation that there are tissue environment factors that are able to influence or modulate CSCs. The main one is hypoxia, which activates the Hypoxia Induced Factor alpha number 1 (HIFα-1) alpha to enhance the self-renewal activity of CD133-positive cells and to inhibit their differentiation (Soeda et al., 2009). This and other signaling systems drive the transformation of normal stem cells, and perhaps of the bulk of tumor cells to cancer stem cells or to maintain the CSC phenotype (Katoh, 2011). For instance, the oxygen level of 7% has been observed to enhance the stem cell–like phenotype of CD133+ in GBM cells (McCord et al., 2009). Furthermore, it has been observed that human glioblastoma cells from tumor biopsies, which were engrafted intracerebrally into nude rats, that CD133 negative glioma cells were tumorgenic in nude rats, and that CD133 positive cells can be obtained from these tumors. Upon the passing of the cell tumors in vivo, CD133 expression is upregulated, coinciding with the onset of angiogenesis and a shorter patient survival (Wang et al., 2008). Furthermore, the bone morphogenic protein BMP4 effectively reduces proliferation of CD133 positive cells in vitro and the tumor growth in vivo. BMP4 may act as a key inhibitory regulator of cancer initiation and therefore may be used in combined stem cell-based therapy as a non-cytotoxic therapeutic agent (Altaner, 2008).

If one accepts that there is a subpopulation of cancer cells with stem cell properties, which is responsible for tumor maintenance and progression, and may contribute to the resistance to anticancer treatments, it is very reasonable to deduce that compounds that target cancer stem-like cells could be effective to impair or even to destroy a neoplasm and nas important therapeutic implications. Various compounds have been investigated as putative influencers of stemness and malignancies in glioma stem-like cells, leading the proposal that stem cell regulatory factors may provide significant targets for therapeutic strategies (Holmberg et al., 2011). Ongoing work aims the identification of unique pathways governing self-renewal of these putative stem cells and their validation as ultimate therapeutic targets (Panagiotakos & Tabar, 2007). Additionally, it is possible to conceive that epigenetic-based drugs that modulate gene expression in CSC possibly constitute a promising alternative resource for target therapy in the treatment of these, thus far, incurable malignancy.

8. References

Altaner, C. 2008. Glioblastoma and stem cells. *Neoplasma*, Vol.55, No.5, pp.369-374.

Braakhuis BJM, Tabor MP, Kummer JA, Leemans CR, Brakenhoff RH. 2003. A genetic explanation of Slaughter's concept of field cancerization: evidence and clinical implications. *Cancer Res*, Vol.63, No.8, pp.1727-1730.

Bruewer, M.; Schmid, K.W.; Krieglstein, C.F.; Senninger, N.; Schuermann, G. 2002. Metallothionein: early marker in the carcinogenesis of ulcerative colitis-associated colorectal carcinoma. *World Journal of Surgery*, 26,6,726-731.

Bulnes-Sesma S, Ullibarri-Ortiz de Zárate N, Lafuente-Sánchez JV. 2006. Tumour induction by ethylnitrosourea in the central nervous system. *Rev Neurol*, Vol.43, No12, pp.733-738.

Castillo, M. 2010. Stem cells, radial glial cells, and a unified origin of brain tumors. *American Journal Neuroradiology*, No.3, Mar, pp.389-390.

Chen, R.; Nishimura, M.C.; Bumbaca, S.M.; Kharbanda, S.; Forrest, W.F.; Kasman, I.M.; Greve, J.M.; Soriano, R.H.; Gilmour, L.L.; Rivers, C.S.; Modrusan, Z.; Nacu, S.; Guerrero, S.; Edgar, K.A.; Wallin, J.J.; Lamszus, K.; Westphal, M.; Heim, S.; James, C.D.; VandenBerg, S.R.; Costello, J.F.; Moorefield, S.; Cowdrey, C.J.; Prados, M.; Phillips, H.S. 2010. A hierarchy of self-renewing tumor-initiating cell types in glioblastoma. *Cancer Cell*, Vol.17, No.4, April, pp.362-375.

Cheng L, Zhang S, Davidson DD, MacLennan GT, Koch MO, Montironi R, Lopez-Beltran A. 2009. Molecular determinants of tumor recurrence in the urinary bladder. *Future Oncology*, Vol.5, No.6, pp. 843-857.

Clément, V.; Dutoit, V.; Marino, D.; Dietrich, P.Y.; Radovanovic, I. 2009. Limits of CD133 as a marker of glioma self-renewing cells. *Int J Cancer*. Jul 1;125(1):244-8.

Collins, V.P. Brain tumours: classification and genes. 2004. *J Neurol Neurosurg Psychiatry*, Vol.75 Suppl 2, pp.2-11.

Cook, A.H.; Williams, D.; Thomas, A.G. 2000. Crypt-restricted metallothionein immunopositivity in murine colon: validation of a model for studies of somatic stem cell mutation. *J Pathology*, Vol.191, No.3, pp.306-312.

Dakubo, G.D.; Jakupciak, J.P.; Birch-Machin, M.A.; Parr, R.L.; 2007. Clinical implications and utility of field cancerization., *Cancer Cell International, Vol.7*, pp.2. ???

Dai, C. & Holland, E.C. 2001. Glioma models. *Biochim Biophys Acta*, Vol.1551, No.1, pp.M19-27.

Das, S.; Srikanth, M.; Kessler, J.A. 2008. Cancer stem cells and glioma. *Nat Clin Pract Neurology*, Vol.4, pp.427–435.

Fernandes da Silva, J.C.; Kanen, V.C.; Turatti, A.; Ribeiro-Silva, A.; Herrero, C.F.S.; Garcia, S.B. 2009. Overexpression of metallothioneins, stem cell niches and field cancerization in experimental gliomagenesis. *COLUNA/COLUMNA*, Vol.8, No.4, pp.428-433.

Frosina, G. 2011. Frontiers in targeting glioma stem cells. *Eur J Cancer*, Vol.47, No.4, Mar, pp.496-507.

Garcia SB, Park HS, Novelli M, Wright NA. 199. Field cancerization, clonality, and epithelial stem cells: the spread of mutated clones in epithelial sheets. *J Pathol*, Vol.187, pp.61-81.

Gilbertson, R.J. 2006. Brain tumors provide new clues to the source of cancer stem cells: does oncology recapitulate ontogeny? *Cell Cycle*, Vol.5, pp.135–137.

Gilbertson, R.J. & Rich, J.N. 2007. Making a tumour's bed: glioblastoma stem cells and the vascular niche. *Nat Rev Cancer*, Vol.7, No.10, pp.733-736.

Hiura, T.; Khalıd, H.; Yamashita, H.; Tokunaga, Y.; Yasunaga, A.; Shibata, S. 1998. Immunohistochemical analysis of metallothionein in astrocytic tumors in relation to tumor grade, proliferative potential, and survival. *Cancer*, Vol.83, No.11, pp.2361-2369.

Holmberg J, He X, Peredo I, Orrego A, Hesselager G, Ericsson C, Hovatta O, Oba-Shinjo SM, Marie SK, Nistér M, Muhr J. 2011. Activation of neural and pluripotent stem cell signatures correlates with increased malignancy in human glioma. *PLoS One*, Vol.6, No.3, pp.e18454.

Huang, Q.; Zhang, Q.B.; Dong, J.; Wu, Y.Y.; Shen, Y.T.; Zhao, Y.D.; Zhu, Y.D.; Diao, Y.; Wang, A.D.; Lan, Q. 2008. Glioma stem cells are more aggressive in recurrent tumors with malignant progression than in the primary tumor, and both can be maintained long-term in vitro, *BMC Cancer*, Vol.8, Oct, pp.304.

Hulleman, E. & Helin, K. Molecular mechanisms in gliomagenesis. 2005. *Adv Cancer Research*, Vol.94, pp.1-27.

Inoue, A.; Takahashi, H.; Harada, H.; Kohno, S.; Ohue, S.; Kobayashi, K.; Yano, H.; Tanaka, Ohnishi, T. 2010. Cancer stem-like cells of glioblastoma characteristically express MMP-13 and display highly invasive activity. *Int Journal of Oncology*, Vol.37, No.5, Nov, pp.1121-1131.

Inoue, T.; Kanamori, M.; Sonoda, Y.; Watanabe, M.; Sasajima, T.; Kamisato, N.; Kumabe, T.; Tominaga, T. 2008. Glioblastoma multiforme developing separately from the initial lesion 9 years after successful treatment for gliomatosis cerebri: a case report. *No Shinkei Geka*, Vol.36, No.8, Aug, pp.709-715.

Kaji, T.; Yamamoto, C.; Tsubaki, S.; Sakamoto, M.; Sato, M.; Kozuka, H. 1993. Metallothionein induction by cadmium, cytokines, thrombin and endothelin-1 in cultured vascular endothelial cells. *Life Sci*, Vol.53, No.15, pp.1185-1191.

Katoh, M. 2011. Network of WNT and other regulatory signaling cascades in pluripotent stem cells and cancer stem cells. *Curr Pharm Biotechnol.* Vol.12, No.2, pp.160-170.

Kattar, M.M.; Kupsky, W.J.; Shimoyama, R.K.; Vo, T.D.; Olson, M.W.; Bargar, G.R.; Sarkar, F.H. 1997. Clonal analysis of gliomas. *Human Pathology,* Vol.28, No.10, Oct, pp.1166-1179.

Koestner, A.; Swenberg, J.A.; Wechsler, W. 1971. Transplacental production with ethylnitrosourea of neoplasms of the nervous system in Sprague-Dawley rats. Am J Pathology, Vol.63, No.1, Apr, pp.37-56. (PMID:4323476)

Koeva, M.; Forsberg, E.C.; Stuart, J.M. 2011 . Computational integration of homolog and pathway gene module expression reveals general stemness signatures. *PLoS One.* Vol.6, No.4, pp.e18968.

Kros, J.M.; Zheng, P.; Dinjens, W.N.; Alers, M; Janeke, C. 2002. Genetic Aberrations in Gliomatosis Cerebri Support Monoclonal Tumorigenesis. *Journal of Neuropathology & Experimental Neurology,* Vol.61, No.9, pp.806–814.

Li, Z.; Bao, S.; Wu, Q.; Wang, H.; Eyler, C.; Sathornsumetee, S.; Shi, Q.; Cao, Y.; Lathia, J.; McLendon, R.E.; Hjelmeland, A.B.; Rich, J.N. 2009. Hypoxia-inducible factors regulate tumorigenic capacity of glioma stem cells. *Cancer Cell,* Vol.15, No.6, Jun, pp.501-513.

Li, Z. & Rich JN. 2010. Hypoxia and hypoxia inducible factors in cancer stem cell maintenance. *Curr Top Microbiol Immunol,* Vol.345, pp.21-30.

Maier, H.; Jones, C.; Jasani, B.; Ofner, D.; Zelger, B.; Schmid, K.W.; Budka, H. 1997. Metallothionein overexpression in human brain tumours. *Acta Neuropathol,* Vol.94, No.6, pp.599-604.

Malatesta, P.; Hack, M.A.; Hartfuss, E.; Kettenmann, H.; Klinkert, W.; Kirchhoff, F.; Götz, M. 2003. Neuronal or glial progeny: regional differences in radial glia fate. *Neuron,* Vol.37, No.5, pp.751-764.

McCord, A.M.; Jamal, M.; Shankavaram, U.T.; Lang, F.F.; Camphausen, K.; Tofilon, P.J. 2009. Physiologic oxygen concentration enhances the stem-like properties of CD133+ human glioblastoma cells in vitro. *Mol Cancer Res,* Vol.7, No.4, Apr, pp.489-497.

Moore, K. A. & Lemischka, I. R. 2006. Stem cells and their niches. *Science,* Vol.311, pp.1880–1885.

Naito, M.; Naito, Y.; Ito, A.; Watanabe, H.; Kawashima, K. 1984. Spinal cord tumors induced by N-ethyl-N-nitrosourea in rats: presence of spinal subpial target cells. *J Natl Cancer Institute,* Vol.2, No.3, pp.715-724.

Niu, C.S.; Li, D.X.; Liu, Y.H.; Fu, X.M.; Tang, S.F.; Li, J. Expression of NANOG in human gliomas and its relationship with undifferentiated glioma cells. 2011. *Oncol Rep*ort, May 13, doi: 10.3892/or.2011.1308. [Epub ahead of print]

Nowell, P.C. 1976. The clonal evolution of tumor cell populations. *Science;* Vol.194, pp. 23–28.

Panagiotakos, G. & Tabar, V. 2007. Brain tumor stem cells. *Current Neurology and Neuroscience Reports,* Vol.7, No.3, pp.215-220.

Park, D.M.; Rich, J.N. 2009. Biology of glioma cancer stem cells. *Mol Cells,* Vol.28, No.1, Jul, pp.7-12.

Penkowa, M.; Carrasco, J.; Giralt, M.; Molinero, A.; Hernández, J.; Campbell, I.L. 2000. Altered central nervous system cytokine-growth factor expression profiles and angiogenesis in metallothionein-I+II deficient mice. *J Cereb Blood Flow Metab*. Vol.20, No.8; pp.1174-1189.

Pérez Castillo, A.; Aguilar-Morante, D.; Morales-García, J.A.; Dorado, J. 2008. Cancer stem cells and brain tumors. *Clin Transl Oncol*, Vol.10, No.5, May, pp.262-267.

Reya, T.; Morrison, S.J.; Clarke, M.F.; Weissman, I.L. 2001. Stem cells, cancer, and cancer stem cells. *Nature.*;414:105–11.

Rich, J.N. & Eyler, C.E. 2008. Cancer stem cells in brain tumor biology. *Cold Spring Harb Symp Quant Biol*, Vol.73, pp.411-420.

Riquelme, P.A.; Drapeau, E.; Doetsch F. 2008. Brain micro-ecologies: neural stem cell niches in the adult mammalian brain. *Philos Trans R Soc Lond B Biol Science*, Vol.363, No.1489, pp.123-137.

Ryan, L.P. 2007. Clinical implications and utility of field cancerization. *Cancer Cell International*, 7:2.

Sanchez-Martin, M. 2008. Brain tumor stem cells: implications for cancer therapy and regenerative medicine. *Curr Stem Cell Res Ther*, Vol.3, No.3, pp.197-207.

Scadden, D. T. 2006. The stem-cell niche as an entity of action. *Nature*, Vol.441, pp.1075–1079.

Singh, S.K.; Clarke, I.D.; Hide, T.; Dirks PB. 2004. Cancer stem cells in nervous system tumors. *Oncogene*, Vol.23, No.43, Sep., pp.7267-7273.

Slaughter, D.P.; Southwick, H.W.; Smejkal, W. 1953. Field cancerization in oral stratified squamous epithelium; clinical implications of multicentric origin. *Cancer*. Vol.6, No.5, Sep., pp.963-968. (PMID:13094644)

Soeda, A.; Park, M.; Lee, D.; Mintz, A, Androutsellis-Theotokis A, McKay RD, Engh J, Iwama T, Kunisada T, Kassam AB, Pollack IF, Park DM. 2009. Hypoxia promotes expansion of the CD133-positive glioma stem cells through activation of HIF-1alpha. *Oncogene*, Vol.28, No.45, pp.3949-3959.

Thirumoorthy, N.M.; Kumar, K.T.; Shyam, S.A.; Panayappan, L.; Chatterjee, M. 2007. Metallothionein: an overview. *World J Gastroenterology*, Vol.13, No.7, pp.993-996.

Vescovi, A.L.; Galli, R.; Reynolds, B.A. 2006. Brain tumor stem cells. *Nat Rev Cancer*, Vol.6, pp.425–436

Wang, J.; Sakariassen, P.O.; Tsinkalovsky, O.; Immervoll, H.; Bøe, S.O.; Svendsen, A.; Prestegarden, L.; Røsland, G.; Thorsen, F.; Stuhr, L.; Molven, A.; Bjerkvig, R.; Enger, P.Ø. 2008. CD133 negative glioma cells form tumors in nude rats and give rise to CD133 positive cells. *Int J Cancer*, Vol.122, No.4, Feb, pp.761-768.

Weiner, L.P. 2008. Definitions and criteria for stem cells. *Methods Mol Biol*. Vol. 438, pp.3-8.

Yan, X.; Ma, L.; Yi, D.; Yoon, J.G.; Diercks, A.; Foltz, G.; Price, N.D.; Hood, L.E.; Tian, Q. 2011. A CD133-related gene expression signature identifies an aggressive glioblastoma subtype with excessive mutations. *Proc Natl Acad Science*, Vol.108, No.4, Jan, pp.1591-1596.

Yao, X.H.; Ping, Y.F.; Chen, J.H.; Xu, C.P.; Chen, D.L.; Zhang, R.; Wang, J.M.; Bian, X.W.
2008. Glioblastoma stem cells produce vascular endothelial growth factor by
activation of a G-protein coupled formylpeptide receptor FPR. *J Pathology*, Vol.215,
No.4, Aug, pp.369-376.
Zeng, J.; Heuchel, R.; Schaffner, W.; Kägi, J.H. 1991. Thionein (apometallothionein) can
modulate DNA binding and transcription activation by zinc finger containing
factor Sp1. *FEBS Lett*, Vol.279, No.2, pp.310-312.

10

Bone Marrow-Derived Cells Support Malignant Transformation of Low-Grade Glioma

Jeffrey P. Greenfield et al.*
Weill Cornell Medical College
USA

1. Introduction

Gliomas, the most common primary brain tumors, exist as a continuum between low-grade and high-grade states. Low grade gliomas are generally found in children and young adults. These tumors are characterized by well-differentiated cellularity which is mildly pleomorphic. These tumors lack mitotic figures and neovascularization and do not enhance on MRI. The average survival of patients after diagnosis is 7-10 years; the morbidity associated with these lesions is largely dependent on progression of these lesions to a higher grade state. High-grade gliomas, conversely, which exist on the other end of the glial neoplasm spectrum, are extremely malignant with poorly differentiated cells that are highly pleomorphic and display numerous mitotic figures. These tumors contain significant vascular proliferation, hemorrhage and necrosis. High grade gliomas enhance brightly on contrast MRI and often exhibit widespread invasion throughout the brain. Prognosis is poor for high grade gliomas, with a median survival of 18 months even with aggressive therapies. One of the key events in the transition from the low-grade to high-grade state has been referred to as the angiogenic switch. This is defined as the period during which the tumor undergoes a transition to an environment capable of rapid blood vessel formation supporting subsequent exponential tumor growth. It is theorized that in the low-grade state, tumor growth may be limited, at least in part, by a lack of blood supply limiting the tumor to linear growth. Once the tumor acquires the ability to recruit or form new blood vessels through this angiogenic switch, exponential growth may occur, which results in rapid clinical progression. It has been well-described in the literature that bone marrow-derived cells (BMDC) participate in the progression of cancer. BMDCs in the local tumor microenvironment have been proposed to be capable of breaking down normal structures thereby promoting vasculogenesis and invasiveness. This, in turn, provides an environment capable of sustaining and promoting tumor growth. The role of BMDC in metastatic disease has been well-documented and recent data suggests that BMDC participate in the growth and progression of brain tumors as well. This chapter will explore the role of BMDC in the transition from low-grade to high-grade gliomas particularly with respect to the angiogenic

---
* William S. Cobb, Caitlin E. Hoffman, Xueying Chen, Prajwal Rajappa,
Chioma Ihunnah, Yujie Huang and David Lyden
Weill Cornell Medical College
USA

switch. The possibility of this pathway as a potential therapeutic target will also be reviewed.

2. Low-grade glioma transformation in adults

Low-grade gliomas (LGG) are a heterogeneously diverse group of tumors with a generally benign histology and an associated variable outcome. This unpredictable course relies, in part, on the potential for malignant transformation to a higher grade. These tumors present a unique therapeutic challenge as they are typically associated with minimal symptoms and benign radiographic appearance. Initially, the majority of LGGs run an indolent clinical course but often ultimately progress into aggressive tumors with a poor prognosis. As a result, significant controversy exists as to appropriate treatment protocols for this disease. The natural history of LGG, and the risk factors for progression, have been one focus of glioma research due to the potential impact on treatment strategy. Many recent studies have helped clarify treatment recommendations including extent of resection, timing and efficacy of radiation therapy, and response to chemotherapy. Significant debate remains, however, regarding standardization of treatment for low-grade glioma given the tremendous diversity in tumor histology, biology, and outcome. While observation of low-grade gliomas was previously considered a valid treatment option to avoid the morbidity of surgery, chemotherapy, and radiation, early intervention has gradually become standard of care as the impact and incidence of malignant progression has become fully realized. Subjecting patients to the morbidity of aggressive treatment in an unpredictable tumor with variable outcome remains controversial, however. Currently, significant effort is focused on identification of risk factors and tumor characteristics that lead to progression. Better appreciation for the molecular and cellular mechanisms of malignant transformation carries the potential to create novel treatment regimens with less morbidity, thereby alleviating the use of radiation and chemotherapy which present significant toxicity to both children and adults. A review of the characteristics of low-grade gliomas, current treatment strategies, their transformation potential, and current efforts to define novel pathways involved in malignant transformation follows.

The term LGG includes World Health Organization Grade I and Grade II tumors, which are typically associated with indolent tumor growth and significantly better prognosis compared to high grade gliomas. Grade I gliomas include pilocytic astrocytoma, desmoplastic neuroectodermal tumors, subependymoma, ganglioglioma, myxopapillary ependymoma, and desmoplastic infantile tumors, which represent a spectrum of typically benign lesions. Within this class, pilocytic histology is the most common (Stieber, 2001). These pilocytic tumors are well-circumscribed, non-infiltrative, and do not generally transform to more malignant, higher grade lesions. While malignant transformation has been reported in WHOI tumors, the primary risk for malignant degeneration exists in Grade II tumors including low-grade or fibrillary astrocytoma, oligodendroglioma, or mixed oligo-astrocytoma. Ependymoma, ganglioglioma, pleomorphic xanthoastrocytoma, and choroid gliomas of the third ventricle are also considered grade II. Fibrillary astrocytomas, which comprise the majority of grade II lesions (Stieber, 2001), have garnered significant attention due to the significant morbidity and mortality of patients with this diagnosis.

While WHO I gliomas are typically well-circumscribed tumors with benign histology, WHO II gliomas are diffuse, infiltrative and have malignant potential (Stieber, 2001). Both classes, however, are associated with slow tumor growth. The incidence of LGG is reported to be between 2,700 and 4,700 cases per year, comprising approximately 30% of all malignant gliomas (Schiff et al., 2007, Wessels et al., 2003). These tumors are most common in Caucasian males, and typically present in the second to fourth decades (Schomas et al., 2009, Wessels et al., 2003). Patients greater than 60 years of age carry a poorer prognosis with generally lower Karnofsky scores and larger tumor burden at diagnosis. In adults, the most common presenting symptom is seizure followed by incidental findings on imaging. Less common presentations include trauma trauma, sinus pathology, and pituitary disorder (Wessels et al., 2003). Thirty percent of patients present with neurological deficit, and only 10% present with symptoms of raised intracranial pressure ICP. Speech and language deficits have been reported in 10% of patients (Prabhu et al., 2010), however, focal deficits are less common (Schomas et al., 2009, Wessels et al., 2003).

In adults, LGGs are generally hemispheric, supratentorial, and typically occur in the frontal and temporal lobes. They may involve eloquent cortex, which limits the capacity for gross total resection due to significant risk of morbidity (Prabhu et al., 2010, Stieber, 2001). LGG are hypointense on T1 weighted magnetic resonance imaging (MRI), hyperintense on FLAIR and T2 sequences, and enhance in 30% of cases. There is often associated vasogenic edema (Prabhu et al., 2010, Wessels et al., 2003).

LGG are typically sporadic tumors, although they can occur in association with Li Fraumeni syndrome and Neurofibromatosis Types 1 and 2 (Prabhu et al., 2010, Wessels et al., 2003). Additional risk factors include previous irradiation and exposure to industrial chemicals (Prabhu et al., 2010, Wessels et al., 2003). Allergy has been reported to lower the risk for LGG, suggesting a possible role for immune surveillance in tumor pathogenesis (Prabhu et al., 2010). Survival is highly variable for LGG as median overall survival (OS) is reported to range from 3 to 40 years. Median progression free survival (PFS) is only 50% at 5 years and 17% at 15 years (Bauman et al., 1999, Berger et al., 1994, Jaeckle et al., Stieber, 2001). Median time to progression is 7.2 years (Schomas et al., 2009). In adults, the overall malignant transformation rate ranges from 35-89% with 74% in primary astrocytoma, 70% with mixed tumors, and 45% with primarily oligodendroglial histology (Jaeckle et al., 2010). Importantly, 50% of low risk adults, defined as patients less than 40 years of age with gross total resection (GTR), underwent transformation within 5 years (Jaeckle et al., 2010, Schiff et al., 2007).

Multiple studies have found that age greater than 40 years, extent of resection, tumor diameter greater than 6cm, tumor crossing midline, neurological deficit at diagnosis, and astrocytic histology are risk factors for poor prognosis in LGG (Bauman et al., 1999, E. G. Shaw et al., 2008, Stieber, 2001, Jaeckle et al., 2010, Schiff et al., 2007, E. G. Shaw & Wisoff, 2003). The NCCTG found that astrocytomas carry a worse prognosis than oligodendroglioma. Other retrospective reports corroborate these finding and further specify gemistocytic astrocytoma as carrying a worse prognosis (Jaeckle et al., 2010, Schomas et al., 2009, Stieber, 2001, Wessels et al., 2003, E. G. Shaw et al., 2008). Contrast enhancement, Karnofsky score, mitotic activity, and genetics have also been identified as risk factors for progression (Schiff et al., 2007, Schomas et al., 2009, E. G. Shaw & Wisoff, 2003, Stieber, 2001). Additionally, a Ki67-MIB1 index greater than 4% is associated with a more rapid rate of transformation.

3. Malignant transformation of pediatric low-grade glioma

The presentation and prognosis of LGG in children differs significantly from that in adults. Overall survival and rate of malignant transformation is significantly different in the pediatric population, leading to the hypothesis that tumor biology in children is inherently different from that in adults. For LGG in children, the overall rate of malignant transformation ranges from 4.3%-38%, which is much lower than in adults (Armstrong et al., 2011, Pollack et al., 1995). This difference may be accounted for in part by the higher rate of pilocytic astrocytomas that comprise the vast majority of pediatric LGG, a histological subset that rarely transforms (Tihan et al., 1999). While no prospective studies have been performed to identify reliable risk factors for transformation in children, radiation therapy is reported to be a possible causative agent (Dirks et al., 1994). Mean time to transformation is relatively short at approximately 6.4 years (Dirks et al., 1994). While the overall rate of progression is certainly lower in children, the risk of transformation in this population is still significant and warrants active and expectant observation.

Despite this risk for malignant degeneration, overall prognosis for children with LGG is significantly better than that for adults. Overall survival in children with LGG 65-90%, however, OS is 51% when pilocytic pathology is excluded (Armstrong et al., 2011, Fisher et al., 2008, Pollack et al., 1995). Following gross total resection, survival is 90-100% with 0% progression, in comparison to the adult transformation rate of 50% even in low risk, young patients with complete resection (Pollack et al., 1995). Progression free survival is between approximately 50% at 10 years, and 53% at 15 years (Armstrong et al., 2011). Gross total resection has been the only factor currently identified to have an impact on progression free survival in children with 0% progression with GTR and 17% progression with near total resection (Pollack et al., 1995). Due to the infiltrative nature of non-pilocytic grade II astrocytomas, this histology in children is more comparable to the adult population and is associated with poorer prognosis (Pollack et al., 1995).

4. Effect of resection and adjuvant therapy on malignant transformation

Currently, initial treatment consists of pharmacologic seizure control if patients present with seizures and steroids for vasogenic edema (Prabhu et al., 2010, Stieber, 2001). For patients with lesions amenable to surgery, the goal is gross total resection as many studies have found overall survival to correlate with extent of initial resection irrespective of adjuvant therapy. At 5 years, OS was 63% with GTR versus 27% OS with STR (Prabhu et al., 2010). Recurrence is also higher with STR (Prabhu et al., 2010). Berger et al. (1994) reported no recurrences within 54 months with GTR, 14.8% recurrence with residual tumor less than 10cm^3, and 46.2% recurrence with residual greater than 10cm^3 (Berger et al., 1994, Stieber, 2001). In some cases, tumor location within or near eloquent cortex limits the extent of resection, therefore, newer methods including functional MRI, fiber tracking with diffuser tensor imaging (DTI), intra-operative stimulation and mapping, or intra-operative MRI have helped reduce morbidity and allow more aggressive surgery. As survival decreases with lower Karnofsky score, while the surgical goal remains complete resection, equally important is the avoidance of new neurological deficit (Gil-Robles & Duffau, 2010, Schomas et al., 2009).

The role of adjuvant therapy following surgical resection remains controversial. Although LGG are fairly slow growing tumors with low or absent mitotic activity, their infiltrative behavior and high rate of recurrence and malignant transformation has caused most centers to institute adjuvant therapy regardless of the extent of resection. Recent prospective trials have addressed the role of radiation therapy (E. Shaw et al., 2002). RT was found to improve PFS but not OS (Stieber, 2001). As a result, early RT is administered to patients at high risk for malignant transformation (defined as age > 40yrs, astrocytic histology, crossing midline, diameter > 6cm, or intractable seizures) or for control of disease at the time of progression (Prabhu et al., 2010). The study also recommended RT to all patients greater than 40 years of age irrespective of resection, as age was the most consistent prognostic factor for malignant transformation (Stieber, 2001). For patients aged 18 to 40, RT was recommended only for patients with incomplete resection. Regardless of these data, treatment protocols vary widely and are often practitioner dependant.

Chemotherapy has also been used as an initial treatment in LGG, most commonly in the setting of unresectable disease, or in patients less than 3 years of age in which RT should be deferred (Prabhu et al., 2010). The response rates to available agents are highly variable, with favorable responses reported between 10 and 60%. Poor response is often associated with low grade tumors as they tend to have lower sensitivity to chemotherapeutic agents due their inherently slow growth and minimal mitosis (Prabhu et al., 2010). The Southwest Oncology Group (SWOG) investigated the use of CCNU in addition to RT following GTR and found no added benefit of CCNU (E. G. Shaw & Wisoff, 2003). The NCCTG found a favorable response using PCV in the treatment of primary disease. Currently, the RTOG is investigating the safety and efficacy of PCV in unfavorable patients following resection and RT. Temozolamide is also under investigation for use in LGG patients at high risk for transformation (Schomas et al., 2009). Clearly, the use of adjuvant therapy requires more investigation before formal recommendations can be defined. Until then, adjuvant therapies will remain controversial and site dependant.

Treatment of pediatric gliomas is subject to a different set of considerations and standards as toxicity of therapy has a greater impact on the developing nervous and skeletal system. Surgery with GTR is the primary mode of therapy as this has been shown to be the most effective method for cure (Fisher et al., 2008, Unal et al., 2008). While rare, malignant transformation does occur so observation is not recommended with lesions that are amenable to surgery. As an exception, optic and hypothalamic gliomas are treated initially with observation and chemotherapy. Due to their slow growth and associated morbidity with surgery or radiotherapy in these locations, conservative management is standard. Ultimately, these tumors are associated with a worse prognosis due to their location and difficulty of surgical intervention in the event of progression. Similarly, first line of therapy for brainstem lesions is observation and potential biopsy only for progression of symptoms or radiographic appearance (Fisher et al., 2008). Based on the 0% progression in the setting of GTR, RT has no role following complete resection in children, as compared to adults (Pollack et al., 1995).

Although standard dose RT (50.4-54 Gy) has been shown to be effective in the pediatric population, RT is deferred in children irrespective of residual tumor burden, recurrence or progression due to the risk of toxicity including endocrine dysfunction, cognitive impairment with decreased memory, lower IQ, attention deficit, cerebrovascular disease, and secondary neoplasms (Fisher et al., 2008, Pollack et al., 1995). Standard dose RT is associated with 34% cognitive dysfunction compared to 8.6% without RT, and 17% endocrine dysfunction compared to 2.9% without RT (Pollack et al., 1995). Overall, the rate of endocrine dysfunction was 10% and cognitive dysfunction was 21%. These findings support the use of repeat surgery and chemotherapy prior to the use of RT for recurrence in children. Chemotherapeutic agents possess significant toxicity as well. While carboplatin and vincristine showed good response rates with 68% 3 year PFS, 40% of patients demonstrated hypersensitivity reactions. CCNU, vincristine, and dibromodulcitol have all been associated with significant hypersensitivity reactions (Fisher et al., 2008). As a result, TPCV is now being tested for efficacy and safety in a prospective pediatric trial (Fisher et al., 2008).

5. Histology of malignant transformation

As mentioned previously, low grade gliomas comprise a histologically diverse group of tumors. The current WHO classification describes four categories for astrocytomas (Kleihues et al., 1995, Louis et al., 2007). While it is theorized that the majority of grade IV glioblastomas (GBM) occur *de novo* (primary GBM), a significant number of lesions result from progression of a low-grade tumor (secondary GBM). Excluding Grade I pilocytic astrocytomas as they rarely progress, low grade (II) and high grade (III and IV) astrocytomas can be viewed to exist along a continuum based on the histological analysis of tumor tissue. Grade II lesions are defined by low or absent mitotic activity and, unlike Grade I gliomas, are infiltrative and invasive and should not be considered benign. Cellular density is low to moderate, and well-differentiated, mildly pleomorphic tumor cells are present. One important feature of low grade astrocytomas is the absence of neovascularization.

This is in distinct comparison to high grade gliomas, grade III anaplastic tumors and grade IV GBMs, which are poorly differentiated, widely infiltrative and display prominent mitotic activity and neovascularization. Both confer a poor prognosis. High-grade lesions display increased cellularity, marked pleomorphism and nuclear atypia and may include multinucleated giant cells. Necrosis is the defining feature of GBM and these areas are typically surrounded by pseudopalisading cells. Most importantly, extensive irregular vascular proliferation is present in GBM as these tumors have adopted the capability of undergoing the angiogenic switch to produce their own vasculature, allowing for exponential tumor growth.

While morbidity is associated with low-grade astrocytomas themselves, it is hypothesized that the majority of morbidity is caused by progression to high-grade tumor. One of the key factors in this progression is the angiogenic switch whereby the tumor adopts the ability to acquire its own vascular supply. This enables explosive growth and precipitates rapid clinical deterioration. While an increased understanding of LGG biology and behavior has led to a more aggressive approach to these tumors, clinical outcome measures still remain poor. This is due mostly in part to our inability to prevent or detect malignant degeneration. A significant amount of research is now focused on understanding the factors involved in the angiogenic switch, which is likely to lead to additional treatment targets and potentially better outcomes. This will be further discussed in the sections to follow.

6. Molecular biology of malignant transformation

While histological characteristics currently determine tumor grade in astrocytoma, important molecular differences also exist between low grade and high-grade gliomas (Table 1) (Godard et al., 2003). These molecular differences are likely to be an important factor in initiating or promoting the angiogenic switch (Wen & Kesari, 2008). Both primary and secondary GBM exhibit elevated VEGF expression and loss of heterozygosity at 10q. The majority of primary GBM show overexpression of EGFR and PTEN mutations. In particular, glioblastomas that express the EGFRvIII genetic variant have a worse prognosis and show resistance to current therapeutic regimens (Furnari et al., 2007, Hatanpaa et al., Johns et al., 2007, Pelloski et al., 2007). While PTEN mutations occur more frequently in primary glioblastoma in adults, PTEN mutations exist in high frequency in pediatric gliomas that have undergone malignant transformation (Broniscer et al., 2007).

Genetic Mutation	Incidence in Grade II Astrocytoma and Secondary GBM	Incidence in Primary GBM
p53 (TP53)	↑↑↑	↑
EGFR	↑	↑↑↑
PTEN	↑↑	↑↑↑
IDH 1&2	↑↑↑	↑↑
PDGF	↑↑↑	↑↑
BRAF	↑	--

Table 1. Various genetic mutations associated with gliomas. EGFR - epidermal growth factor receptor, PTEN - phosphatase and tensin homolog, IDH - isocitrate deyhdrogenase, PDGFR – platelet derived growth factor receptor.

In contrast, secondary GBMs often have p53 mutations and overexpress PDGF. Mutations of p53 frequently are associated with low-grade gliomas occurring in 53% of astrocytoma, 44% of oligoastrocytoma, and 13% of oligodendroglioma (Okamoto et al., 2004). Therefore, p53 may be an important molecular event involved in the malignant progression of low-grade gliomas (Louis et al., 2007). Interestingly, in children, the rate of p53 mutations is reported as only 10% in progressive pediatric LGG. While this alteration may seem to possibly explain the improved survival in pediatric gliomas, the 1p19q deletion, an indicator of a favorable response to specific chemotherapies in adults, is not found in pediatric gliomas (Fisher et al., 2008).
Other molecular changes have also been identified (Ichimura et al., 2009, Watanabe et al., 2009). IDH1 abnormalities exist in 59-88% of diffuse astrocytomas, 68-82% of oligodendrogliomas, 50-78% of anaplastic astrocytomas, 49-75% of anaplastic oligodendrogliomas, and 50-88% of secondary glioblastomas and often co-exist with p53 mutated lesions or 1p19q co-deleted tumors (Hartmann et al., 2009, Ichimura et al., 2009, Parsons et al., 2008, Sanson et al., 2009, Watanabe et al., 2009, Yan et al., 2009). While the presence of IDH mutations in low-grade tumors and secondary GBMs suggests a role for IDH in malignant progression , the literature suggests that the presence of IDH1 or IDH2 mutations correlates with better outcomes in patients (De Carli et al., 2009, Yan et al., 2009). PDGFR and the p16ink4a /RB1 pathway have also been implicated in gliomagenesis as hypermethylation of the RB1 gene may result in uncontrolled cell cycle progression, which may then drive tumor formation (Sathornsumetee et al., 2007). Both primary and secondary GBMs express PDGF, but increased RB1 gene promoter methylation appears to occur more frequently in secondary GBMs (43%) than primary GBMs (14%) (Nakamura et al., 2001).
The expression of MGMT, a DNA repair enzyme, has also been implicated in glioblastoma and low-grade gliomas (Bourne & Schiff, 2010). Of particular interest is the methylation

status of MGMT as it may correlate to resistance to alkylating therapy in some patients (Hegi et al., 2005).

Finally, chromosomal e 7 (7q34) gene BRAF mutations and overexpression of B-raf, which stimulates the mitogen-activated protein kinase (MAPK) pathway, is a major factor in tumorigenesis of pilocytic astrocytomas (Pfister et al., 2008). This mutation is also present in 23-38% of adult grade II astrocytomas. The role of BRAF mutation in progression to high-grade tumors, however, has yet to be elucidated.

Defining molecular differences amongst glioma subpopulations offers an exciting new dynamic in understanding the behaviors of this highly diverse tumor although much work is required before the variability observed is completely delineated. Already, studies are underway to target tumors at the molecular level in hopes of providing better treatment options (Johns et al., 2007). As it is apparent that the angiogenic switch is important in the progression of low-grade to high-grade glioma, defining the molecular changes that promote this event may offer additional treatment benefits. Animal studies have already shown that preventing the angiogenic switch in other solid tumors reduces tumor growth (Lyden et al., 2001). Therefore, further understanding of how specific molecular changes in tumor cells promote angiogenesis may offer promising new treatment options in gliomas.

7. Advancing imaging of low-grade gliomas

MRI is the initial imaging modality of choice in brain tumors. Low-grade gliomas usually appear as well defined lesions with little mass effect. They have low-signal on T1- and high-signal on T2-weighted imaging - particularly on fluid attenuated inversion recovery (FLAIR) sequences where low-grade gliomas are very hyperintense (Kates et al., 1996). Currently, the absence of gadolinium enhancement is used to differentiate low grade versus high grade glioma (Fig. 2) (Castillo, 1994), however, a significant portion of the low-grade gliomas defined by MRI were found to be high-grade after biopsy (Kondziolka et al., 1993). As a result, MRI is not sensitive enough to definitively diagnose low-grade gliomas as there are frequently small areas within the tumor that have already undergone malignant progression. Therefore, advanced imaging technologies, such as perfusion imaging, diffusion-weighted and diffusion tensor imaging, MR spectroscopy, and position emission tomography (PET), are currently being employed to more accurately identify low-grade versus high-grade gliomas. These modalities provide exciting insight into tumor vascularity, cellularity, metabolism, and proliferation and may prove more effective in differentiating low-grade from high-grade glioma particularly in regions within a given tumor.

Since the degree of vascularity correlates with tumor grade in gliomas, (Daumas-Duport et al., 1997) perfusion MRI and MRI with gradient echo differentiates low-grade versus high-grade gliomas based on relative cerebral blood volume (rCBV) (Boxerman et al., 2006, Law et al., 2003, Law et al., 2004, Shin et al., 2002, Sugahara et al., 1998, Sugahara et al., 2001). While promising, it has been difficult to establish a reliable threshold based on rCBV for low- versus high-grade state. Diffusion-weighted MRI has also been utilized based on the apparent diffusion coefficient, which inversely correlates with tumor cellularity (Gauvain et al., 2001, Kono et al., 2001, Sugahara et al., 1999). Again, it has been difficult to reliably predict tumor grade using diffusion MRI (Bulakbasi et al., 2003, Stieber, 2001). Diffusion tensor imaging (DTI) is a modification of diffusion-weighted imaging and measures fractional anisotropy (FA), which correlated with tumor cellularity and vascularity (Price, 2010). DTI is a promising new modality as one study reports the ability to distinguish between low- and high-grade gliomas using a threshold FA value of 0.188 (Inoue et al., 2005).

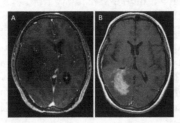

Fig. 1. Serial imaging of malignant progression of glioma. A, T1-weighted MRI with contrast. Patient presented with headache. MRI revealed hypointense lesion in right hemisphere. Note edema and mass effect but lack of contrast enhancement. Pt underwent gross total surgical resection and pathology revealed grade II astrocytoma. B, T1-weighted MRI with contrast. Subsequent imaging revealed recurrent tumor seen as a contrast enhancing lesion in the previous resection cavity. Pathology revealed progression to grade IV astrocytoma (GBM).

MR spectroscopy (MRS) also can potentially differentiate low-grade versus high-grade gliomas in the brain. All gliomas have an increased choline peak and a reduced N-acetyl aspartate peak (NAA) which are markers of membrane turnover and neuronal cell death respectively. Levels of lipid and lactate are markers of necrosis and hypoxia respectively and are decidedly elevated in high-grade compared to low-grade gliomas (McBride et al., 1995, Nafe et al., 2003, Negendank et al., 1996). Creatine (Cr), which serves as a marker of energy metabolism, is decreased in brain tumors (Meyerand et al., 1999, Moller-Hartmann et al., 2002), however, this reduction does not appear to correlate with tumor grade by itself (Moller-Hartmann et al., 2002). Using the choline/Cr ratio may be more effective, however, as low-grade gliomas tend to have a lower ratio of choline/Cr (McBride et al., 1995, Murphy et al., 2002, Sijens & Oudkerk, 2002), as well as an increase in NAA/Cr ratio (Law et al., 2003, McKnight et al., 2002, Murphy et al., 2002, Nafe et al., 2003, Negendank et al., 1996). MRS is a promising technique in differentiating low- from high-grade gliomas with sensitivity between 73% and 92% and specificity between 63% and 100% (Astrakas et al., 2004, Fayed & Modrego, 2005, Law et al., 2003, Nafe et al., 2003, Setzer et al., 2007). MRS may also be capable of identifying regions that have undergone malignant transformation within a given tumor that may not be identifiable by other imaging techniques although one such study attempting to detect malignant transformation within low-grade glioma yielded a specificity of only 57.1% (Alimenti et al., 2007).

Positron emission tomography (PET) imaging has been employed to examine gliomas in the brain by measuring the metabolic activity of tissue. Fluorinated glucose analogue 2-[18F]-fluoro-2-deoxy-D-glucose (FDG), which is administered to patients intravascularly, has high sensitivity for identifying areas of increased tumor metabolism and has been used as an index to predict tumor aggressiveness. While low-grade gliomas tend to have the same or even lower uptake of FDG than normal brain matter, high-grade gliomas demonstrate increased uptake of FDG on PET imaging (Derlon et al., 1997, Tamura et al., 1998), Studies have shown that it is possible to differentiate low- from high-grade gliomas with a sensitivity of 94% and specificity of 77% using a tumor-to-white-matter ratio of greater than 1.5 and tumor-to-grey-matter ratio of greater than 0.6 (Delbeke et al., 1995).

In addition to FDG, other tracers have been utilized in attempts to further characterize these tumors such as carbon 11 and fluorine 18 (18F)-labeled amino acid (Isselbacher, 1972). Methionine PET appears to have a higher sensitivity than FDG PET in detecting low-grade versus high-grade gliomas (Derlon et al., 1997, Giammarile et al., 2004, Ogawa et al., 1993). In particular, methionine PET exhibits a heightened sensitivity in detecting radiation necrosis from recurrent tumors, as inflammatory cells in radiation necrosis have little uptake of methionine (Thiel et al., 2000). Perhaps the most promising technique for diagnosing low-grade gliomas is 18F-FDOPA PET imaging. 18F-FDOPA PET is more accurate that FDG PET and has been shown to be highly predictive in determining tumor grade on initial diagnosis and may help differentiate tumor necrosis from recurrence (Chen et al., 2006, Fueger et al., Tripathi et al., 2009).

While there currently is no one imaging modality capable of definitively determining low-grade from high-grade tumors on its own, advanced imaging technology continues to develop and complement standard MRI. As we come to understand the behavior and variability of these tumors, advance imaging techniques provide exciting new possibilities for more precise treatments. Given the variability within a given tumor, advanced imaging techniques may allow for more precise targets for biopsy, vigilant monitoring of malignant transformation, and improved prognostic power in the management of low- and high-grade gliomas.

8. The Role of bone-marrow derived cells in malignant transformation

The vast majority of brain tumor research, molecular profiling, histological characteristics, diagnostic imaging modalities and treatment targets have focused on the actual tumor cells themselves. As mentioned earlier, one of the key events in the transition from the low-grade to the high-grade state is the angiogenic switch. It is theorized that in the low-grade state, tumor growth may be limited, at least in part, by a lack of blood supply. In this state, the tumor is only capable of a steady-state or linear growth (Mandonnet et al., 2003). Once the tumor acquires the ability to recruit or form new blood vessels, exponential growth occurs (Rees et al., 2009) resulting in rapid clinical decline. While there is considerable evidence that tumor cells undergo continued molecular changes that increase their malignant potential, these changes also allow these cells to initiate the angiogenic switch. It must also be noted that while recent evidence suggests that tumor cells may be capable of directly forming new blood vessels (Ricci-Vitiani et al., Wang et al.), a considerable body of evidence suggests that tumor cells do not do this completely on their own. While the exact details of this process still remain to be fully elucidated, tumor cells acquire the ability to transition the local tumor niche to an environment capable of rapid blood vessel formation. A variety of growth factors, signaling pathways, and indigenous populations of cells is hypothesized to participate in this process. If this theory proves to be correct, this population of cells forms an additional therapeutic target that may be as important as the tumor cells themselves. As current therapies directed at neoplastic cells are limited in part to their toxicity, elucidating other potential treatment pathways may further benefit patient outcome.

Neovascularization is a normal process in tissues and the brain during ischemia. In low oxygen states, cells release signals such as VEGF, PDGF, PlGF and HIF-1 that recruit from local existing vessels within the tissue itself (angiogenesis.) In addition, this can activate distant processes that facilitate neovascularization and may even form *de novo* blood vessels (vasculogenesis). These factors mobilize bone marrow precursor cells which then travel to the site of ischemia via the bloodstream. It is theorized that these cells facilitate vasculogenesis by breaking down existing structures and creating an environment that promotes new blood vessel growth.

Tumors are capable of adopting this machinery to increase growth and invasiveness by activating the angiogenic switch (Bergers & Benjamin, 2003, Rafii & Lyden, 2008). During early tumor development, neoplastic cells rely on existing blood flow and grow in a slow linear fashion (Mandonnet et al., 2003). Once the switch is initiated and neovascularization brings more oxygen and nutrients, tumor cells grow at a much faster rate and tumor size increases significantly (Rees et al., 2009). This initial process is thought to occur mostly by angiogenesis (Kioi, 2010). The release of proteases and proangiogenic factors causes pericytes to detach from existing vessels creating a defect in the extracellular matrix in the environment surrounding the vessel wall (Bergers & Benjamin, 2003). Endothelial cells proliferate locally and sprout outward into the tumor bed creating newly formed blood vessels feeding the tumor. While angiogenesis is an important factor in the angiogenic switch, vasculogenesis and the contribution of BMDC play a critical role as well. For example, when recruitment of BMDC is impaired in an animal model of lymphoma and lung carcinoma, tumor angiogenesis and growth is significantly decreased (Lyden et al., 2001) suggesting that BMDCs contribute significantly to neovascularization and growth in solid tumors.

In metastatic disease, the contribution of BMDC has been well described (Wels et al., 2008). Endothelial (EPCs) and hematopoietic precursor cells (HPC), mesenchymal stem cells (MSC), myeloid-derived suppressor cells (MDSCs), Tie-2 expressing monocytes (TEM) and tumor associated macrophages (TAM) all are mobilized from the bone marrow to future metastatic sites prior to tumor formation. It should be noted that these primitive cells are prominent during embryology and that a significant population of these cells is not present under normal conditions. While the exact role of each cell type has yet to be fully elucidated, their basic function is to break down normal structures and promote vasculogenesis and tumor invasiveness. The net result is a tumor friendly environment capable of sustaining tumor growth. This has been demonstrated experimentally in a murine model of metastatic disease by implanting m-cherry labeled melanoma cells into the flank of mice with GFP-labeled bone marrow and examining the lungs of these animals over time (Kaplan et al., 2005). It was observed that the first cells to arrive in future metastases were not tumor cells, but actual BMDC. This suggested, at least in metastatic disease, that the environment in future metastatic sites is primed by cells from the bone marrow before tumors can begin to grow in these distant areas (Rafii & Lyden, 2008). This also supports the hypothesis by Stephen Paget over 100 years ago that the tumor microenvironment may play as important a role as the tumor cells themselves.

In the brain, the role of BMDC has only recently garnered attention. One of the basic histological differences between low-grade and high-grade gliomas is a lack of neovascularization. Thus, activation of the angiogenic switch is a key element in the transformation of low-grade to high-grade glioma. Two elements are likely to contribute to this process. Genetic changes in tumor cells that occur during progression of disease activate pro-angiogenic factors. This has been observed in human tumor samples whereby genes involved in angiogenesis are upregulated in glioblastoma as compared to low grade astrocytoma (Godard et al., 2003). Kioi et al. also showed in their animal model that release of soluble factors by tumor cells or cells within the tumor microenvironment including

VEGF, FGF and EGF stimulates local angiogenesis (Kioi, 2010). Secondly, hypoxia is an additional critical event in triggering the switch (Kioi, 2010). As tumor size grows and metabolic demand exceeds local perfusion, hypoxic conditions occur. Release of hypoxia inducible factor-1 (HIF-1α) by tumor cells or cells within the hypoxic tumor environment, combined with stromal cell-derived factor-1 (SDF-1) and CXCR-4 receptor activation, mobilizes BMDCs to the tumor site and promotes vasculogenesis in gliomas (Du et al., 2008, Greenfield et al., 2010, Kioi, 2010).

In an attempt to further understand these processes in gliomas, Du et al. utilized an orthotopic model of GBM in mice to demonstrate recruitment of BMDC in gliomas (Du et al., 2008). Based on their results they theorize that hypoxia and the subsequent release of HIF-1α is the key event in tumor progression. Elevation of VEGF, and subsequent SDF-1 release and CXCR-4 receptor activation, mobilizes BMDC and recruits EPC and myeloid cells to the tumor. The net effect tips the balance to a pro-angiogenic state and neovascularization within the tumor bed. Kioi et al also further theorized that radiation treatment may exacerbate the vasculogenesis process and boost eventual tumor recurrence observed in current treatment regimens (Greenfield et al., 2010, Kioi, 2010). The endothelial-mesenchymal transition and MSC have also been described in metastatic disease (Singh & Settleman). MSC exist within the brain and mobilize to the tumor site as well (Hata et al., Kang et al.). The exact roles of these particular BMDC remain elusive and require more study before they are fully delineated.

In our laboratory, we have begun to investigate the correlation of BMDC mobilization and tumor grade in gliomas (unpublished data.) We used a PDGF-driven mouse model of GBM within which tumors develop slowly from low-grade to high-grade. Low-grade tumors have a clear absence of neovascularization and BMDC are not present within these lesions. In high-grade tumors, however, we have observed a profound increase in larger, irregularly shaped, hemorrhagic vessels and a significant population of BMDC exists that is not observed in low grade tumors. In addition, these cells are located near newly forming blood vessels in the perivascular niche. We have also observed that BMDC are mobilized in the bone marrow and are elevated in the peripheral blood of tumor bearing animals versus controls. In addition, a significant difference in this population of cells in the blood exists between low-grade and high-grade animals. While much work is yet to be done before this process is fully elucidated, it appears that the presence of BMDC correlates with tumor grade and the process of neovascularization. Thus, BMDC have a potential role in the angiogenic switch as tumors progress from low-grade to high-grade tumors.

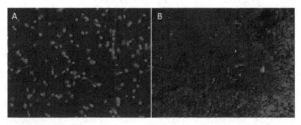

Fig. 2. Bone marrow-derived cells in human glioma. A, Immunofluorescence in grade II astrocytoma shows normal blood vessels (red, VE Cadherin) and a paucity of CD11b+ myeloid suppressor cells (Green). B, GBM shows abnormal vessel formation and an influx of CD11b+ cells (unpublished data.)

Mobilization of BMDC in peripheral blood samples has similarly been observed in patients with astrocytomas. Circulating CD133+ and VEGFR2+ EPC were measured in patients with different grade gliomas. This population of cells was significantly elevated in brain tumor patients versus controls, correlated with tumor grade, and predicted survival. In one patient, this population also predicted recurrence prior to detection by serial radiographic study. Currently, patients are followed with serial imaging in order to diagnose recurrence or malignant progression. While advances in imaging technology show promise in earlier more accurate diagnosis, the critical event has already occurred and prognosis worsens considerably. Therefore, the identification of a potential surrogate biomarker that measures tumor angiogenicity and aggressiveness may potentially serve as an index for ongoing treatment effectiveness or recurrence.

As histological and molecular differences between low-grade and high-grade gliomas are further defined and it becomes apparent that tumors cannot be loosely classified, specific treatments based on the particular characteristics of each individual tumor can potentially be designed. In addition, the presence of particular populations of BMDC in these tumors may also provide additional information on tumor behavior and serve as an additional treatment target along with tumor cells themselves. It has already been shown that the presence of BMDC in the blood correlates with tumor grade and initial animal studies suggest that BMDC are present in high-grade tumors only (Greenfield et al., 2009). In addition, TAM have been associated with poorer prognosis in metastatic lesions and other solid tumors (Wels et al., 2008). Thus histological stains aimed at identifying this population of cells may provide more accurate diagnosis and prognosis. Likewise, the molecular markers of this particular population of cells may offer an even more specific therapeutic target. Based on data collected in glioma patients, EPC can be identified by cell surface markers including CD133 and VEGFR2. Knocking down this population with specifically designed drug therapies has the potential for preventing recurrence by decreasing migration of these cells and reducing vasculogenesis within the tumor bed. Finally, one can also envision a role for advanced imaging technologies for improved diagnosis and treatment. For instance, PET has been used to specifically measure VEGF that has been labeled with copper in an orthotropic mouse model of GBM (Cai et al., 2006). If one could identify and label molecular targets that are specific to individual tumors subtypes and sensitive to new imaging techniques, this provides exciting non-invasive possibilities for tumor specific identification and treatment for each individual patient.

9. Conclusions

In summary, one of the primary factors predicting outcome in patients with low-grade glioma is malignant progression to high-grade tumor and it is evident that the angiogenic switch is an important event in this process. Initial management often entails surgical resection while adjuvant therapy for low-grade gliomas remains a controversial topic. Tumor grade is determined by histological analysis of tumor specimens, but the molecular fingerprint of these tumors is now being analyzed more thoroughly and holds promise for more exciting targeted treatment options. In addition, distinct, but as yet undefined, populations of cells are recruited to the tumor site and participate in neovascularization and promote tumor growth and invasiveness. Therefore, this population may represent an important therapeutic target in combating these tumors. Since survival is directly correlated with tumor grade, preventing tumor progression is imperative. While BMDC certainly are not the only factor in progression of disease and neovascularization, blocking recruitment of these cells to tumors has been shown to reduce growth in animal models of other tumor types. Therefore, a greater understanding of this process may define a role for targeting this population of cells. In addition, BMDC exist in the periphery, and make for an easier therapeutic target than tumor cells within the blood brain barrier. Lastly, current management of tumor recurrence relies on serial imaging studies. Therefore, an effective and accurate biomarker capable of predicting progression of disease may allow for earlier detection and better treatment outcomes. This makes the case for monitoring BMDC in the periphery in addition to therapy aimed at this population of cells as potential adjuvant therapy in glioma.

10. References

Alimenti, A., Delavelle, J., Lazeyras, F., Yilmaz, H., Dietrich, P. Y., de Tribolet, N. & Lovblad, K. O. (2007). Monovoxel 1H magnetic resonance spectroscopy in the progression of gliomas. *Eur Neurol*, Vol. 58, No. 4, pp. (198-209)

Armstrong, G. T., Conklin, H. M., Huang, S., Srivastava, D., Sanford, R., Ellison, D. W., Merchant, T. E., Hudson, M. M., Hoehn, M. E., Robison, L. L., Gajjar, A. & Morris, E. B. (2011). Survival and long-term health and cognitive outcomes after low-grade glioma. *Neuro Oncol*, Vol. 13, No. 2, pp. (223-34)

Astrakas, L. G., Zurakowski, D., Tzika, A. A., Zarifi, M. K., Anthony, D. C., De Girolami, U., Tarbell, N. J. & Black, P. M. (2004). Noninvasive magnetic resonance spectroscopic imaging biomarkers to predict the clinical grade of pediatric brain tumors. *Clin Cancer Res*, Vol. 10, No. 24, pp. (8220-8)

Bauman, G., Lote, K., Larson, D., Stalpers, L., Leighton, C., Fisher, B., Wara, W., MacDonald, D., Stitt, L. & Cairncross, J. G. (1999). Pretreatment factors predict overall survival for patients with low-grade glioma: a recursive partitioning analysis. *Int J Radiat Oncol Biol Phys*, Vol. 45, No. 4, pp. (923-9)

Berger, M. S., Deliganis, A. V., Dobbins, J. & Keles, G. E. (1994). The effect of extent of resection on recurrence in patients with low grade cerebral hemisphere gliomas. *Cancer*, Vol. 74, No. 6, pp. (1784-91)

Bergers, G. & Benjamin, L. E. (2003). Tumorigenesis and the angiogenic switch. *Nat Rev Cancer*, Vol. 3, No. 6, pp. (401-10)

Bourne, T. D. & Schiff, D. (2010). Update on molecular findings, management and outcome in low-grade gliomas. *Nat Rev Neurol*, Vol. 6, No. 12, pp. (695-701)

Boxerman, J. L., Schmainda, K. M. & Weisskoff, R. M. (2006). Relative cerebral blood volume maps corrected for contrast agent extravasation significantly correlate with glioma tumor grade, whereas uncorrected maps do not. *AJNR Am J Neuroradiol*, Vol. 27, No. 4, pp. (859-67)

Broniscer, A., Baker, S. J., West, A. N., Fraser, M. M., Proko, E., Kocak, M., Dalton, J., Zambetti, G. P., Ellison, D. W., Kun, L. E., Gajjar, A., Gilbertson, R. J. & Fuller, C. E. (2007). Clinical and molecular characteristics of malignant transformation of low-grade glioma in children. *J Clin Oncol*, Vol. 25, No. 6, pp. (682-9)

Bulakbasi, N., Kocaoglu, M., Ors, F., Tayfun, C. & Ucoz, T. (2003). Combination of single-voxel proton MR spectroscopy and apparent diffusion coefficient calculation in the evaluation of common brain tumors. *AJNR Am J Neuroradiol*, Vol. 24, No. 2, pp. (225-33)

Cai, W., Chen, K., Mohamedali, K. A., Cao, Q., Gambhir, S. S., Rosenblum, M. G. & Chen, X. (2006). PET of vascular endothelial growth factor receptor expression. *J Nucl Med*, Vol. 47, No. 12, pp. (2048-56)

Castillo, M. (1994). Contrast enhancement in primary tumors of the brain and spinal cord. *Neuroimaging Clin N Am*, Vol. 4, No. 1, pp. (63-80)

Chen, W., Silverman, D. H., Delaloye, S., Czernin, J., Kamdar, N., Pope, W., Satyamurthy, N., Schiepers, C. & Cloughesy, T. (2006). 18F-FDOPA PET imaging of brain tumors: comparison study with 18F-FDG PET and evaluation of diagnostic accuracy. *J Nucl Med*, Vol. 47, No. 6, pp. (904-11)

Daumas-Duport, C., Tucker, M. L., Kolles, H., Cervera, P., Beuvon, F., Varlet, P., Udo, N., Koziak, M. & Chodkiewicz, J. P. (1997). Oligodendrogliomas. Part II: A new grading system based on morphological and imaging criteria. *J Neurooncol*, Vol. 34, No. 1, pp. (61-78)

De Carli, E., Wang, X. & Puget, S. (2009). IDH1 and IDH2 mutations in gliomas. *N Engl J Med*, Vol. 360, No. 21, pp. (2248; author reply 2249)

Delbeke, D., Meyerowitz, C., Lapidus, R. L., Maciunas, R. J., Jennings, M. T., Moots, P. L. & Kessler, R. M. (1995). Optimal cutoff levels of F-18 fluorodeoxyglucose uptake in the differentiation of low-grade from high-grade brain tumors with PET. *Radiology*, Vol. 195, No. 1, pp. (47-52)

Derlon, J. M., Petit-Taboue, M. C., Chapon, F., Beaudouin, V., Noel, M. H., Creveuil, C., Courtheoux, P. & Houtteville, J. P. (1997). The in vivo metabolic pattern of low-grade brain gliomas: a positron emission tomographic study using 18F-fluorodeoxyglucose and 11C-L-methylmethionine. *Neurosurgery*, Vol. 40, No. 2, pp. (276-87; discussion 287-8)

Dirks, P. B., Jay, V., Becker, L. E., Drake, J. M., Humphreys, R. P., Hoffman, H. J. & Rutka, J. T. (1994). Development of anaplastic changes in low-grade astrocytomas of childhood. *Neurosurgery*, Vol. 34, No. 1, pp. (68-78)

Du, R., Lu, K. V., Petritsch, C., Liu, P., Ganss, R., Passegue, E., Song, H., Vandenberg, S., Johnson, R. S., Werb, Z. & Bergers, G. (2008). HIF1alpha induces the recruitment of bone marrow-derived vascular modulatory cells to regulate tumor angiogenesis and invasion. *Cancer Cell*, Vol. 13, No. 3, pp. (206-20)

Fayed, N. & Modrego, P. J. (2005). The contribution of magnetic resonance spectroscopy and echoplanar perfusion-weighted MRI in the initial assessment of brain tumours. *J Neurooncol*, Vol. 72, No. 3, pp. (261-5)

Fisher, P. G., Tihan, T., Goldthwaite, P. T., Wharam, M. D., Carson, B. S., Weingart, J. D., Repka, M. X., Cohen, K. J. & Burger, P. C. (2008). Outcome analysis of childhood low-grade astrocytomas. *Pediatr Blood Cancer*, Vol. 51, No. 2, pp. (245-50)

Fueger, B. J., Czernin, J., Cloughesy, T., Silverman, D. H., Geist, C. L., Walter, M. A., Schiepers, C., Nghiemphu, P., Lai, A., Phelps, M. E. & Chen, W. Correlation of 6-18F-fluoro-L-dopa PET uptake with proliferation and tumor grade in newly diagnosed and recurrent gliomas. *J Nucl Med*, Vol. 51, No. 10, pp. (1532-8)

Furnari, F. B., Fenton, T., Bachoo, R. M., Mukasa, A., Stommel, J. M., Stegh, A., Hahn, W. C., Ligon, K. L., Louis, D. N., Brennan, C., Chin, L., DePinho, R. A. & Cavenee, W. K.

(2007). Malignant astrocytic glioma: genetics, biology, and paths to treatment. *Genes Dev*, Vol. 21, No. 21, pp. (2683-710)

Gauvain, K. M., McKinstry, R. C., Mukherjee, P., Perry, A., Neil, J. J., Kaufman, B. A. & Hayashi, R. J. (2001). Evaluating pediatric brain tumor cellularity with diffusion-tensor imaging. *AJR Am J Roentgenol*, Vol. 177, No. 2, pp. (449-54)

Giammarile, F., Cinotti, L. E., Jouvet, A., Ramackers, J. M., Saint Pierre, G., Thiesse, P., Jouanneau, E., Guyotat, J., Pelissou-Guyotat, I., Setiey, A., Honnorat, J., Le Bars, D. & Frappaz, D. (2004). High and low grade oligodendrogliomas (ODG): correlation of amino-acid and glucose uptakes using PET and histological classifications. *J Neurooncol*, Vol. 68, No. 3, pp. (263-74)

Gil-Robles, S. & Duffau, H. (2010). Surgical management of World Health Organization Grade II gliomas in eloquent areas: the necessity of preserving a margin around functional structures. *Neurosurg Focus*, Vol. 28, No. 2, pp. (E8)

Godard, S., Getz, G., Delorenzi, M., Farmer, P., Kobayashi, H., Desbaillets, I., Nozaki, M., Diserens, A. C., Hamou, M. F., Dietrich, P. Y., Regli, L., Janzer, R. C., Bucher, P., Stupp, R., de Tribolet, N., Domany, E. & Hegi, M. E. (2003). Classification of human astrocytic gliomas on the basis of gene expression: a correlated group of genes with angiogenic activity emerges as a strong predictor of subtypes. *Cancer Res*, Vol. 63, No. 20, pp. (6613-25)

Greenfield, J. P., Jin, D. K., Young, L. M., Christos, P. J., Abrey, L., Rafii, S. & Gutin, P. H. (2009). Surrogate markers predict angiogenic potential and survival in patients with glioblastoma multiforme. *Neurosurgery*, Vol. 64, No. 5, pp. (819-26; discussion 826-7)

Greenfield, J. P., Cobb, W. S. & Lyden, D. (2010). Resisting arrest: a switch from angiogenesis to vasculogenesis in recurrent malignant gliomas. *J Clin Invest*, Vol. 120, No. 3, pp. (663-7)

Hartmann, C., Meyer, J., Balss, J., Capper, D., Mueller, W., Christians, A., Felsberg, J., Wolter, M., Mawrin, C., Wick, W., Weller, M., Herold-Mende, C., Unterberg, A., Jeuken, J. W., Wesseling, P., Reifenberger, G. & von Deimling, A. (2009). Type and frequency of IDH1 and IDH2 mutations are related to astrocytic and oligodendroglial differentiation and age: a study of 1,010 diffuse gliomas. *Acta Neuropathol*, Vol. 118, No. 4, pp. (469-74)

Hata, N., Shinojima, N., Gumin, J., Yong, R., Marini, F., Andreeff, M. & Lang, F. F. Platelet-derived growth factor BB mediates the tropism of human mesenchymal stem cells for malignant gliomas. *Neurosurgery*, Vol. 66, No. 1, pp. (144-56; discussion 156-7)

Hatanpaa, K. J., Burma, S., Zhao, D. & Habib, A. A. Epidermal growth factor receptor in glioma: signal transduction, neuropathology, imaging, and radioresistance. *Neoplasia*, Vol. 12, No. 9, pp. (675-84)

Hegi, M. E., Diserens, A. C., Gorlia, T., Hamou, M. F., de Tribolet, N., Weller, M., Kros, J. M., Hainfellner, J. A., Mason, W., Mariani, L., Bromberg, J. E., Hau, P., Mirimanoff, R. O., Cairncross, J. G., Janzer, R. C. & Stupp, R. (2005). MGMT gene silencing and benefit from temozolomide in glioblastoma. *N Engl J Med*, Vol. 352, No. 10, pp. (997-1003)

Ichimura, K., Pearson, D. M., Kocialkowski, S., Backlund, L. M., Chan, R., Jones, D. T. & Collins, V. P. (2009). IDH1 mutations are present in the majority of common adult gliomas but rare in primary glioblastomas. *Neuro Oncol*, Vol. 11, No. 4, pp. (341-7)

Inoue, T., Ogasawara, K., Beppu, T., Ogawa, A. & Kabasawa, H. (2005). Diffusion tensor imaging for preoperative evaluation of tumor grade in gliomas. *Clin Neurol Neurosurg*, Vol. 107, No. 3, pp. (174-80)

Isselbacher, K. J. (1972). Sugar and amino acid transport by cells in culture--differences between normal and malignant cells. *N Engl J Med*, Vol. 286, No. 17, pp. (929-33)

Jaeckle, K. A., Decker, P. A., Ballman, K. V., Flynn, P. J., Giannini, C., Scheithauer, B. W., Jenkins, R. B. & Buckner, J. C. (2010). Transformation of low grade glioma and correlation with outcome: an NCCTG database analysis. *J Neurooncol*, Vol. No. pp.

Johns, T. G., Perera, R. M., Vernes, S. C., Vitali, A. A., Cao, D. X., Cavenee, W. K., Scott, A. M. & Furnari, F. B. (2007). The efficacy of epidermal growth factor receptor-specific antibodies against glioma xenografts is influenced by receptor levels, activation status, and heterodimerization. *Clin Cancer Res*, Vol. 13, No. 6, pp. (1911-25)

Kang, S. G., Shinojima, N., Hossain, A., Gumin, J., Yong, R. L., Colman, H., Marini, F., Andreeff, M. & Lang, F. F. Isolation and perivascular localization of mesenchymal stem cells from mouse brain. *Neurosurgery*, Vol. 67, No. 3, pp. (711-20)

Kaplan, R. N., Riba, R. D., Zacharoulis, S., Bramley, A. H., Vincent, L., Costa, C., MacDonald, D. D., Jin, D. K., Shido, K., Kerns, S. A., Zhu, Z., Hicklin, D., Wu, Y., Port, J. L., Altorki, N., Port, E. R., Ruggero, D., Shmelkov, S. V., Jensen, K. K., Rafii, S. & Lyden, D. (2005). VEGFR1-positive haematopoietic bone marrow progenitors initiate the pre-metastatic niche. *Nature*, Vol. 438, No. 7069, pp. (820-7)

Kates, R., Atkinson, D. & Brant-Zawadzki, M. (1996). Fluid-attenuated inversion recovery (FLAIR): clinical prospectus of current and future applications. *Top Magn Reson Imaging*, Vol. 8, No. 6, pp. (389-96)

Kioi, M., et al. (2010). Inhibition of vasculogenesis, but not angiogenesis, prevents the recurrencec of glioblastoma following irradiation in mice. *J Clin Invest*, Vol. 120, No. pp. (XXX-YYY)

Kleihues, P., Soylemezoglu, F., Schauble, B., Scheithauer, B. W. & Burger, P. C. (1995). Histopathology, classification, and grading of gliomas. *Glia*, Vol. 15, No. 3, pp. (211-21)

Kondziolka, D., Lunsford, L. D. & Martinez, A. J. (1993). Unreliability of contemporary neurodiagnostic imaging in evaluating suspected adult supratentorial (low-grade) astrocytoma. *J Neurosurg*, Vol. 79, No. 4, pp. (533-6)

Kono, K., Inoue, Y., Nakayama, K., Shakudo, M., Morino, M., Ohata, K., Wakasa, K. & Yamada, R. (2001). The role of diffusion-weighted imaging in patients with brain tumors. *AJNR Am J Neuroradiol*, Vol. 22, No. 6, pp. (1081-8)

Law, M., Yang, S., Wang, H., Babb, J. S., Johnson, G., Cha, S., Knopp, E. A. & Zagzag, D. (2003). Glioma grading: sensitivity, specificity, and predictive values of perfusion MR imaging and proton MR spectroscopic imaging compared with conventional MR imaging. *AJNR Am J Neuroradiol*, Vol. 24, No. 10, pp. (1989-98)

Law, M., Yang, S., Babb, J. S., Knopp, E. A., Golfinos, J. G., Zagzag, D. & Johnson, G. (2004). Comparison of cerebral blood volume and vascular permeability from dynamic susceptibility contrast-enhanced perfusion MR imaging with glioma grade. *AJNR Am J Neuroradiol*, Vol. 25, No. 5, pp. (746-55)

Louis, D. N., Ohgaki, H., Wiestler, O. D., Cavenee, W. K., Burger, P. C., Jouvet, A., Scheithauer, B. W. & Kleihues, P. (2007). The 2007 WHO classification of tumours of the central nervous system. *Acta Neuropathol*, Vol. 114, No. 2, pp. (97-109)

Lyden, D., Hattori, K., Dias, S., Costa, C., Blaikie, P., Butros, L., Chadburn, A., Heissig, B., Marks, W., Witte, L., Wu, Y., Hicklin, D., Zhu, Z., Hackett, N. R., Crystal, R. G., Moore, M. A., Hajjar, K. A., Manova, K., Benezra, R. & Rafii, S. (2001). Impaired recruitment of bone-marrow-derived endothelial and hematopoietic precursor cells blocks tumor angiogenesis and growth. *Nat Med*, Vol. 7, No. 11, pp. (1194-201)

Mandonnet, E., Delattre, J. Y., Tanguy, M. L., Swanson, K. R., Carpentier, A. F., Duffau, H., Cornu, P., Van Effenterre, R., Alvord, E. C., Jr. & Capelle, L. (2003). Continuous growth of mean tumor diameter in a subset of grade II gliomas. *Ann Neurol*, Vol. 53, No. 4, pp. (524-8)

McBride, D. Q., Miller, B. L., Nikas, D. L., Buchthal, S., Chang, L., Chiang, F. & Booth, R. A. (1995). Analysis of brain tumors using 1H magnetic resonance spectroscopy. *Surg Neurol*, Vol. 44, No. 2, pp. (137-44)

McKnight, T. R., von dem Bussche, M. H., Vigneron, D. B., Lu, Y., Berger, M. S., McDermott, M. W., Dillon, W. P., Graves, E. E., Pirzkall, A. & Nelson, S. J. (2002). Histopathological validation of a three-dimensional magnetic resonance spectroscopy index as a predictor of tumor presence. *J Neurosurg*, Vol. 97, No. 4, pp. (794-802)

Meyerand, M. E., Pipas, J. M., Mamourian, A., Tosteson, T. D. & Dunn, J. F. (1999). Classification of biopsy-confirmed brain tumors using single-voxel MR spectroscopy. *AJNR Am J Neuroradiol*, Vol. 20, No. 1, pp. (117-23)

Moller-Hartmann, W., Herminghaus, S., Krings, T., Marquardt, G., Lanfermann, H., Pilatus, U. & Zanella, F. E. (2002). Clinical application of proton magnetic resonance spectroscopy in the diagnosis of intracranial mass lesions. *Neuroradiology*, Vol. 44, No. 5, pp. (371-81)

Murphy, M., Loosemore, A., Clifton, A. G., Howe, F. A., Tate, A. R., Cudlip, S. A., Wilkins, P. R., Griffiths, J. R. & Bell, B. A. (2002). The contribution of proton magnetic resonance spectroscopy (1HMRS) to clinical brain tumour diagnosis. *Br J Neurosurg*, Vol. 16, No. 4, pp. (329-34)

Nafe, R., Herminghaus, S., Raab, P., Wagner, S., Pilatus, U., Schneider, B., Schlote, W., Zanella, F. & Lanfermann, H. (2003). Preoperative proton-MR spectroscopy of gliomas--correlation with quantitative nuclear morphology in surgical specimen. *J Neurooncol*, Vol. 63, No. 3, pp. (233-45)

Nakamura, M., Yonekawa, Y., Kleihues, P. & Ohgaki, H. (2001). Promoter hypermethylation of the RB1 gene in glioblastomas. *Lab Invest*, Vol. 81, No. 1, pp. (77-82)

Negendank, W. G., Sauter, R., Brown, T. R., Evelhoch, J. L., Falini, A., Gotsis, E. D., Heerschap, A., Kamada, K., Lee, B. C., Mengeot, M. M., Moser, E., Padavic-Shaller, K. A., Sanders, J. A., Spraggins, T. A., Stillman, A. E., Terwey, B., Vogl, T. J., Wicklow, K. & Zimmerman, R. A. (1996). Proton magnetic resonance spectroscopy in patients with glial tumors: a multicenter study. *J Neurosurg*, Vol. 84, No. 3, pp. (449-58)

Ogawa, T., Shishido, F., Kanno, I., Inugami, A., Fujita, H., Murakami, M., Shimosegawa, E., Ito, H., Hatazawa, J., Okudera, T. & et al. (1993). Cerebral glioma: evaluation with methionine PET. *Radiology*, Vol. 186, No. 1, pp. (45-53)

Okamoto, Y., Di Patre, P. L., Burkhard, C., Horstmann, S., Jourde, B., Fahey, M., Schuler, D., Probst-Hensch, N. M., Yasargil, M. G., Yonekawa, Y., Lutolf, U. M., Kleihues, P. & Ohgaki, H. (2004). Population-based study on incidence, survival rates, and genetic alterations of low-grade diffuse astrocytomas and oligodendrogliomas. *Acta Neuropathol*, Vol. 108, No. 1, pp. (49-56)

Parsons, D. W., Jones, S., Zhang, X., Lin, J. C., Leary, R. J., Angenendt, P., Mankoo, P., Carter, H., Siu, I. M., Gallia, G. L., Olivi, A., McLendon, R., Rasheed, B. A., Keir, S., Nikolskaya, T., Nikolsky, Y., Busam, D. A., Tekleab, H., Diaz, L. A., Jr., Hartigan, J., Smith, D. R., Strausberg, R. L., Marie, S. K., Shinjo, S. M., Yan, H., Riggins, G. J., Bigner, D. D., Karchin, R., Papadopoulos, N., Parmigiani, G., Vogelstein, B., Velculescu, V. E. & Kinzler, K. W. (2008). An integrated genomic analysis of human glioblastoma multiforme. *Science*, Vol. 321, No. 5897, pp. (1807-12)

Pelloski, C. E., Ballman, K. V., Furth, A. F., Zhang, L., Lin, E., Sulman, E. P., Bhat, K., McDonald, J. M., Yung, W. K., Colman, H., Woo, S. Y., Heimberger, A. B., Suki, D., Prados, M. D., Chang, S. M., Barker, F. G., 2nd, Buckner, J. C., James, C. D. & Aldape, K. (2007). Epidermal growth factor receptor variant III status defines clinically distinct subtypes of glioblastoma. *J Clin Oncol*, Vol. 25, No. 16, pp. (2288-94)

Pfister, S., Janzarik, W. G., Remke, M., Ernst, A., Werft, W., Becker, N., Toedt, G., Wittmann, A., Kratz, C., Olbrich, H., Ahmadi, R., Thieme, B., Joos, S., Radlwimmer, B., Kulozik, A., Pietsch, T., Herold-Mende, C., Gnekow, A., Reifenberger, G., Korshunov, A., Scheurlen, W., Omran, H. & Lichter, P. (2008). BRAF gene duplication constitutes a mechanism of MAPK pathway activation in low-grade astrocytomas. *J Clin Invest*, Vol. 118, No. 5, pp. (1739-49)

Pollack, I. F., Claassen, D., al-Shboul, Q., Janosky, J. E. & Deutsch, M. (1995). Low-grade gliomas of the cerebral hemispheres in children: an analysis of 71 cases. *J Neurosurg*, Vol. 82, No. 4, pp. (536-47)

Prabhu, V. C., Khaldi, A., Barton, K. P., Melian, E., Schneck, M. J., Primeau, M. J. & Lee, J. M. (2010). Management of diffuse low-grade cerebral gliomas. *Neurol Clin*, Vol. 28, No. 4, pp. (1037-59)

Price, S. J. (2010). Advances in imaging low-grade gliomas. *Adv Tech Stand Neurosurg*, Vol. 35, No. pp. (1-34)

Rafii, S. & Lyden, D. (2008). Cancer. A few to flip the angiogenic switch. *Science*, Vol. 319, No. 5860, pp. (163-4)

Rees, J., Watt, H., Jager, H. R., Benton, C., Tozer, D., Tofts, P. & Waldman, A. (2009). Volumes and growth rates of untreated adult low-grade gliomas indicate risk of early malignant transformation. *Eur J Radiol*, Vol. 72, No. 1, pp. (54-64)

Ricci-Vitiani, L., Pallini, R., Biffoni, M., Todaro, M., Invernici, G., Cenci, T., Maira, G., Parati, E. A., Stassi, G., Larocca, L. M. & De Maria, R. Tumour vascularization via endothelial differentiation of glioblastoma stem-like cells. *Nature*, Vol. 468, No. 7325, pp. (824-8)

Sanson, M., Marie, Y., Paris, S., Idbaih, A., Laffaire, J., Ducray, F., El Hallani, S., Boisselier, B., Mokhtari, K., Hoang-Xuan, K. & Delattre, J. Y. (2009). Isocitrate dehydrogenase 1 codon 132 mutation is an important prognostic biomarker in gliomas. *J Clin Oncol*, Vol. 27, No. 25, pp. (4150-4)

Sathornsumetee, S., Reardon, D. A., Desjardins, A., Quinn, J. A., Vredenburgh, J. J. & Rich, J. N. (2007). Molecularly targeted therapy for malignant glioma. *Cancer*, Vol. 110, No. 1, pp. (13-24)

Schiff, D., Brown, P. D. & Giannini, C. (2007). Outcome in adult low-grade glioma: the impact of prognostic factors and treatment. *Neurology*, Vol. 69, No. 13, pp. (1366-73)

Schomas, D. A., Laack, N. N., Rao, R. D., Meyer, F. B., Shaw, E. G., O'Neill, B. P., Giannini, C. & Brown, P. D. (2009). Intracranial low-grade gliomas in adults: 30-year experience with long-term follow-up at Mayo Clinic. *Neuro Oncol*, Vol. 11, No. 4, pp. (437-45)

Setzer, M., Herminghaus, S., Marquardt, G., Tews, D. S., Pilatus, U., Seifert, V., Zanella, F. & Lanfermann, H. (2007). Diagnostic impact of proton MR-spectroscopy versus image-guided stereotactic biopsy. *Acta Neurochir (Wien)*, Vol. 149, No. 4, pp. (379-86)

Shaw, E., Arusell, R., Scheithauer, B., O'Fallon, J., O'Neill, B., Dinapoli, R., Nelson, D., Earle, J., Jones, C., Cascino, T., Nichols, D., Ivnik, R., Hellman, R., Curran, W. & Abrams, R. (2002). Prospective randomized trial of low- versus high-dose radiation therapy in adults with supratentorial low-grade glioma: initial report of a North Central Cancer Treatment Group/Radiation Therapy Oncology Group/Eastern Cooperative Oncology Group study. *J Clin Oncol*, Vol. 20, No. 9, pp. (2267-76)

Shaw, E. G. & Wisoff, J. H. (2003). Prospective clinical trials of intracranial low-grade glioma in adults and children. *Neuro Oncol*, Vol. 5, No. 3, pp. (153-60)

Shaw, E. G., Berkey, B., Coons, S. W., Bullard, D., Brachman, D., Buckner, J. C., Stelzer, K. J., Barger, G. R., Brown, P. D., Gilbert, M. R. & Mehta, M. (2008). Recurrence following neurosurgeon-determined gross-total resection of adult supratentorial low-grade glioma: results of a prospective clinical trial. *J Neurosurg*, Vol. 109, No. 5, pp. (835-41)

Shin, J. H., Lee, H. K., Kwun, B. D., Kim, J. S., Kang, W., Choi, C. G. & Suh, D. C. (2002). Using relative cerebral blood flow and volume to evaluate the histopathologic grade of cerebral gliomas: preliminary results. *AJR Am J Roentgenol*, Vol. 179, No. 3, pp. (783-9)

Sijens, P. E. & Oudkerk, M. (2002). 1H chemical shift imaging characterization of human brain tumor and edema. *Eur Radiol*, Vol. 12, No. 8, pp. (2056-61)

Singh, A. & Settleman, J. EMT, cancer stem cells and drug resistance: an emerging axis of evil in the war on cancer. *Oncogene*, Vol. 29, No. 34, pp. (4741-51)

Stieber, V. W. (2001). Low-grade gliomas. *Curr Treat Options Oncol*, Vol. 2, No. 6, pp. (495-506)

Sugahara, T., Korogi, Y., Kochi, M., Ikushima, I., Hirai, T., Okuda, T., Shigematsu, Y., Liang, L., Ge, Y., Ushio, Y. & Takahashi, M. (1998). Correlation of MR imaging-determined cerebral blood volume maps with histologic and angiographic determination of vascularity of gliomas. *AJR Am J Roentgenol*, Vol. 171, No. 6, pp. (1479-86)

Sugahara, T., Korogi, Y., Kochi, M., Ikushima, I., Shigematu, Y., Hirai, T., Okuda, T., Liang, L., Ge, Y., Komohara, Y., Ushio, Y. & Takahashi, M. (1999). Usefulness of diffusion-weighted MRI with echo-planar technique in the evaluation of cellularity in gliomas. *J Magn Reson Imaging*, Vol. 9, No. 1, pp. (53-60)

Sugahara, T., Korogi, Y., Kochi, M., Ushio, Y. & Takahashi, M. (2001). Perfusion-sensitive MR imaging of gliomas: comparison between gradient-echo and spin-echo echo-planar imaging techniques. *AJNR Am J Neuroradiol*, Vol. 22, No. 7, pp. (1306-15)

Tamura, M., Shibasaki, T., Zama, A., Kurihara, H., Horikoshi, S., Ono, N., Oriuchi, N. & Hirano, T. (1998). Assessment of malignancy of glioma by positron emission tomography with 18F-fluorodeoxyglucose and single photon emission computed tomography with thallium-201 chloride. *Neuroradiology*, Vol. 40, No. 4, pp. (210-5)

Thiel, A., Pietrzyk, U., Sturm, V., Herholz, K., Hovels, M. & Schroder, R. (2000). Enhanced accuracy in differential diagnosis of radiation necrosis by positron emission tomography-magnetic resonance imaging coregistration: technical case report. *Neurosurgery*, Vol. 46, No. 1, pp. (232-4)

Tihan, T., Fisher, P. G., Kepner, J. L., Godfraind, C., McComb, R. D., Goldthwaite, P. T. & Burger, P. C. (1999). Pediatric astrocytomas with monomorphous pilomyxoid features and a less favorable outcome. *J Neuropathol Exp Neurol*, Vol. 58, No. 10, pp. (1061-8)

Tripathi, M., Sharma, R., D'Souza, M., Jaimini, A., Panwar, P., Varshney, R., Datta, A., Kumar, N., Garg, G., Singh, D., Grover, R. K., Mishra, A. K. & Mondal, A. (2009). Comparative evaluation of F-18 FDOPA, F-18 FDG, and F-18 FLT-PET/CT for metabolic imaging of low grade gliomas. *Clin Nucl Med*, Vol. 34, No. 12, pp. (878-83)

Unal, E., Koksal, Y., Cimen, O., Paksoy, Y. & Tavli, L. (2008). Malignant glioblastomatous transformation of a low-grade glioma in a child. *Childs Nerv Syst*, Vol. 24, No. 12, pp. (1385-9)

Wang, R., Chadalavada, K., Wilshire, J., Kowalik, U., Hovinga, K. E., Geber, A., Fligelman, B., Leversha, M., Brennan, C. & Tabar, V. Glioblastoma stem-like cells give rise to tumour endothelium. *Nature*, Vol. 468, No. 7325, pp. (829-33)

Watanabe, T., Nobusawa, S., Kleihues, P. & Ohgaki, H. (2009). IDH1 mutations are early events in the development of astrocytomas and oligodendrogliomas. *Am J Pathol*, Vol. 174, No. 4, pp. (1149-53)

Wels, J., Kaplan, R. N., Rafii, S. & Lyden, D. (2008). Migratory neighbors and distant invaders: tumor-associated niche cells. *Genes Dev*, Vol. 22, No. 5, pp. (559-74)

Wen, P. Y. & Kesari, S. (2008). Malignant gliomas in adults. *N Engl J Med*, Vol. 359, No. 5, pp. (492-507)

Wessels, P. H., Weber, W. E., Raven, G., Ramaekers, F. C., Hopman, A. H. & Twijnstra, A. (2003). Supratentorial grade II astrocytoma: biological features and clinical course. *Lancet Neurol*, Vol. 2, No. 7, pp. (395-403)

Yan, H., Parsons, D. W., Jin, G., McLendon, R., Rasheed, B. A., Yuan, W., Kos, I., Batinic-Haberle, I., Jones, S., Riggins, G. J., Friedman, H., Friedman, A., Reardon, D.,

Herndon, J., Kinzler, K. W., Velculescu, V. E., Vogelstein, B. & Bigner, D. D. (2009). IDH1 and IDH2 mutations in gliomas. *N Engl J Med*, Vol. 360, No. 8, pp. (765-73)

Permissions

The contributors of this book come from diverse backgrounds, making this book a truly international effort. This book will bring forth new frontiers with its revolutionizing research information and detailed analysis of the nascent developments around the world.

We would like to thank Dr. Anirban Ghosh, for lending his expertise to make the book truly unique. He has played a crucial role in the development of this book. Without his invaluable contribution this book wouldn't have been possible. He has made vital efforts to compile up to date information on the varied aspects of this subject to make this book a valuable addition to the collection of many professionals and students.

This book was conceptualized with the vision of imparting up-to-date information and advanced data in this field. To ensure the same, a matchless editorial board was set up. Every individual on the board went through rigorous rounds of assessment to prove their worth. After which they invested a large part of their time researching and compiling the most relevant data for our readers. Conferences and sessions were held from time to time between the editorial board and the contributing authors to present the data in the most comprehensible form. The editorial team has worked tirelessly to provide valuable and valid information to help people across the globe.

Every chapter published in this book has been scrutinized by our experts. Their significance has been extensively debated. The topics covered herein carry significant findings which will fuel the growth of the discipline. They may even be implemented as practical applications or may be referred to as a beginning point for another development. Chapters in this book were first published by InTech; hereby published with permission under the Creative Commons Attribution License or equivalent.

The editorial board has been involved in producing this book since its inception. They have spent rigorous hours researching and exploring the diverse topics which have resulted in the successful publishing of this book. They have passed on their knowledge of decades through this book. To expedite this challenging task, the publisher supported the team at every step. A small team of assistant editors was also appointed to further simplify the editing procedure and attain best results for the readers.

Our editorial team has been hand-picked from every corner of the world. Their multi-ethnicity adds dynamic inputs to the discussions which result in innovative outcomes. These outcomes are then further discussed with the researchers and contributors who give their valuable feedback and opinion regarding the same. The feedback is then collaborated with the researches and they are edited in a comprehensive manner to aid the understanding of the subject.

Apart from the editorial board, the designing team has also invested a significant amount of their time in understanding the subject and creating the most relevant covers. They scrutinized every image to scout for the most suitable representation of the subject and create an appropriate cover for the book.

The publishing team has been involved in this book since its early stages. They were actively engaged in every process, be it collecting the data, connecting with the contributors or procuring relevant information. The team has been an ardent support to the editorial, designing and production team. Their endless efforts to recruit the best for this project, has resulted in the accomplishment of this book. They are a veteran in the field of academics and their pool of knowledge is as vast as their experience in printing. Their expertise and guidance has proved useful at every step. Their uncompromising quality standards have made this book an exceptional effort. Their encouragement from time to time has been an inspiration for everyone.

The publisher and the editorial board hope that this book will prove to be a valuable piece of knowledge for researchers, students, practitioners and scholars across the globe.

List of Contributors

Jimmy T. Efird
Center for Health Disparities Research, Department of Public Health, Brody School of Medicine
Greenville, North Carolina, USA

Esperanza García Mendoza and Julio Sotelo
Neuroimmunology Unit, Instituto Nacional de Neurología y Neurocirugía, México

Alfonso Marhx-Bracho
Neurosurgery Department, Instituto Nacional de Pediatría, México

Roberto García-Navarrete
Neuroimmunology Unit, Instituto Nacional de Neurología y Neurocirugía, México
Neurosurgery Department, Instituto Nacional de Pediatría, México
Hospital General Naval de Alta Especialidad, Armada de México, México

Kimberly Ng.
Department of Radiation Oncology, Dana-Farber Cancer Institute, Boston, MA, USA

Santosh Kesari
Department of Neurology, Moores UCSD Cancer Center, UCSD, USA

Bob Carter
Center for Theoretic and Applied Neuro-Oncology, University of California San Diego, San
Diego, CA, USA Department of Surgery, Division of Neurosurgery, USA

Clark C. Chen
Department of Radiation Oncology, Dana-Farber Cancer Institute, Boston, MA, USA
Division of Neurosurgery, Beth Israel Deaconess Medical Center, Boston, MA, USA

Kerrie L. McDonald
Cure For Life Neuro-oncology Group, University of NSW, Australia

Giovanny Pinto
Federal University of Piauí, Parnaíba, Brazil

France Yoshioka, Fábio Motta and Renata Canalle
Federal University of Piauí, Parnaíba, Brazil

Aline Custódio and Cacilda Casartelli
University of São Paulo, Ribeirão Preto, Brazil

Rommel Burbano
Federal University of Pará, Belém, Brazil

Juan Rey
University Hospital La Paz, Madrid, Spain

Franz-Josef Klinz, Sergej Telentschak and Klaus Addicks
Department of Anatomy I, University of Cologne, Germany

Roland Goldbrunner
Department of Neurosurgery, University of Cologne, Germany

Maria Beatrice Morelli
School of Pharmacy, Section of Experimental Medicine, University of Camerino, Italy
Department of Molecular Medicine, Sapienza University, Rome, Italy

Consuelo Amantini, Giorgio Santoni, Matteo Santoni and Massimo Nabissi
School of Pharmacy, Section of Experimental Medicine, University of Camerino, Italy

Ivana Magnani, Chiara Novielli and Lidia Larizza
Università degli Studi di Milano, Italy

Sergio Garcia, Vinicius Kannen and Luciano Neder
Faculty of Medicine of Ribeirao Preto, University of Sao Paulo, Brazil

Jeffrey P. Greenfield, William S. Cobb, Caitlin E. Hoffman, Xueying Chen, Prajwal Rajappa, Chioma Ihunnah, Yujie Huang and David Lyden
Weill Cornell Medical College, USA

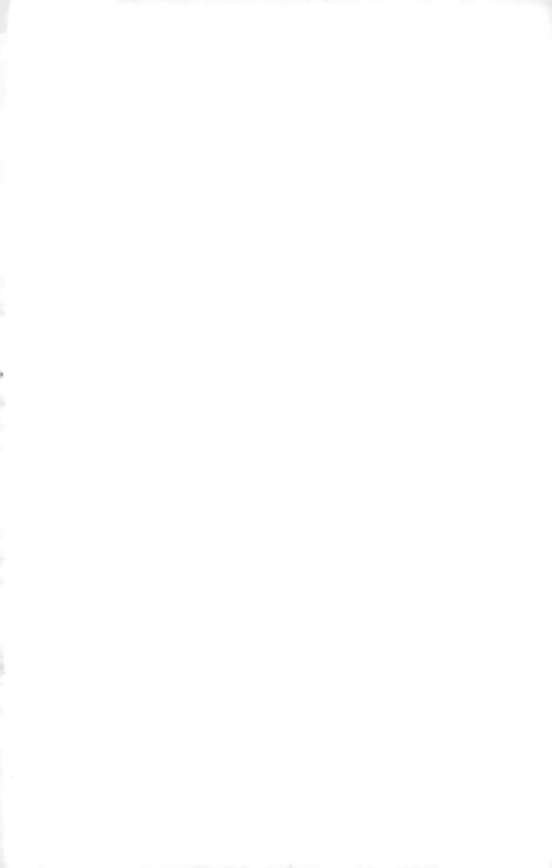